Pocket Guide to Diagnostic Hematopathology

AF213299

S. David Hudnall • Melissa A. Much
Alexa J. Siddon

Pocket Guide to Diagnostic Hematopathology

Springer

S. David Hudnall
Professor of Pathology and Laboratory Medicine
Yale School of Medicine
New Haven, CT
USA

Melissa A. Much
Department of Pathology
Yale School of Medicine
New Haven, CT
USA

Alexa J. Siddon
Department of Laboratory Medicine
Yale School of Medicine
New Haven, CT
USA

ISBN 978-3-030-10628-7 ISBN 978-3-030-10630-0 (eBook)
https://doi.org/10.1007/978-3-030-10630-0

© Springer Nature Switzerland AG 2019
This work is subject to copyright. All rights are reserved by the Publisher, whether the whole or part of the material is concerned, specifically the rights of translation, reprinting, reuse of illustrations, recitation, broadcasting, reproduction on microfilms or in any other physical way, and transmission or information storage and retrieval, electronic adaptation, computer software, or by similar or dissimilar methodology now known or hereafter developed.
The use of general descriptive names, registered names, trademarks, service marks, etc. in this publication does not imply, even in the absence of a specific statement, that such names are exempt from the relevant protective laws and regulations and therefore free for general use.
The publisher, the authors, and the editors are safe to assume that the advice and information in this book are believed to be true and accurate at the date of publication. Neither the publisher nor the authors or the editors give a warranty, expressed or implied, with respect to the material contained herein or for any errors or omissions that may have been made. The publisher remains neutral with regard to jurisdictional claims in published maps and institutional affiliations.

This Springer imprint is published by the registered company Springer Nature Switzerland AG
The registered company address is: Gewerbestrasse 11, 6330 Cham, Switzerland

Preface

With the rapid advances in molecular diagnosis, the field of diagnostic hematopathology has become increasingly complex. This complexity is reflected in the increasing girth of the standard WHO classification *Blue Book*. Over a 10-year period (2007–2017), the WHO *Blue Book*[1] has grown from 335 to 452 pages of text—an increase of 117 pages. This complexity has made it all the more challenging to apply this vast wealth of information to our cases in a timely fashion. To address this issue, three hematopathology faculty at Yale School of Medicine have collaborated in preparing this pocket guide to diagnostic hematopathology.

The *Pocket Guide to Diagnostic Hematopathology* is designed not as a comprehensive textbook, but instead as a short practical guide to the diagnosis of neoplastic and non-neoplastic diseases of blood, bone marrow, and lymphoid tissues.

Major diagnostic features of each disease entity are outlined in a single page of text and accompanied by a single figure page. This simple format was chosen to provide essential information that may quickly be reviewed at the microscope. Each entry begins with a one-line *Snapshot* description, followed by short descriptions of clinical, morphologic, immunohistochemical, and genetic features, and ending with *Caveats and Pearls* and *Differential Diagnosis*.

---

[1] Swerdlow SH; International Agency for Research on Cancer; World Health Organization; et al. WHO classification of tumours of haematopoietic and lymphoid tissues. Lyon: International Agency for Research on Cancer; 2017.

For more in-depth reading, several excellent comprehensive texts and recently published review articles are listed in the reference section.

New Haven, CT, USA

S. David Hudnall
Melissa A. Much
Alexa J. Siddon

Contents

Contributors

S. David Hudnall Professor of Pathology and Laboratory Medicine, Yale School of Medicine, New Haven, CT, USA

Melissa A. Much Department of Pathology, Yale School of Medicine, New Haven, CT, USA

Alexa J. Siddon Department of Laboratory Medicine, Yale School of Medicine, New Haven, CT, USA

Center for Biomedical Data Science, Yale School of Medicine, New Haven, CT, USA

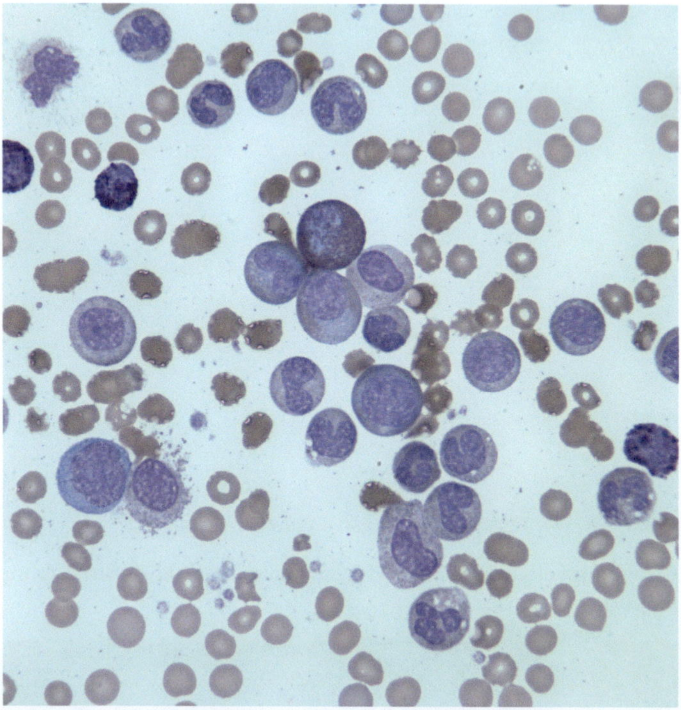

Chronic myeloid leukemia. Increased basophils and eosinophils (peripheral blood smear)

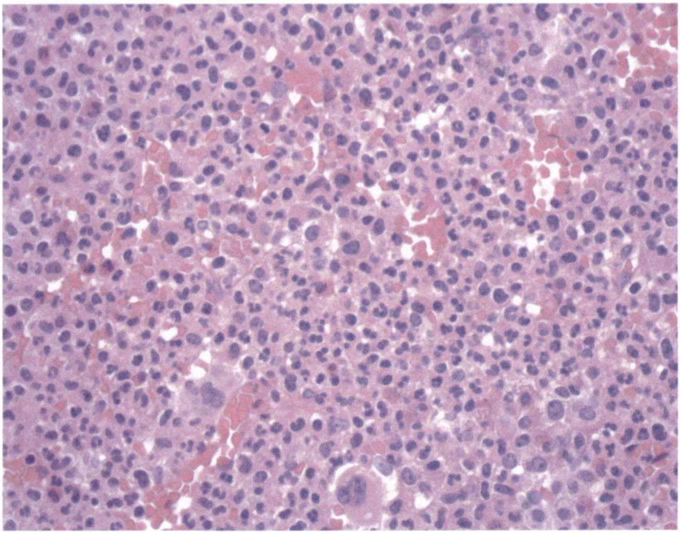

Chronic myeloid leukemia. Hypercellular myeloid marrow (core biopsy)

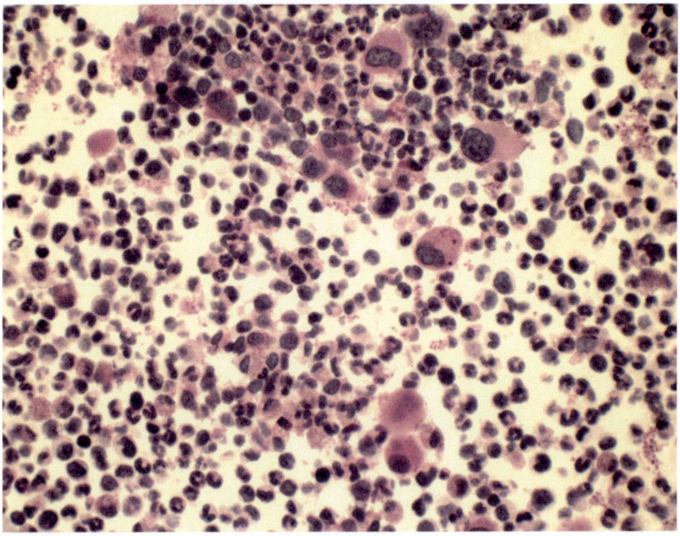

Chronic myeloid leukemia. Increased small hypolobated megakaryocytes

Chronic Neutrophilic Leukemia[2]

Snapshot

- Persistent nonreactive neutrophilia with hypercellular neutrophil-rich bone marrow and *CSF3R1* mutation

Clinical Features

- Absolute neutrophilia ($\geq 25 \times 10^9$/L)
- $\geq$80% segmented neutrophils and bands (WBC count)
- Hepatosplenomegaly
- Mucosal bleeding (some cases)

Marrow Morphology

- Neutrophil-rich marrow without myeloid left shift (<5% blasts)
- No dysplasia and no reticulin fibrosis (most cases)

Genetics

- POSITIVE: *CSF3R* mutation, often with *SETBP1* or *ASXL1* mutation
- NEGATIVE: (9;22) *BCR/ABL* translocation

Differential Diagnosis

- *Chronic myeloid leukemia, neutrophilic variant* (positive for p230 fusion protein)
- *Reactive neutrophilia* (acute infection, acute inflammation, drug effect [G-CSF, corticosteroids, others], underlying neoplasm [including plasma cell neoplasm], stress, toxin exposure)

---

[2] Note: Adapted from Table 2.02 from Swerdlow SH; International Agency for Research on Cancer; World Health Organization; et al. WHO classification of tumours of haematopoietic and lymphoid tissues. Lyon: International Agency for Research on Cancer; 2017.

Caveats and Pearls

- Development of myelodysplasia may herald progression to acute myeloid leukemia

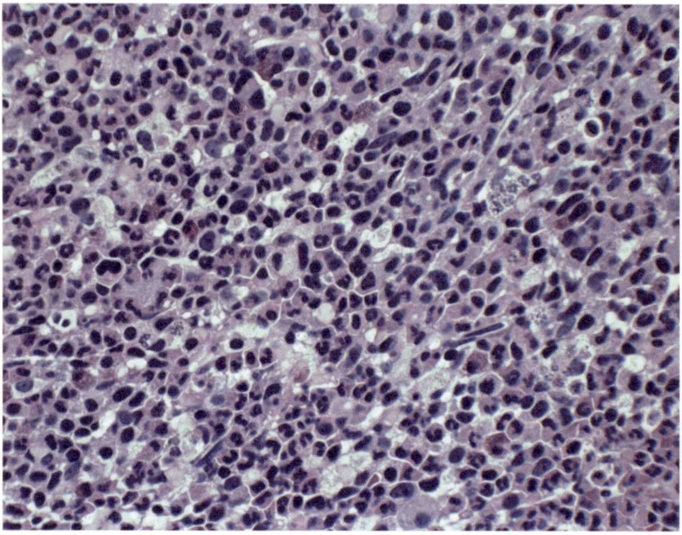

Chronic neutrophilic leukemia. Hypercellular neutrophil-rich marrow

Polycythemia Vera

Snapshot

- Persistent nonreactive *JAK2*-positive polycythemia (elevated hemoglobin or hematocrit) with panmyelosis

Clinical Features

- Symptoms may include thrombosis, headache, blurred vision, dizziness, pruritis, splenomegaly

Morphology

- Hypercellular marrow with trilineage proliferation (panmyelosis), increased pleomorphic (not atypical) megakaryocytes, absent stainable iron, and absent-minimal reticulin fibrosis (in most cases)

Diagnostic Criteria

Polycythemia vera

1. Elevated hemoglobin (>16.5 g/dL males, >16 g/dL females) or hematocrit (>49% males, >48% females)
2. Hypercellular marrow with panmyelosis and pleomorphic megakaryocytes
3. *JAK2* mutation or low serum EPO level

NOTE: If hemoglobin or hematocrit is markedly elevated (HGB: >18.5 g/dL males, >16.5 g/dL females; HCT: >55.5% males, 49.5% females), and criteria 3 and 4 are met, criterion 2 may not be required

Post-PV myelofibrosis

1. Prior history of PV
2. Myelofibrosis (moderate to severe)

3. At least two of the following: anemia, leukoerythroblastosis, increasing splenomegaly, constitutional symptoms (fever, weight loss, night sweats)

Genetics

- *JAK2 V617F* or *JAK2 exon 12* mutation (nearly all cases)

Differential Diagnosis

- *Prefibrotic myelofibrosis* (abnormal megakaryocytes with irregular hyperchromatic nuclei)

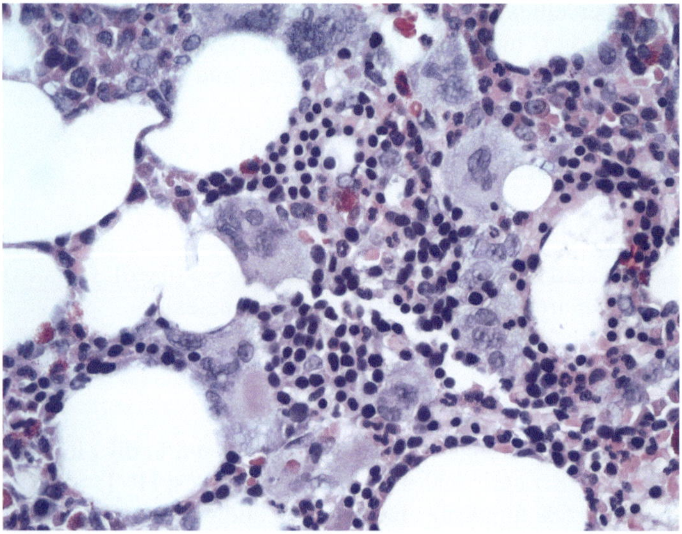

Polycythemia vera. Hypercellular erythroid-predominant marrow with numerous pleomorphic megakaryocytes

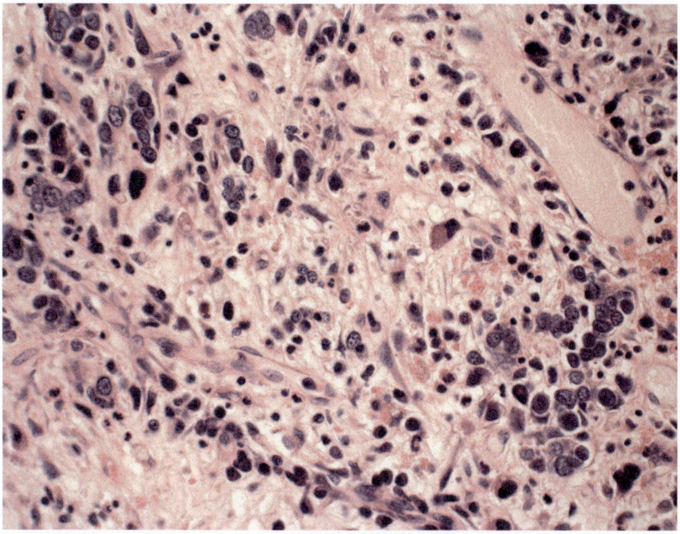

Polycythemia vera (PV). Post-PV myelofibrosis

Primary Myelofibrosis

Snapshot

- Hypercellular marrow with increased abnormal megakaryocytes in clusters, fibrosis, osteosclerosis, and splenomegaly with extramedullary hematopoiesis

Clinical Features

- Blood smear with leukocytosis, left shift, nucleated red cells, and dacrocytes (leukoerythroblastosis), thrombocytosis, splenomegaly

Diagnosis

Must have all of the following:

1. Increased abnormal megakaryocytes (large irregular hyperlobated forms in clusters)
2. Moderate to marked reticulin fibrosis with or without collagen fibrosis
3. Does not meet criteria for another myeloproliferative neoplasm
4. Presence of a mutation in *JAK2, CALR,* or *MPL* (if not detected, search for abnormal karyotype or another mutation)
5. At least one of the following: leukocytosis ($\geq 11 \times 10^9$/L), anemia (not attributable to an unrelated condition), splenomegaly, leukoerythroblastosis, elevated lactate dehydrogenase (LDH)

Prefibrotic Myelofibrosis

- Early stage of disease with no significant fibrosis (absent to mild)
- Leukoerythroblastosis and splenomegaly may be absent

Genetics

- Mutations of *JAK2 V617F* (most common), *CALR*, or *MPL* in nearly all cases
- Up to 30% of cases have an abnormal karyotype

Differential Diagnosis

- *Essential thrombocythemia* (difficult to distinguish from prefibrotic PMF, enlarged megakaryocytes without irregular hyperchromatic nuclei)
- *Reactive thrombocytosis or leukoerythroblastosis* (absence of clonal genetic abnormality, findings secondary to infection, inflammation, growth factor therapy, metastatic disease, splenic disease)

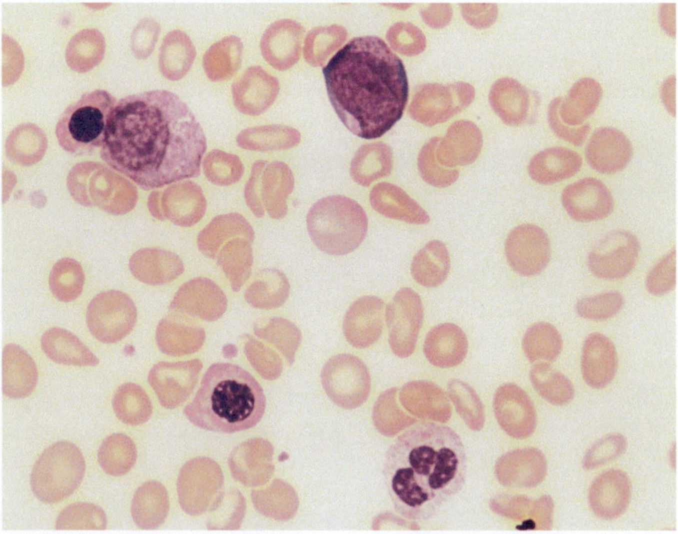

Primary myelofibrosis. Peripheral blood exhibited leukoerythroblastosis with neutrophils, immature myeloid precursors, and nucleated red blood cells

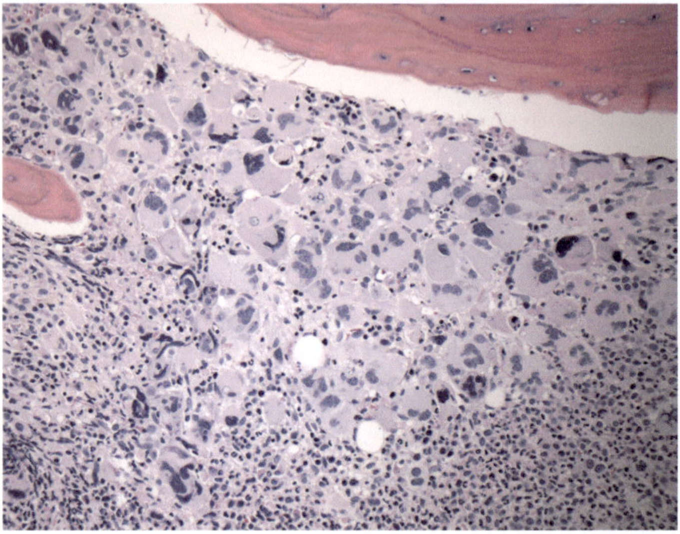

Primary myelofibrosis. Hypercellular marrow with markedly increased enlarged, bizarre megakaryocytes

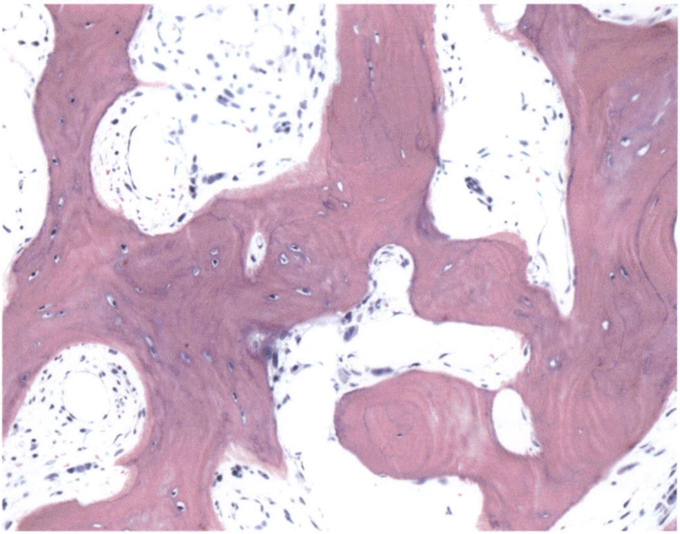

Primary myelofibrosis. Osteosclerosis of bone

Essential Thrombocythemia

Snapshot

- Hypercellular marrow with increased enlarged megakaryocytes

Clinical Features

- Often asymptomatic thrombocytosis
- May present with thrombosis or hemorrhage
- No significant extramedullary hematopoiesis

Diagnostic Criteria[3]

1. Platelet count $\geq 450 \times 10^9/L$
2. Hypercellular marrow with numerous enlarged megakaryocytes with hyperlobated nuclei
3. Does not meet criteria for another myeloproliferative neoplasm
4. Presence of a *JAK2*, *CALR*, or *MPL* mutation
   - If not identified, another clonal marker should be identified, or all reactive causes of thrombocytosis excluded

Post-Essential Thrombocythemia Myelofibrosis

Diagnostic criteria:

- Previous diagnosis of ET
- Increased reticulin fibrosis (2/3 or 3/3)
- Other findings: leukoerythroblastosis, splenomegaly, anemia, elevated LDH, and the development of constitutional symptoms

Genetics

- *JAK2 V617F*, *CALR*, or *MPL* mutation
- Only few cases have an abnormal karyotype

---

[3] Note: Diagnostic criteria adapted from Tables 2.12 and 2.13 from Swerdlow SH; International Agency for Research on Cancer; World Health Organization; et al. WHO classification of tumours of haematopoietic and lymphoid tissues. Lyon: International Agency for Research on Cancer; 2017.

Differential Diagnosis

- *Polycythemia vera* (panmyelosis, nearly all cases with *JAK2 V617F* mutation)
- *Myelodysplastic syndrome* (erythroid or granulocytic dysplasia usually present, may have increased blasts)
- *Reactive thrombocytosis* (normal genetics, secondary causes include infection, inflammation, bleeding)

Caveats and Pearls

- There should be no significant proliferation of erythroid or granulocyte lineages

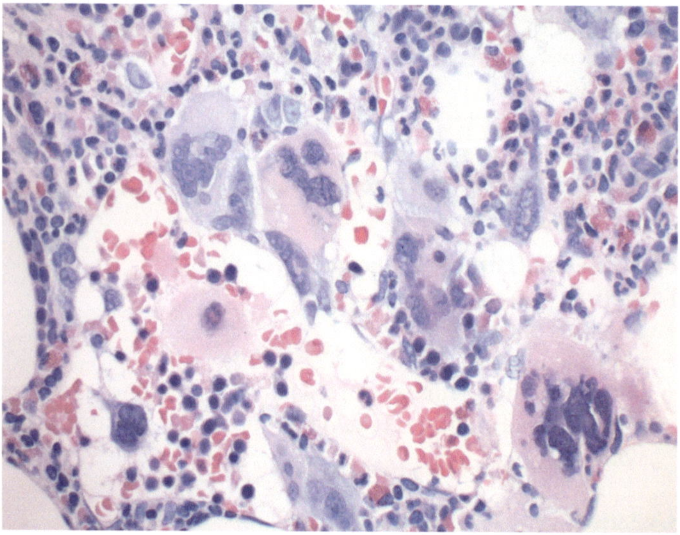

Essential thrombocythemia. Increased, enlarged, hyperlobated megakaryocytes in clusters

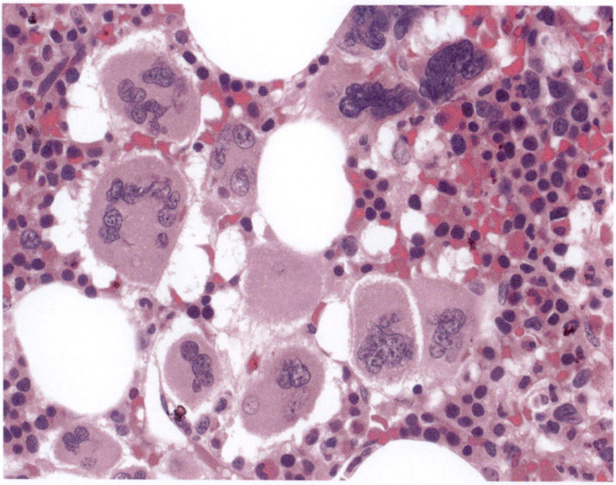

Essential thrombocythemia. Another example of clustered megakaryocytes, many with hyperlobated nuclei

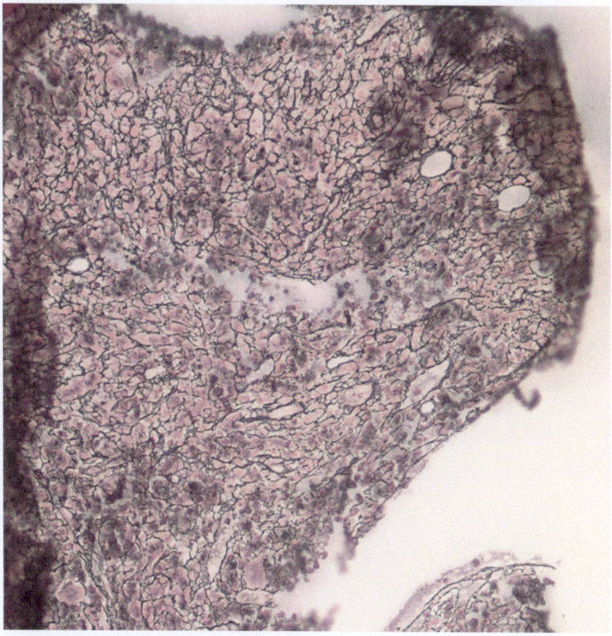

Essential thrombocythemia (ET). Marked increase in reticulin found in post-ET myelofibrosis

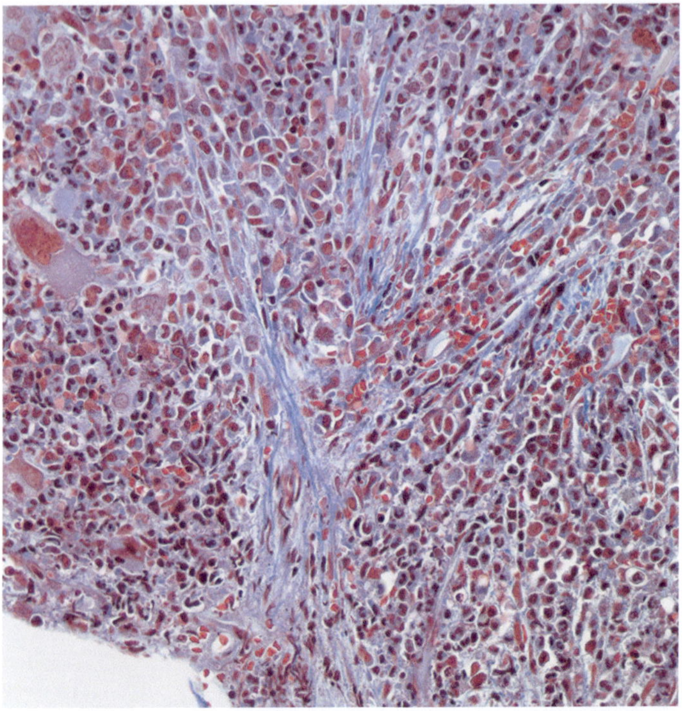

Essential thrombocythemia. Masson trichrome stain showing focal collagen fibrosis

Chronic Eosinophilic Leukemia

Snapshot

- Chronic myeloproliferative neoplasm leading to a persistent eosinophilia

Clinical Features

- Very rare
- Marrow and blood are always involved
- Frequent involvement of skin, GI tract, heart, lungs, and CNS
- Can cause end-organ damage due to eosinophil infiltration
- May be an incidental finding, however may have constitutional symptoms

Diagnosis

- Eosinophils range from morphologically normal to abnormal, with abnormal granulation, abnormal nuclear segmentation, or increased size

Diagnostic criteria[4]

1. Peripheral blood eosinophilia of $\geq 1.5 \times 10^9$/L
2. Blasts are <20% of marrow and blood
3. Does not meet criteria for acute leukemia, another myeloproliferative neoplasm, or a myeloid/lymphoid neoplasm with eosinophilia and *PDGFRA/B*, *FGFR1*, or *PCM1-JAK2* rearrangement
4. Definitive clonal abnormality by cytogenetic or molecular studies (not CHIP)

[4] Note: Diagnostic criteria adapted from Table 2.14 from Swerdlow SH; International Agency for Research on Cancer; World Health Organization; et al. WHO classification of tumours of haematopoietic and lymphoid tissues. Lyon: International Agency for Research on Cancer; 2017.

Genetics

- May have mutations of *ASXL1*, *TET2*, or *EZH2*
- Rarely with *JAK2* or *KIT* mutations

Differential Diagnosis

- *Myeloid/lymphoid neoplasms with eosinophilia and PDGFRA/B, FGFR1, or PCM1-JAK2 rearrangement* (specific cytogenetic finding)
- *Reactive eosinophilia* (parasitic or fungal infection, allergic conditions, immune disorders, drug hypersensitivity, lymphoid neoplasms, carcinoma)

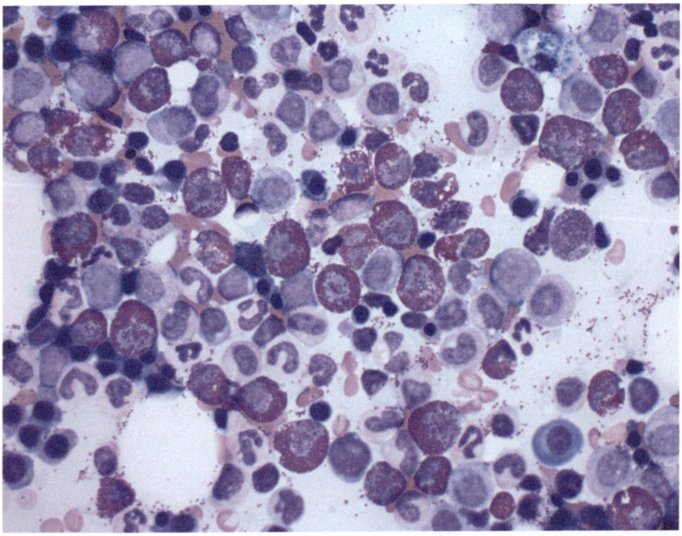

Chronic eosinophilic leukemia. Increased mature eosinophils throughout the marrow

Myeloproliferative Neoplasm, Unclassifiable

Snapshot

- A chronic myeloproliferative neoplasm that does not meet strict criteria for any specific MPN type (PV, ET, CML, PMF)

Diagnostic Criteria

- MPN cases with prepolycythemic PV, prefibrotic MPN, or early ET features that do not meet strict diagnostic criteria
- MPN cases with portal/splanchnic thrombosis
- Advanced stage MPN cases with marked fibrosis, increased blasts, and/or myelodysplasia in which the underlying disorder cannot be determined

Genetics

- Negative: *BCR/ABL*, *PDGFRA/B*, *FGFR1*, or *PCM1-JAK2* rearrangement
- Variable positivity for *JAK2*, CALR, or MPL mutation
- Variable positivity for other myeloid neoplasm-associated mutations

Differential Diagnosis

- *Reactive non-neoplastic conditions* (chronic inflammatory disease, chronic infection) *with leukocytosis, erythrocytosis, and/or thrombocytosis*

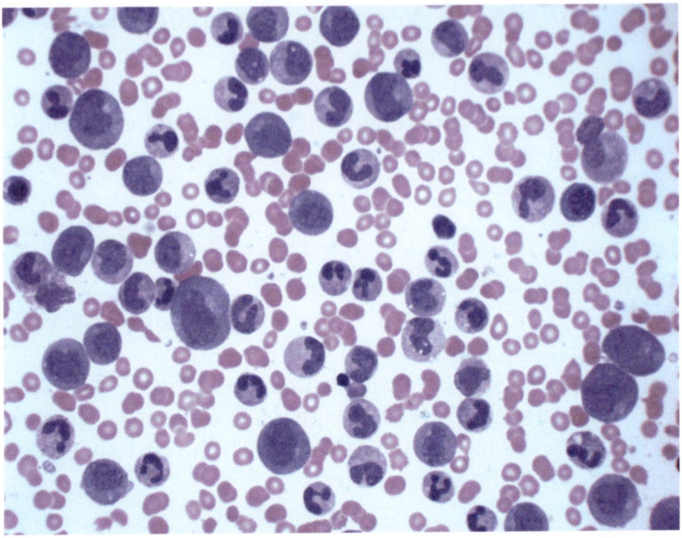

Myeloproliferative neoplasm, unclassifiable. Peripheral blood showing leukocytosis with significant myeloid left shift. No *BCR-ABL1* translocation, no *JAK2, MPL*, or *CALR* mutation

Myelodysplastic/Myeloproliferative Neoplasms

Chronic Myelomonocytic Leukemia

Snapshot

- Clonal myeloid neoplasm with of both a myeloproliferative neoplasm and a myelodysplastic neoplasm, in a setting of sustained absolute monocytosis

Clinical Features

- At least half of cases present with leukocytosis
- Remaining cases white count is normal or mildly decreased (dysplastic type, WBC $<13 \times 10^9$/L; proliferative type, WBC $\geq 13 \times 10^9$/L)
- Splenomegaly and hepatomegaly are more frequent in patients with leukocytosis
- Involves blood and marrow; sometimes involves skin, spleen, liver, and lymph nodes

Diagnosis/Immunophenotype[5]

- Persistent monocytosis ($\geq 1 \times 10^9$/L), monocytes account for >10% of blood leukocytes, dysplastic morphology is common
- <20% blasts in marrow and blood
- Monocytic cells are increased in marrow but may be difficult to identify (CD14, CD64, CD68, or lysozyme IHC on biopsy sections may help)

[5] Note: Diagnostic criteria adapted from Table 5.01 from Swerdlow SH; International Agency for Research on Cancer; World Health Organization; et al. WHO classification of tumours of haematopoietic and lymphoid tissues. Lyon: International Agency for Research on Cancer; 2017.

Genetics

- *TET2, SRSF2, SETBP1, or ASXL1* mutation seen in most cases (supportive but nondiagnostic)
- No specific cytogenetic defect; however, trisomy 8 and monosomy 7 are relatively common

CMML Subtypes

- *CMML-0* (<5% blasts in marrow, <2% blasts in blood, no Auer rods identified in blood or marrow)
- *CMML-1* (5–9% blasts in marrow or 2–4% blasts in blood, no Auer rods identified in blood or marrow)
- *CMML-2* (10–19% blasts in marrow or 5–19% blasts in blood, or Auer rods identified in blood or marrow)

Differential Diagnosis

- *Chronic myeloproliferative neoplasms* (see specific criteria for each; usually little dysplasia)
- *Myelodysplastic syndromes* (usually lack monocytosis, cytopenia always present)
- *Myeloid/lymphoid neoplasms with PDGFRB rearrangement* (eosinophilia with specific genetic findings)

Caveats and Pearls

- Dysplasia in all three lineages may be observed
- May have increased reticulin fibrosis
- Clusters of mature plasmacytoid dendritic cells can be seen in marrow

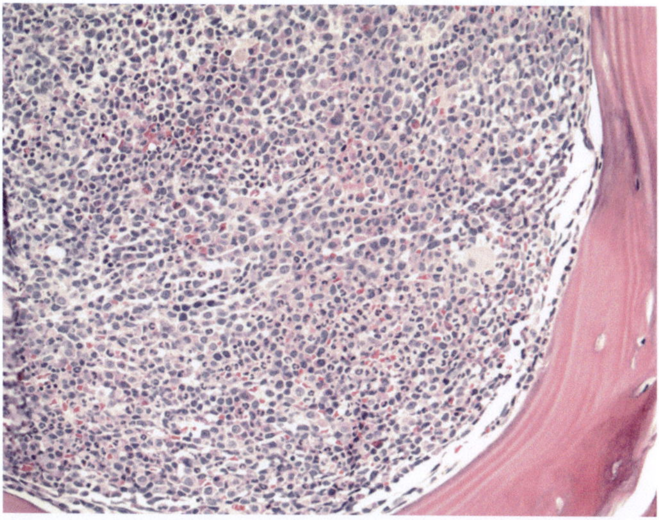

Chronic myelomonocytic leukemia. Hypercellular marrow for age

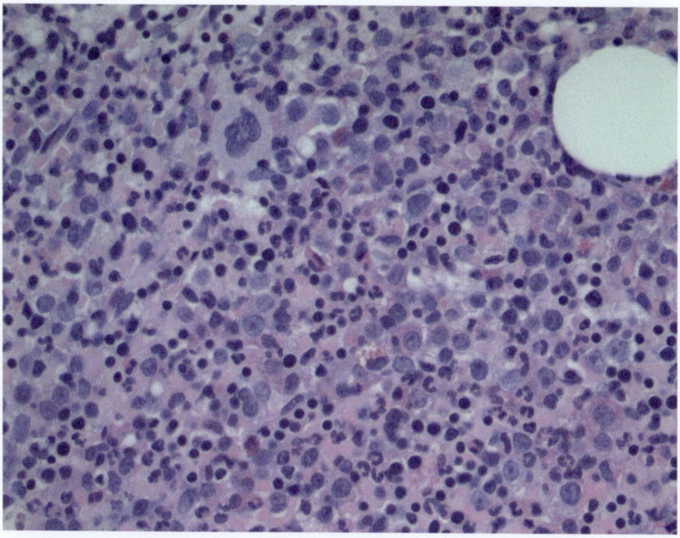

Chronic myelomonocytic leukemia. Hypercellular marrow with abundant myeloid cells

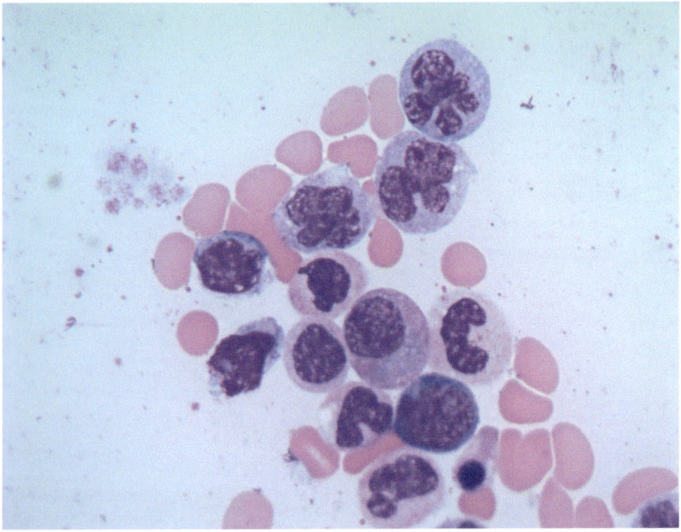

Chronic myelomonocytic leukemia. Aspirate showing increased monocytes, many of which are dysplastic

Atypical Chronic Myeloid Leukemia, BCR-ABL1-Negative

Snapshot

- A myeloid neoplasm with features of a myeloproliferative neoplasm and a myelodysplastic neoplasm, as well as leukocytosis

Clinical Features

- Generally presents in elderly patients
- Involves blood and marrow; can involve spleen and liver

Diagnosis[6]

- Leukocytosis $\geq 13 \times 10^9$/L
- Granulocytic dysplasia most prominent; can have multilineage dysplasia
- <20% blasts in the marrow or blood
- Does not meet criteria for other myeloproliferative neoplasms

Genetics

- Absence of *BCR-ABL1*, *PDGFRA*, *PDGFRB*, *FGFR1*, or *PCM1-JAK2 rearrangement*
- Absence of *JAK2, MPL, or CALR mutation*

Differential Diagnosis

- *Chronic myeloid leukemia* (*BCR-ABL1*-positive)
- *Other chronic myeloproliferative neoplasms* (see specific criteria for each*)*
- *Myelodysplastic syndromes* (peripheral cytopenia)

---

[6] Note: Diagnostic criteria adapted from Table 5.02 from Swerdlow SH; International Agency for Research on Cancer; World Health Organization; et al. WHO classification of tumours of haematopoietic and lymphoid tissues. Lyon: International Agency for Research on Cancer; 2017.

- *Other myelodysplastic/myeloproliferative overlap syndromes* (see specific criteria for each)
- *Myeloid/lymphoid neoplasms with eosinophilia and rearrangement* of *PDGFRA, PDGFRB OR FGFR1,* or with *PCM1-JAK2*

Caveats and Pearls

- No significant basophilia or monocytosis

Juvenile Myelomonocytic Leukemia

Snapshot

- Clonal myeloid neoplasm of children with granulocytic and monocytic proliferation and molecular abnormalities involving the *RAS* pathway

Clinical Features

- Majority diagnosed before 3 years of age
- Male:female ratio is 2:1
- 15% of cases associated with Noonan syndrome (*CBL* mutation)
- 10% of cases associated with neurofibromatosis type 1
- Generally present with leukocytosis, anemia, and thrombocytopenia

Diagnosis

- Splenomegaly
- Persistent monocytosis ($\geq 1 \times 10^9$/L)
- Blasts are <20% of marrow or blood
- No *BCR-ABL1*

Genetics

Must have one of:

- Mutation in *PTPN11*, *KRAS*, or *NRAS*
- Germline *CBL* mutation
- *NF1* mutation

Rarely, a different chromosomal abnormality such as monosomy 7 is present

Differential Diagnosis

- Childhood myelodysplastic syndrome (lack the monocytosis and genetic findings of JMML)
- Other myelodysplastic/myeloproliferative neoplasms (generally present in older patients)

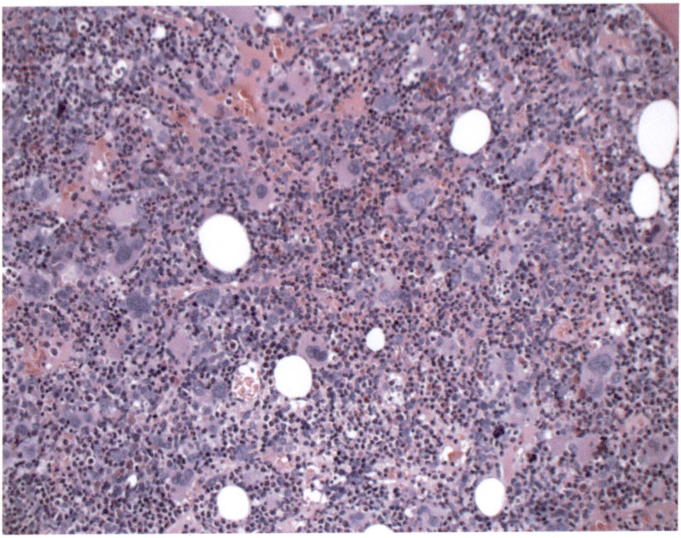

Juvenile myelomonocytic leukemia. Cellular marrow with abundant megakaryocytes

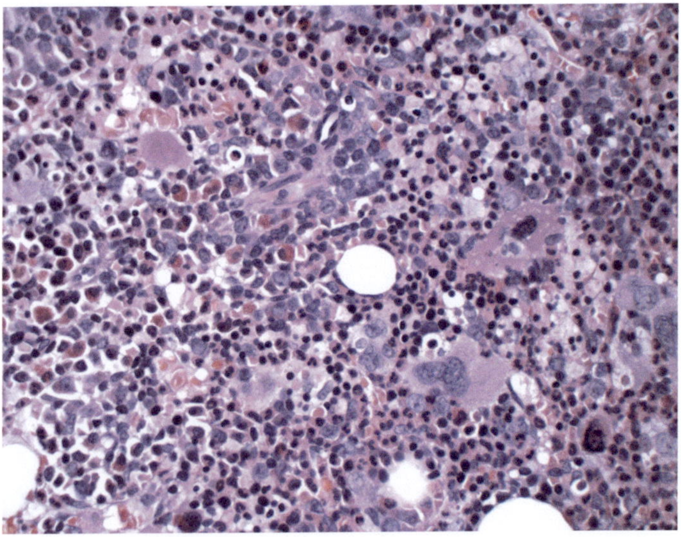

Juvenile myelomonocytic leukemia. Scattered dysplastic megakaryocytes are apparent in *JMML*

Myelodysplastic/Myeloproliferative Neoplasm with Ring Sideroblasts and Thrombocytosis

Snapshot

- A clonal myeloid neoplasm with myelodysplastic and myeloproliferative features including ring sideroblasts and increased platelets

Clinical Features

- Generally diagnosed in elderly patients
- Blood and marrow are always involved
- Often splenomegaly, with or without hepatomegaly

Diagnosis/Immunophenotype[7]

- Persistent thrombocytosis of $\geq 450 \times 10^9$/L
- Blasts are <5% of marrow and <1% in blood
- Anemia and dyserythropoiesis with ≥15% ring sideroblasts using iron stain
- Can have multilineage dysplasia

Genetics

- *SF3B1* mutation is seen in the majority of cases
- Can have *JAK2 V617F* or, rarely, *MPL* or *CALR* mutations

Differential Diagnosis

- *Myelodysplastic syndrome with ring sideroblasts* (lacks thrombocytosis)
- *Essential thrombocythemia* (no ring sideroblasts)

---

[7] Note: Diagnostic criteria adapted from Table 5.04 from Swerdlow SH; International Agency for Research on Cancer; World Health Organization; et al. WHO classification of tumours of haematopoietic and lymphoid tissues. Lyon: International Agency for Research on Cancer; 2017.

Caveats and Pearls

- Should not have a history of a myeloproliferative or myelodysplastic syndrome
- Does not meet criteria for another myeloid neoplasm

Myelodysplastic/Myeloproliferative Neoplasm, Unclassifiable

Snapshot

- A myeloid neoplasm with both myelodysplastic and myeloproliferative features, not meeting the criteria for other MDS/MPN

Clinical Features

- Blood and marrow are always involved
- Often splenomegaly, with or without hepatomegaly

Diagnosis/Immunophenotype[8]

- Should have increased peripheral counts of white blood cells or platelets
- Blasts are <5% of marrow and <1% in blood
- Dysplasia of at least one cell lineage

Genetics

- Can have genetic abnormalities; however, should not have any that are diagnostic of another disease entity

Differential Diagnosis

- *Other myelodysplastic/myeloproliferative neoplasms* (see specific criteria for each)

> **Caveats and Pearls**
> - Should not have a history of an antecedent myeloproliferative or myelodysplastic syndrome
> - Does not meet criteria for another myeloid neoplasm

---

[8] Note: Diagnostic criteria adapted from Table 5.05 from Swerdlow SH; International Agency for Research on Cancer; World Health Organization; et al. WHO classification of tumours of haematopoietic and lymphoid tissues. Lyon: International Agency for Research on Cancer; 2017.

Myelodysplastic Syndromes

Myelodysplastic Syndrome with Single Lineage Dysplasia

Snapshot

- Myelodysplastic syndrome with cytopenia (one to two lineages) and ≥10% dysplastic cells in a single myeloid lineage

Clinical Features

- More common in older adults
- Usually presents with anemia or bicytopenia

Diagnosis

- <5% blasts in marrow and <1% in blood
- Hypercellular marrow

Dysplastic cells comprise ≥10% of the lineage:

- *Erythroid lineage*—Megaloblastoid change (nuclear-cytoplasmic dyssynchrony), nuclear budding, intranuclear bridges, multinucleation, ring sideroblasts, PAS positivity
- *Granulocytic lineage*—Pseudo-Pelger-Huët cells (bilobated neutrophils), abnormal nuclear size, nuclear hypersegmentation, cytoplasmic hypogranularity, Auer rods
- *Megakaryocytic lineage*—Hypolobated nuclei, separated nuclei, micromegakaryocytes

Genetics[9]

- Driver mutations in *ASXL1*, *TET2*, and *RUNX1*, among others
- Often with cytogenetic abnormalities, including monosomy 7, del(7q), del(5q), trisomy 8, and del(20q)

[9] For a comprehensive list of cytogenetic abnormalities in MDS see Table 6.03 of Swerdlow SH; International Agency for Research on Cancer; World Health Organization; et al. WHO classification of tumours of haematopoietic and lymphoid tissues. Lyon: International Agency for Research on Cancer; 2017.

Differential Diagnosis

- *Other myelodysplastic syndromes* (do not meet genetic criteria)
- *Secondary reactive myelodysplasia* (nutritional disorders, chronic viral infections, chronic inflammation, drugs, toxins, PNH, etc.)

Caveats and Pearls

- In the absence of morphologic dysplasia and an MDS-defining cytogenetic abnormality, idiopathic cytopenia is best classified as *idiopathic cytopenia of undetermined significance (ICUS)*
- If the dysplastic lineage is erythroid and there are ≥15% ring sideroblasts (or ≥5% and a pathogenic *SF3B1* mutation), then the diagnosis is *myelodysplastic syndrome with ring sideroblasts and single lineage dysplasia*

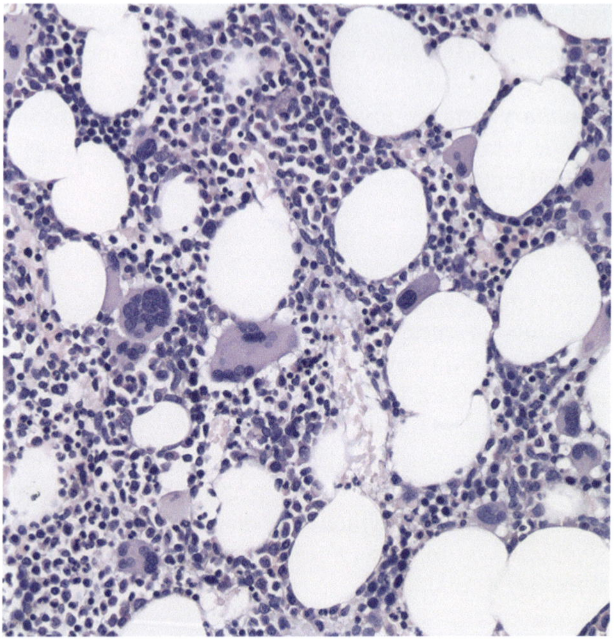

Myelodysplastic syndrome with single lineage dysplasia. Dysmegakaryopoiesis with some hypolobated forms as well as forms with separated nuclear lobes

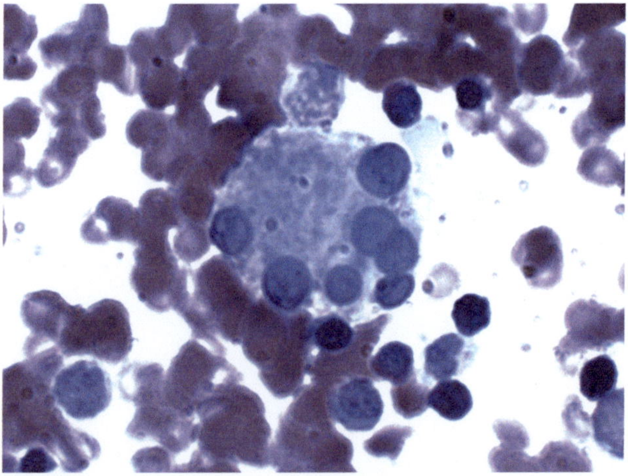

Myelodysplastic syndrome with single lineage dysplasia. Classic Pawn-Ball megakaryocytes with split nuclear lobes

Myelodysplastic Syndrome with Ring Sideroblasts

Snapshot

- Myelodysplastic syndrome with one or more peripheral cytopenias, erythroid dysplasia, and ring sideroblasts comprising ≥15% of erythroid precursors (or 5% with a concurrent *SF3B1* mutation)

Clinical Features

- More common in older adults
- Generally presents with anemia

Diagnosis

- Less than 5% blasts in marrow and 1% in blood
- Marrow is normocellular or hypercellular
- Ring sideroblasts (seen on iron stain) comprise ≥15% of erythroid precursors (or 5% with a concurrent *SF3B1* mutation)

Can present with either single lineage or multilineage dysplasia:

- *Erythroid lineage*—Megaloblastoid change (nuclear-cytoplasmic dyssynchrony), nuclear budding, intranuclear bridges, multinucleation, ring sideroblasts, PAS positivity
- *Granulocytic lineage*—Pseudo-Pelger-Huët cells (bilobated neutrophils), abnormal nuclear size, nuclear hypersegmentation, cytoplasmic hypogranularity, Auer rods
- *Megakaryocytic lineage*—Hypolobated nuclei, separated nuclei, micromegakaryocytes

Genetics

- Majority of cases have a pathogenic mutation in *SF3B1*
- Can have other MDS-associated cytogenetic abnormalities

Differential Diagnosis

- *Other myelodysplastic syndromes* (other types of MDS may have few [<5%] ring sideroblasts)

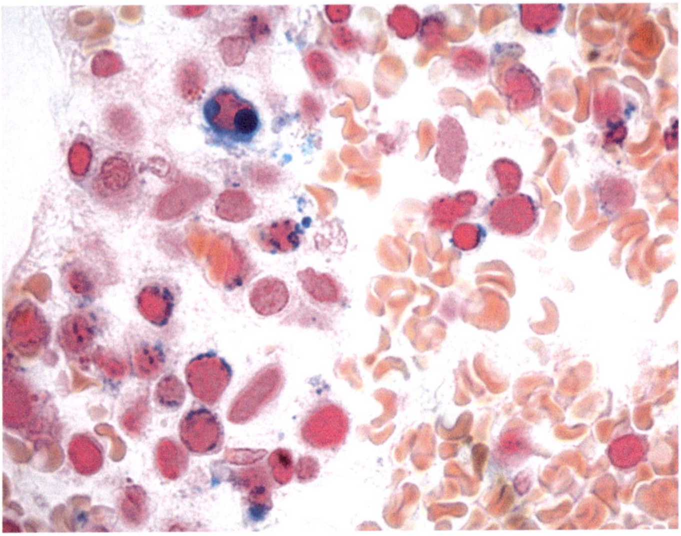

Myelodysplastic syndrome with ring sideroblasts. Iron stains showing numerous ring sideroblasts

Myelodysplastic Syndrome with Multilineage Dysplasia

Snapshot

- Myelodysplastic syndrome with peripheral cytopenia and ≥10% dysplastic cells in at least two myeloid lineages (erythroid, granulocytic, megakaryocytic)

Clinical Features

- More common in older adults

Diagnosis

- <5% blasts in marrow; <1% in blood
- Hypercellular marrow

Dysplastic cells comprise ≥10% of involved lineage:

- *Erythroid*—Megaloblastoid change, nuclear budding, intranuclear bridging, multiple nuclei, ring sideroblasts, PAS positivity
- *Granulocytic*—Bilobed pseudo-Pelger-Huët neutrophils, abnormal nuclear size, hypersegmented forms, hypogranular cytoplasm, Auer rods
- *Megakaryocytic*—Nuclear hypolobation, multiple nuclei, micromegakaryocytes

Genetics

- Driver mutations in *ASXL1*, *SRSF2*, *CBL*, *TET2*, and *RUNX1*, among others
- Often with cytogenetic abnormalities, including monosomy 7, del(7q), del(5q), trisomy 8, del(20q), and complex karyotypes

Differential Diagnosis

- *Other myelodysplastic syndromes* (see specific criteria)
- *Secondary* (*nonclonal*) myelodysplasia (nutritional disorders, chronic viral infections, chronic inflammation, drugs, growth factors, toxins, etc.)

Caveats and Pearls

- Cytopenic lineages may not match the dysplastic lineages
- Erythroid dysplasia with ≥15% ring sideroblasts (or ≥5% if *SF3B1* mutation present) and no increase in blasts is classified as *myelodysplastic syndrome with ring sideroblasts and single lineage dysplasia (MDS-RS-SLD)*

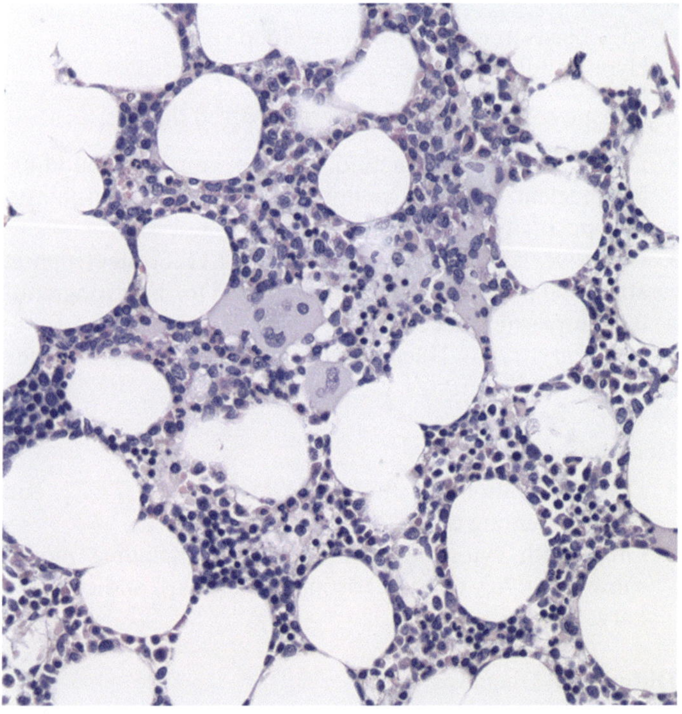

Myelodysplastic syndrome with multilineage dysplasia. Erythroid-predominant marrow with dysplastic megakaryocytes

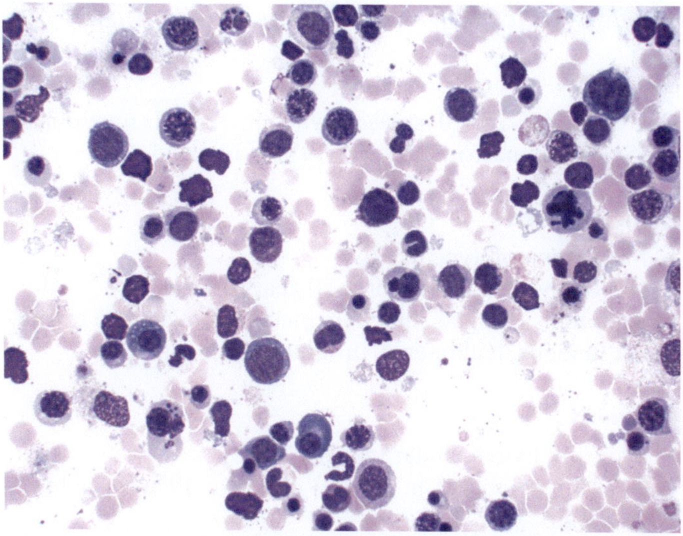

Myelodysplastic syndrome with multilineage dysplasia. Aspirate showing marked erythroid dysplasia including nuclear budding and megaloblastoid changes, as well as scattered hypogranular neutrophils

Myelodysplastic Syndrome with Excess Blasts

Snapshot

- Cytopenia and dysplasia with increased myeloblasts (5–19% in marrow and/or 2–19% in blood)

Clinical Features

- Most common type of MDS
- Generally seen in patients >50 years of age
- Symptoms (fatigue, infection, bleeding) related to cytopenia (anemia, leukopenia, thrombocytopenia)

Diagnosis

- Typically, hypercellular marrow
- 5–19% myeloblasts in marrow and/or 2–19% myeloblasts in blood
- Abnormal localization of immature precursors (beyond paratrabecular region)
- Variable dysplasia of erythroid, granulocytic, and megakaryocytic lineages (usually multilineage)

Subtypes and Variants

- *MDS-EB1* (5–9% blasts in marrow or 2–4% blasts in blood, with no Auer rods)
- *MDS-EB2* (10–19% blasts in marrow, 5–19% blasts in blood, or with Auer rods)
- *MDS-EB and erythroid predominance* (>50% erythroblasts with >20% nonerythroid cells)
- *MDS-EB with fibrosis* (MF grade 2–3)

Genetics

- Up to 50% of cases will have at least one MDS-related cytogenetic abnormality (e.g., monosomy 7, del(5q), del(7q), trisomy 8, and others)
- May have complex karyotype (>3 cytogenetic defects)
- Mutations can be seen in genes *SRSF2*, *ASXL1*, *IDH1*, *IDH2*, and others

Differential Diagnosis

- *Other myelodysplastic syndromes* (<5% blasts)
- *Acute myeloid leukemia* (at least 20% blasts or blast equivalents, or presence of an AML-defining cytogenetic defect, namely, t[8;21], t[5;17], t[17;17], or inv[16])

Caveats and Pearls

- Blasts often found in aggregates (rather than single cells)
- Blasts are counted as a percentage of all nucleated cells in the marrow (preferably by aspirate morphology)
- All cases of MDS with Auer rods are classified as MDS-EB

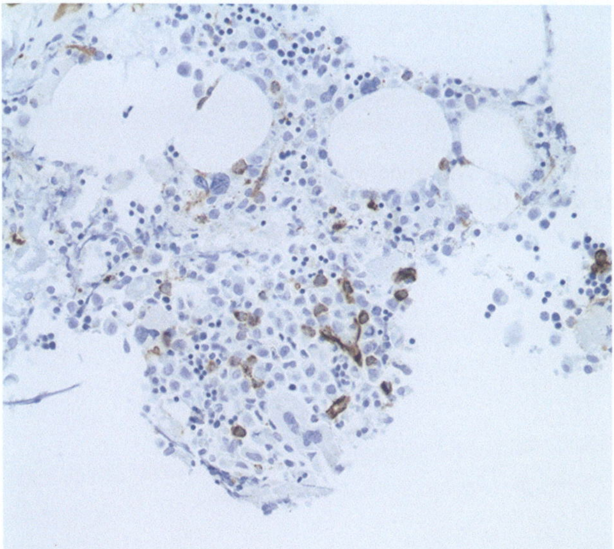

Myelodysplastic syndrome with excess blasts. CD34 stain showing a mild increase in myeloblasts (MDS-EB-1)

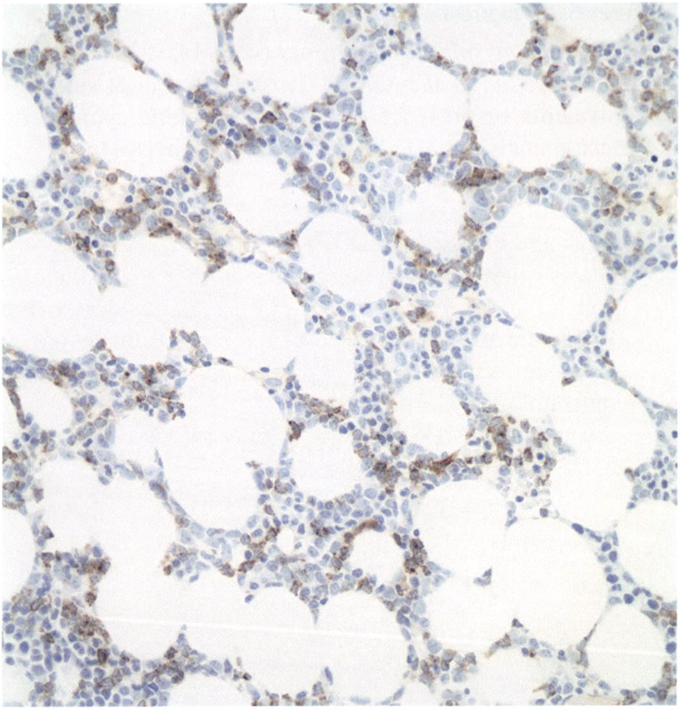

Myelodysplastic syndrome with excess blasts. CD34 stain showing a more substantial increase in blasts (MDS-EB-2)

Myelodysplastic Syndrome with Isolated del(5q)

Snapshot

- Myelodysplastic syndrome with numerous small hypolobated megakaryocytes and del(5q)

Clinical Features

- More common in women
- Anemia and thrombocytosis (common)

Diagnosis

- Normocellular or hypercellular marrow
- Increased megakaryocytes—often smaller in size with small hypolobated nuclei
- Less than 5% blasts in marrow and 1% in blood

Genetics

- del(5q) in all cases
- May have one additional cytogenetic abnormality (but not del[7q] or monosomy 7)
- No complex karyotypes

Differential Diagnosis

- *Other myelodysplastic syndromes* (without isolated del[5q])
- *Myelodysplastic/myeloproliferative neoplasm with ring sideroblasts and thrombocytosis* (generally lacks numerous hypolobated megakaryocytes and del [5q])
- *Chronic myeloid leukemia* (*BCR-ABL-positive*)

Caveats and Pearls

- Ring sideroblasts are occasionally seen
- Morphologic dysplasia of granulocytes and erythroid precursors may be subtle

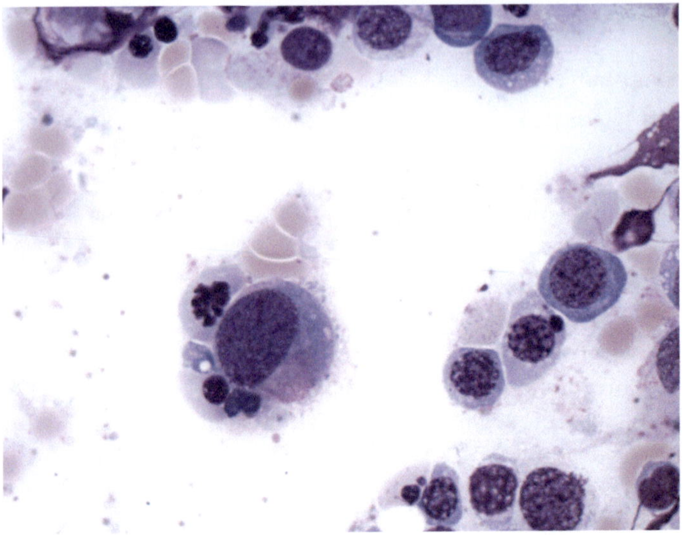

Myelodysplastic syndrome with isolated del(5q). An aspirate smear showing a hypolobated megakaryocyte in a patient with confirmed loss of 5q by karyotype and FISH

Myelodysplastic Syndrome, Unclassifiable

Snapshot

- A myelodysplastic syndrome that does not meet criteria for a specific MDS category

Diagnostic Criteria

Meets at least one of the following criteria:

1. 1% circulating blasts on at least 2 occasions
2. Pancytopenia with single lineage dysplasia
3. No diagnostic morphologic dysplasia but with at least one persistent cytopenia and a diagnostic MDS-related cytogenetic abnormality

MDS Genetics

- Most common: trisomy 8, del(5q), −7, del(7q), del20q, −Y, i(17q), t(17p)

Differential Diagnosis

- *Other myelodysplastic syndromes* (see specific criteria for each MDS type)

Childhood Myelodysplastic Syndrome

Snapshot

- Peripheral blood cytopenia with myelodysplasia in childhood

Clinical Features

- may be idiopathic, or secondary to inherited marrow failure disorders, prior cytotoxic therapy, autoimmune disease, aplastic anemia, PNH, nutritional deficiency, metabolic conditions, mitochondrial defects, or infection
- neutropenia and/or thrombocytopenia more common than anemia
- at least 10% dysplastic cells in at least one lineage, or multilineage dysplasia

Refractory Cytopenia of Childhood[10]

- no increase in blasts (<5%in marrow and <1% in blood)
- marrow is often significantly hypocellular

Differential Diagnosis

- *Other myelodysplastic syndromes* (see specific criteria)
- *Secondary (nonclonal) myelodysplasia* (nutritional disorders, chronic viral infections, chronic inflammation, drugs, growth factors, toxins, etc.)

Caveats and Pearls

- In patients with *primary childhood* MDS, consider germline predisposition

[10] Note: Adapted from Table 6.07 in Swerdlow SH; International Agency for Research on Cancer; World Health Organization; et al. WHO classification of tumours of haematopoietic and lymphoid tissues. Lyon: International Agency for Research on Cancer; 2017.

Chapter 2
Myeloid Neoplasms with Germline Predisposition

Snapshot[1]

Acute myeloid leukemia or myelodysplastic syndrome developing in one of the following settings:

1. Germline mutation of *CEBPA, DDX41, RUNX1, ANKRD26, ETV6*, or *GATA2* gene
2. Inherited bone marrow failure syndromes:
   (a) *Fanconi anemia* (pancytopenia due to *FANC* gene mutations)
   (b) *Severe congenital neutropenia*
   (c) *Diamond-Blackfan anemia* (pure red cell aplasia with *RPS19* mutation)
   (d) *Shwachman-Diamond syndrome* (pancreatic insufficiency and cytopenia with *SBDS* mutation)
   (e) Telomere maintenance disorders (*dyskeratosis congenita*, *TERC* mutation, *TERT* mutation)

---

[1] Note: Adapted from Table 7.01 in Swerdlow SH; International Agency for Research on Cancer; World Health Organization; et al. WHO classification of tumours of haematopoietic and lymphoid tissues. Lyon: International Agency for Research on Cancer; 2017.

© Springer Nature Switzerland AG 2019
S. D. Hudnall et al., *Pocket Guide to Diagnostic Hematopathology*, https://doi.org/10.1007/978-3-030-10630-0_2

Mutation Phenotype

CEBPA
- Children and young adults with AML
- No preexisting hematologic disease

DDX41
- Older adults with MDS, AML, CML, CMML, or lymphoma
- No preexisting hematologic disease

ETV6
- Thrombocytopenia with small hyposegmented megakaryocytes
- MDS, AML, CMML, B-LBL, or myeloma

ANKRD26
- Thrombocytopenia with small hyposegmented megakaryocytes
- AML, MDS, CMML, or CLL

RUNX1
- Variable thrombocytopenia and abnormal platelet function
- Young adults with MDS, AML, CMML, T-LBL, or B-cell neoplasm

GATA2
- MDS or AML, sometimes associated with immunodeficiency, viral/atypical mycobacterial infection, or lymphedema

Chapter 3
Acute Myeloid Leukemia and Related Precursor Neoplasms

Acute Myeloid Leukemia with Recurrent Genetic Abnormalities

Snapshot

- AML with specific balanced translocations or inversions

Morphology

- Clues include promyelocytic maturation, myeloid dysplasia, dysmegakaryopoiesis, abnormal eosinophils, basophilia, and monocytic or megakaryoblastic maturation

Genetic Subtypes

t(15;17)(q22;q12) *PML-RARA* translocation

- *Acute promyelocytic leukemia*
- DIC, ATRA sensitivity
- Negative for CD34 and HLA-DR

© Springer Nature Switzerland AG 2019

S. D. Hudnall et al., *Pocket Guide to Diagnostic Hematopathology*, https://doi.org/10.1007/978-3-030-10630-0_3

t(8;21)(q22;q22) *RUNX1*
- Large myeloblasts with prominent azurophilic granules, granulocytic dysmaturation
- Aberrant expression of CD19 and PAX-5
- Favorable prognosis

inv(16)(p13.1q22) and t(16;16)(p13.1;q22) *CBFB*
- Monocytic and granulocytic maturation with abnormal eosinophils

t(9;11)(p22;q23) KMT2A (*MLL*)
- Monocytic features

t(6;9)(p23;q34) *DEK-NUP214*
- Basophilia and myelodysplasia

***EVI1*(3)(q21q26.2) or t(3;3)(q21;q26.2) EVI1**
- Dysplastic changes with small hypolobated megakaryocytes
- May be acquired during CML in accelerated phase

t(1;22)(p13;q13) *MKL1*
- *Acute megakaryoblastic leukemia*
- Infants without Down syndrome
- Marrow fibrosis
- CD34/myeloperoxidase (MPO)-negative, CD41/CD61-positive blasts

t(9;22) *BCR-ABL1*
- No history of CML
- Additional cytogenetic defects often present
- Aberrant expression of CD7, CD19, TdT

Caveats and Pearls
- AML with a recurrent genetic abnormality arising after chemotherapy or radiation therapy should be classified as *therapy-related AML*
- Cases with t(8;21), t(15;17), inv(16), and t(16;16) are considered AML regardless of the blast count

Acute Promyelocytic Leukemia

Snapshot

- Sheets of abnormal MPO-positive promyelocytes (hypergranular or microgranular)

Clinical Features

- Leukocytosis (in microgranular form)
- Often presents with disseminated intravascular coagulation (DIC)

Morphology

- Hypergranular variant—irregular nuclei with numerous granules and Auer rods
- Microgranular variant—lobulated nuclei with inconspicuous granules and few Auer rods

Immunophenotype

- Hypergranular variant—MPO++, variable CD34 and HLA-DR
- Microgranular variant—MPO++, variable CD2 and CD34

Cytochemical Stains

- Strongly MPO-positive

Genetics

- *PML-RARA* translocation [t(15;17)(q22;q12)]

Differential Diagnosis

- *AML with maturation* (CD34+, HLA-DR+, no *PML-RARA* translocation)

Caveats and Pearls

- Cases with a variant *RARA* translocation should be labeled as AML with variant *RARA* translocation—not as acute promyelocytic leukemia
- Promyelocytes may be prominent in early G-CSF-mediated marrow recovery

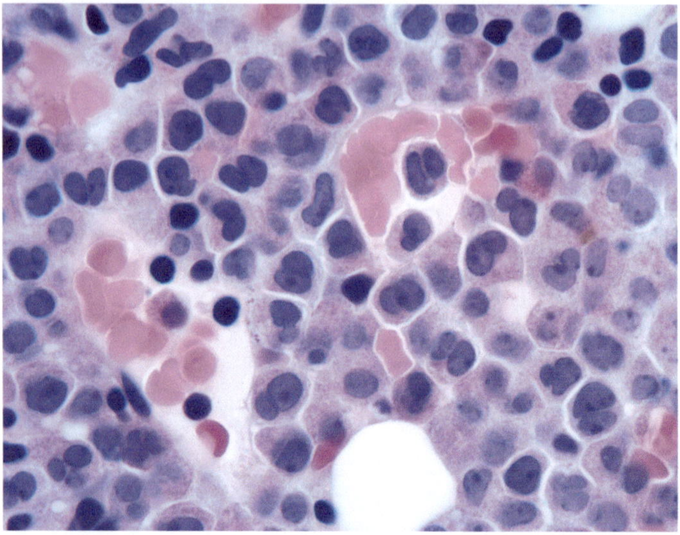

Acute promyelocytic leukemia. Sheets of abnormal promyelocytes in marrow

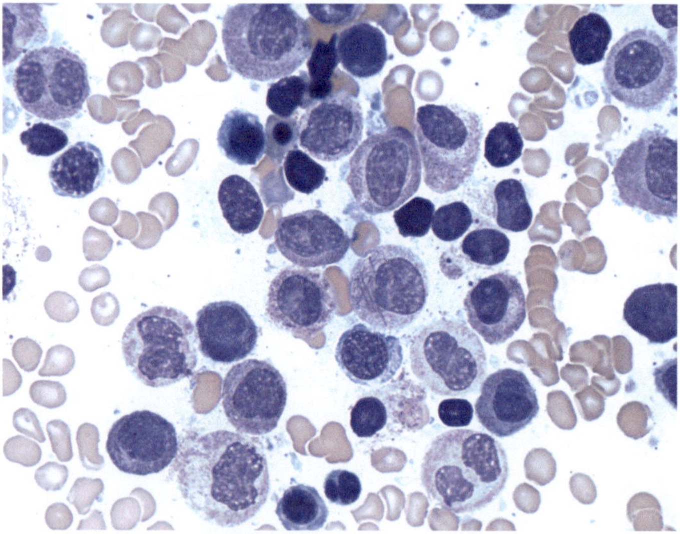

Acute promyelocytic leukemia. Abnormal hypergranular promyelocytes with numerous Auer rods

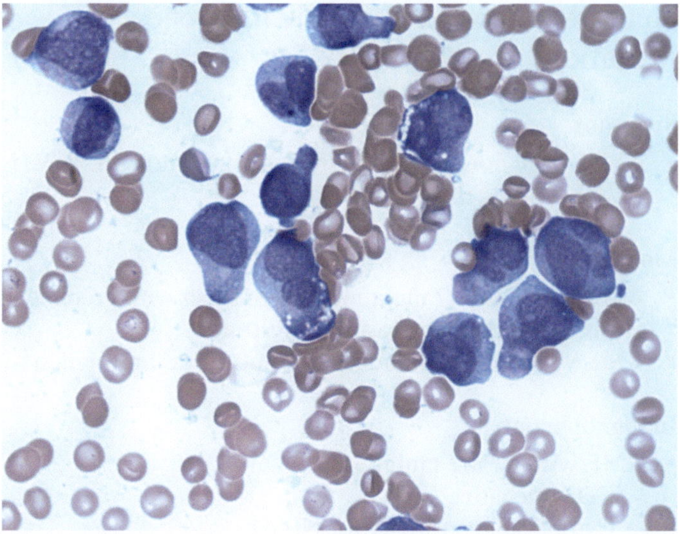

Acute promyelocytic leukemia. Abnormal microgranular promyelocytes

Acute Myeloid Leukemia with Gene Mutations

Snapshot

- AML with normal karyotype and mutation of *NPM1, RUNX1*, or *CEBPA* (biallelic)

Morphology

- AML with *RUNX1* mutation—large blasts with prominent azurophilic granules; mast cell infiltrates
- AML with *NPM1* mutation—monocytic differentiation

Immunophenotype

- AML with *NPM1* mutation
  - CD34-negative
  - Cytoplasmic positivity for NPM1

Genetics

- *FLT3* mutation with internal tandem duplications (*FLT3 ITD*)
- *FLT3* mutation in tyrosine kinase domain (*FLT3 TKD*)
- *NPM1 exon 12* mutation
- Biallelic *CEBPA* mutation

Prognostic Factors

- *FLT3—ITD* mutations—adverse outcome
- Normal karyotype AML with *NPM1* or *CEBPA* mutations in the absence of *FLT3—ITD* is associated with a favorable outcome

Differential Diagnosis

- AML (or MDS) with *RUNX1* mutation is associated with prior radiation or alkylating chemotherapy—if del(7q) or –7 present, best classified as *therapy-related AML*

Caveats and Pearls

- Cytoplasmic *NPM1* positivity by IHC is a surrogate for *NPM1* mutation
- Acute monocytic and myelomonocytic leukemias often have *NPM1* mutations

Acute Myeloid Leukemia with Myelodysplasia-Related Changes

Snapshot

Acute myeloid leukemia with presence of *at least one* of the following:

- Prior history of MDS or MDS/MPN
- MDS-related cytogenetic defect
- Multilineage dysplasia (≥50% of cells in affected lineages)

And absence of *all* of the following:

- Recurrent AML-related genetic defect
- *NPM1* or biallelic *CEBPA* mutation
- History of prior cytotoxic or radiation therapy for unrelated disease

Clinical Features

- Elderly adults with severe pancytopenia

Morphology

- Marrow or blood with ≥20% blasts, often with significant multilineage dysplasia defined as ≥50% dysplastic cells in at least two lineages

Immunophenotype

- Myeloblasts with variable expression of CD34, CD117, TdT, CD7, and CD56

Genetics

- MDS-related defects [del(5q) and del(7q) most common]

Differential Diagnosis

- *Therapy-related AML* (prior cytotoxic or radiation therapy)
- *MDS with excess blasts* (<20% blasts)
- *AML with NPM1 mutation*
- *AML with biallelic CEBPA mutation*

Caveats and Pearls

- More stringent criteria for dysplasia is required for AML-MRC (≥50% in at least 2 lines) than MDS (≥10%)
- The presence of significant multilineage dysplasia together with MDS-related cytogenetic defects takes diagnostic precedence over AML, NOS

Therapy-Related Myeloid Neoplasms

Snapshot

- Myeloid neoplasms other than MPN occurring as a complication of cytotoxic chemotherapy or radiotherapy for a prior neoplastic or non-neoplastic disease

Clinical Features

- MDS, AML, or MDS/MPN seen 5–10 years after alkylating agent chemotherapy or radiotherapy
- AML seen 1–5 years after topoisomerase II inhibitor therapy

Morphology

- Multilineage dysplasia is common

Genetics

- −5, −7 in alkylating agent/radiotherapy-related type disease
- 11q23 (*KMT2A*) and 21q22 (*RUNX1*) rearrangements in topoisomerase-related type

Caveats and Pearls

- This category does not apply to cases of MPN with prior therapy
- This category trumps all other alternative myeloid neoplasm designations, such as acute promyelocytic leukemia and AML with t(9;11)

Acute Myeloid Leukemia with Minimal Differentation

Snapshot

- CD34-positive MPO-negative myeloblasts without maturation

Clinical Features

- Older adults or infants with pancytopenia or leukocytosis with blasts

Morphology

- Sheets of medium-sized agranular blasts, often resembling lymphoblasts
- Auer rods are absent

Cytochemical Stains

- NEGATIVE: MPO, Sudan black B, chloroacetate esterase
- VARIABLE WEAK POSITIVE: Alpha-naphthyl acetate or butyrate esterase

Immunophenotype

- OFTEN POSITIVE: CD13, CD34, CD117, CD33, TdT
- NEGATIVE: MPO (−/+), cCD3, cCD79a, cCD22

Differential Diagnosis

- *Acute lymphoblastic leukemia* (cCD3 or cCD79a/cCD22-positive)
- *Mixed phenotype acute leukemia* (expression of lineage-specific lymphoid and myelomonocytic antigens)
- *Acute undifferentiated leukemia* (MPO-negative, CD34-positive, and CD13 or CD33-positive)

Acute Myeloid Leukemia Without Maturation

Snapshot

- Predominance of MPO+ myeloblasts without granulocytic maturation

Clinical Features

- Middle-aged adults with pancytopenia
- Leukocytosis with numerous blasts sometimes seen

Morphology

- Myeloblastic predominance with only few maturing granulocytic cells (<10% promyelocytes, myelocytes, metamyelocytes, bands, and neutrophils)

Immunophenotype

- POSITIVE: MPO, CD13, CD33, CD117, CD34+/−
- NEGATIVE: cCD3, cCD79a, cCD22

Cytochemical Stains

- Positive for MPO and Sudan black B (≥3% of blasts)

Differential Diagnosis

- *Acute lymphoblastic leukemia* (TdT, cCD19, cCD3)
- *AML with maturation* (≥10% maturing myeloid cells)

Caveats and Pearls

- Blasts with azurophilic granules and Auer rods may be seen
- Blasts may express CD2, CD19

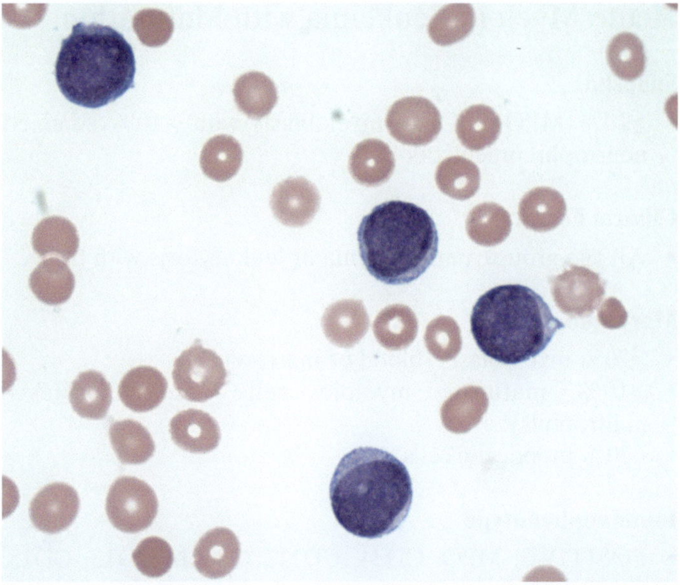

Acute myeloid leukemia without maturation. Agranular myeloblasts

Acute Myeloid Leukemia with Maturation

Snapshot

- ≥20% MPO+ CD34+ myeloblasts with ≥10% admixed neutrophil precursors

Clinical Features

- All age groups; pancytopenia or leukocytosis with blasts

Morphology

- ≥20% myeloblasts (blood or marrow)
- ≥10% maturing myeloid cells (promyelocytes—neutrophils)
- <20% monocytic cells

Immunophenotype

- POSITIVE: MPO, CD34, CD117, CD11b, CD13, CD15, CD33, CD65
- USUALLY NEGATIVE: Monocyte and lymphoid markers

Cytochemical Stains

- Positive for MPO and Sudan black B

Differential Diagnosis

- *MDS-EB* (<20% blasts)
- *AML without maturation* (<10% maturing myeloid cells)
- *AMML* (≥20% monocyte lineage cells)
- *AML with eosinophilia and PDGFRA or FGFR1 rearrangement*

Caveats and Pearls

- Auer rods frequently seen
- Dysplasia sometimes seen
- Eosinophil precursors sometimes increased

Acute Myelomonocytic Leukemia

Snapshot

- ≥20% myeloblasts and promonocytes with admixed neutrophil and monocyte precursors

Clinical Features

- Older adults with anemia and thrombocytopenia; leukocytosis with blasts and promonocytes is common

Morphology

- ≥20% blasts and promonocytes in blood or marrow with:
  - ≥20% neutrophils and precursors
  - ≥20% monocytes and precursors
- Monoblasts have round nuclei with prominent nucleoli
- Promonocytes have delicately folded nuclei with indistinct nucleoli

Immunophenotype

- Mixed blast phenotype—myeloid (MPO, CD13, CD15, CD33); monocytic (CD11b, CD11c, CD14, CD64, CD68, CD163); and blastic (CD34, CD117)

Cytochemical Stains

- Admixed MPO/chloroacetate esterase (CAE, Leder) positive myeloblasts and alpha-naphthyl butyrate esterase (ANBE)/nonspecific esterase (NSE) positive monocytic cells

Differential Diagnosis

- *Acute myeloid leukemia with maturation* (<20% monocytic cells)
- *Acute monocytic leukemia* (<20% myeloblasts)
- *Chronic myelomonocytic leukemia* (absolute monocytosis with <20% blasts and promonocytes, dysplasia)

Caveats and Pearls
- Absolute monocytosis may be seen in AMML—not confined to CMML

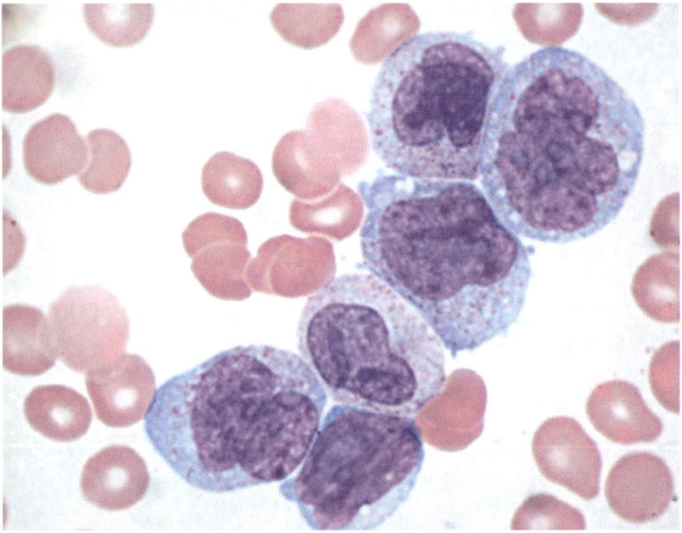

Acute myelomonocytic leukemia. Admixed myeloblasts and monoblast/promonocytes

Acute Monocytic/Monoblastic Leukemia

Snapshot

- Leukemic infiltrate (marrow, extramedullary) with ≥20% monoblasts and promonocytes (in varying proportion)

Clinical Features

- Acute monoblastic leukemia—more frequent in young persons
- Acute monocytic leukemia—more frequent in adults
- Extramedullary involvement is common (skin, gingiva, CNS)

Morphology

- ≥80% monocytic cells (monoblasts, promonocytes, monocytes) in blood or marrow
- In monoblastic leukemia, most of the monocytic cells are *monoblasts*
- In monocytic leukemia, most of the monocytic cells are *promonocytes*
- Monoblasts have round nuclei and prominent nucleoli; promonocytes have folded nuclei and indistinct nucleoli

Immunophenotype

- POSITIVE: ≥2 monocytic markers (CD4, CD11b, CD11c, CD14, CD36, CD64, CD68, lysozyme)
- VARIABLY POSITIVE: CD34, CD117, HLA-DR

Cytochemical Stains

- Usual strong positive nonspecific esterase (NSE) and negative MPO
- Monoblasts may sometimes be NSE-negative
- Promonocytes may be weakly MPO-positive

Genetics

- Erythrophagocytosis associated with t(8;16)(p11.2;p13.3)

Differential Diagnosis

Acute monoblastic leukemia

- *AML without maturation* (no monoblasts)
- *AML with minimal differentiation* (no monoblasts)

Acute monocytic leukemia

- *CMML* (<20% blasts and promonocytes)
- *AMML* (≥20% neutrophil lineage cells)
- *APML, microgranular variant* (strong MPO-positive promyelocytes)

Caveats and Pearls

- MPO may be positive in acute monocytic leukemia

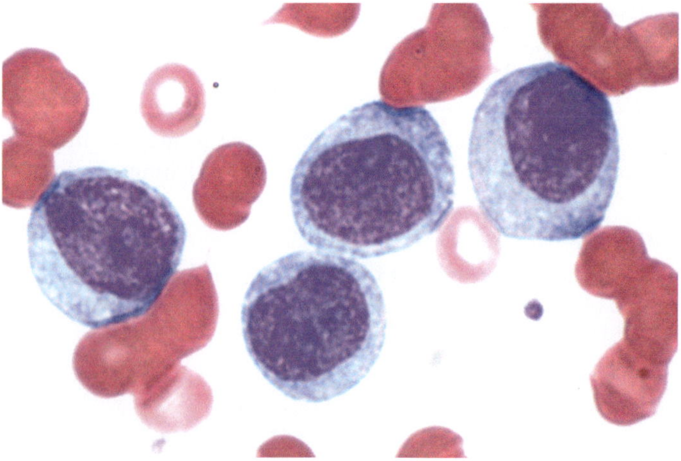

Acute monoblastic leukemia

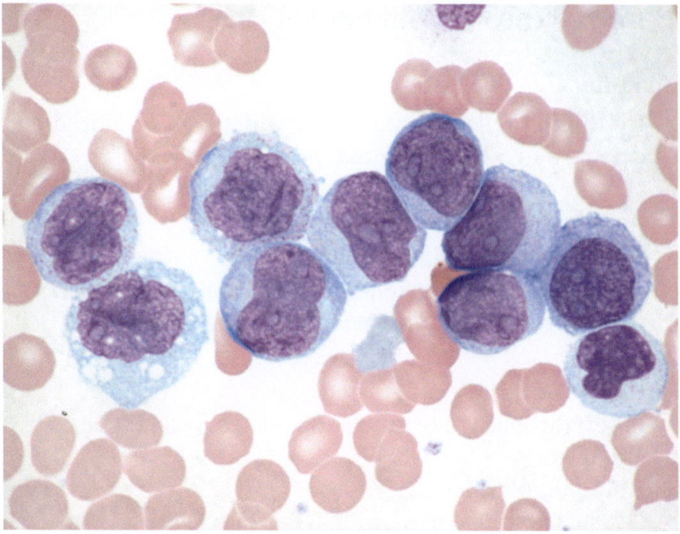

Acute monocytic leukemia

Pure Erythroid Leukemia

Snapshot

- Erythroid predominant marrow with >80% erythroid precursors and >30% abnormal proerythroblasts

Clinical Features

- Anemia with circulating erythroblasts
- Often represents leukemic progression of prior MDS or therapy-related myeloid neoplasm (t-AML)

Morphology

- Proerythroblasts are often vacuolated with PAS-positive granules
- Ring sideroblasts
- Dysmegakaryopoiesis

Immunophenotype

Suggested IHC panel (CD34, CD117, CD71, e-cadherin, glycophorin A, hemoglobin A, MPO, CD61):

- POSITIVE: CD117, e-cadherin, CD71 [+/−], glycophorin A [+/−], hemoglobin A [+/−]
- NEGATIVE: MPO, CD34 (−/+), CD41/61 (−/+)
- ALERT: CD71 may be expressed by highly proliferative nonerythroid cells

Cytochemistry

- MPO-negative, PAS-positive cytoplasmic inclusions

Genetics

- Complex karyotypes; 5q-, 7q- are common

Differential Diagnosis

- *Erythroid hyperplasia* (EPO-induced)
- *Megaloblastic anemia* (deficiency of B12, folate, copper, excess zinc, chemotherapy)

- *Acute megakaryoblastic* leukemia (large cells with cytoplasmic blebs, positive for CD31, CD41, or CD61)
- *Myelodysplastic syndrome* (<20% myeloblasts)
- *Lymphoblastic leukemia* (TdT+, CD19+ or cCD3+, CD99+)

Caveats and Pearls

- An erythroid predominant marrow with >20% myeloblasts in the nonerythroid population, but <20% myeloblasts total (previously classified as erythroleukemia; myeloid/erythroid) should be classified as *myelodysplastic syndrome with excess blasts and erythroid predominance*

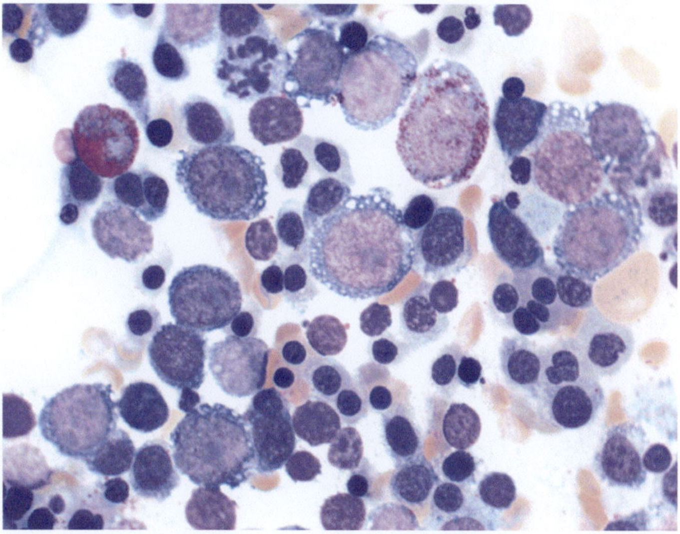

Pure erythroid leukemia. Proerythroblasts with multiple cytoplasmic vacules

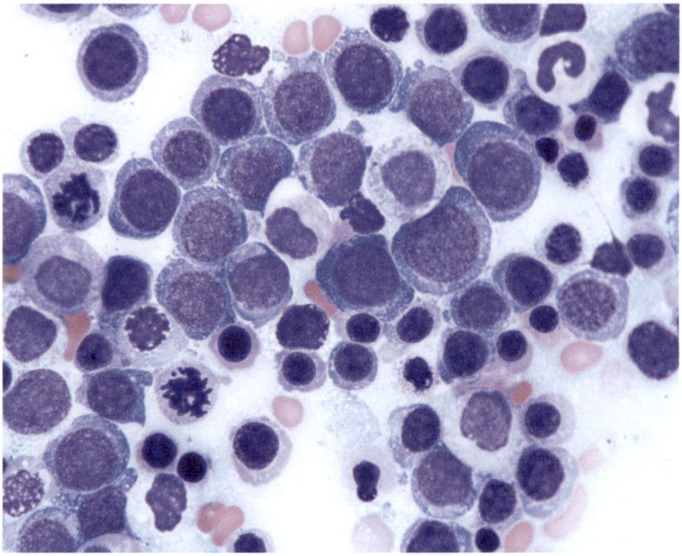

Pure erythroid leukemia. Cluster of proerythroblasts

Acute Megakaryoblastic Leukemia

Snapshot

- Blastic infiltrate in marrow (≥20% blasts) with ≥50% megakaryoblasts and a variable admixture of dysplastic megakaryocytes

Clinical Features

- Peripheral blood cytopenia often with dysplasia, micromegakaryocytes and megakaryocyte fragments, sometimes thrombocytosis

Morphology

- Medium-large blasts with basophilic agranular cytoplasm and cytoplasmic blebs, variable reticulin fibrosis, and variable number of dysplastic megakaryocytes

Cytochemical Stains

- MPO-negative

Immunophenotype

- VARIABLY POSITIVE: CD31, CD41, CD61, VWF
- NEGATIVE: MPO, CD71; often negative for CD45, CD34, HLA-DR

Differential Diagnosis

- *AML-MRC* (with MDS-related cytogenetic defects)
- *Acute panmyelosis with myelofibrosis* (with trilineage proliferation)
- *Rhabdomyosarcoma* (desmin-positive)
- *AML with t(1;22), inv(3), or t(3;3)*
- *Down syndrome–related AML*

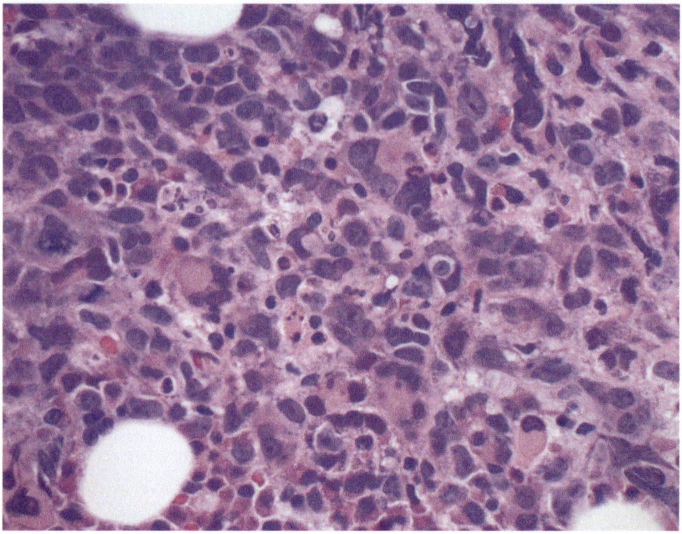

Acute megakaryoblastic leukemia. Hypercellular marrow with sheets of megakaryoblasts

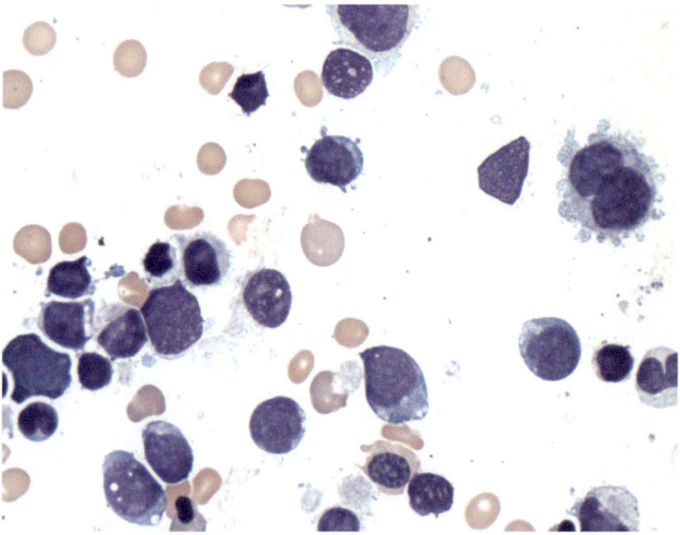

Acute megakaryoblastic leukemia. Bone marrow aspirate with abnormal megakaryoblasts

Acute Basophilic Leukemia

Snapshot

- Mast cell tryptase-negative blasts with basophilic granules

Clinical Features

- Peripheral blood cytopenia +/− circulating blasts
- Allergic hypersensitivity symptoms may be present

Morphology

- >20% blasts with basophilic granules in cytoplasm

Cytochemical Stains

- Toluidine blue–positive granules
- Typically, negative for other cytochemical stains (Sudan black, MPO, CAE, NSE)

Immunophenotype

- POSITIVE: CD13, CD33, CD34
- NEGATIVE: CD117, mast cell tryptase

Differential Diagnosis

- *AML with t(6;9)* (MPO-positive with mature basophils)
- *Mast cell leukemia* (positive for mast cell tryptase and CD117)
- *ALL with cytoplasmic granules* (TdT-positive)
- *CML in basophilic transformation* (BCR-ABL-positive)

Acute Panmyelosis with Myelofibrosis

Snapshot

- Hypercellular marrow with fibrosis, increased myeloblasts, and trilineage proliferation

Clinical Features

- Rapidly progressive pancytopenia with weakness, fever, and bone pain

Morphology

- Hypercellular marrow with diffuse reticulin fibrosis, numerous small hypolobated megakaryocytes, and increased myeloblasts

Immunophenotype

- POSITIVE: CD13, CD33, CD34, CD117
- NEGATIVE: MPO
- Panmyelosis can be highlighted by staining for CD61, CD71, and MPO

Differential Diagnosis

- *AML with myelofibrosis* (no panmyelosis)
- *Acute megakaryocytic leukemia* (≥50% CD41/CD61/VWF positive megakaryoblasts)
- *Refractory anemia with excess blasts and fibrosis (RAEB-F)* (<20% blasts, less acute clinical presentation)
- *Primary myelofibrosis* (<20% blasts, large abnormal megakaryocytes with irregular hyperchromatic nuclei)
- *AML with myelodysplasia-related changes* (dysplasia, MDS-defining cytogenetic defect)

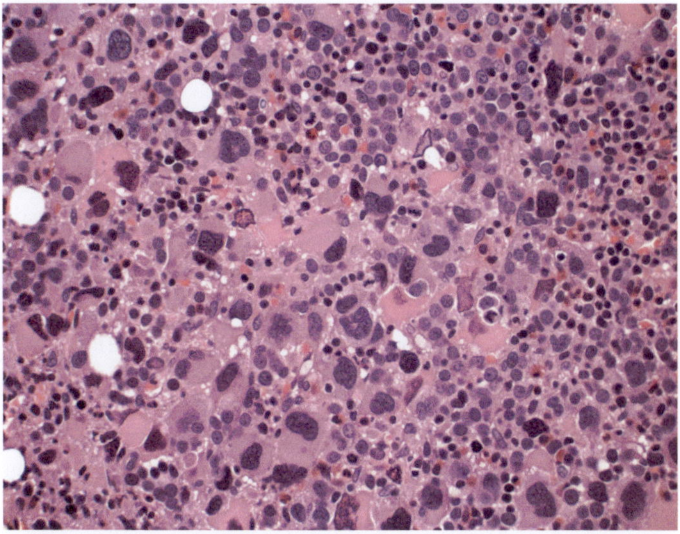

Acute panmyelosis with myelofibrosis

Myeloid Sarcoma

Snapshot

- Myeloblastic/monoblastic tumor in an extramedullary site

Clinical Features

- Mass in skin, node, GI tract, bone, soft tissue, and testis (most common sites)
- May occur de novo, or preceding, coinciding, or following AML
- May occur as blast transformation of MDS or MPN

Morphology

- Effacement of normal architecture by sheets of myeloblasts or monoblasts with or without maturation, often with scattered admixed eosinophils

Immunophenotype

- POSITIVE: CD68 (Kp1), MPO, and CD117

Cytochemical Stains

- Variably positive for MPO, CAE, ANBE

Genetics

- A variety of defects are described, including −7, +8, and inv(16)

Differential Diagnosis

- *Lymphoma*
- *Small round cell tumors*
- *Blastic plasmacytoid dendritic cell neoplasm*

Caveats and Pearls

- Myeloid sarcoma may express BPDCN markers CD4, CD56, and CD123
- Myeloid sarcoma may express TdT and aberrantly express cytokeratin and/or lymphoid markers

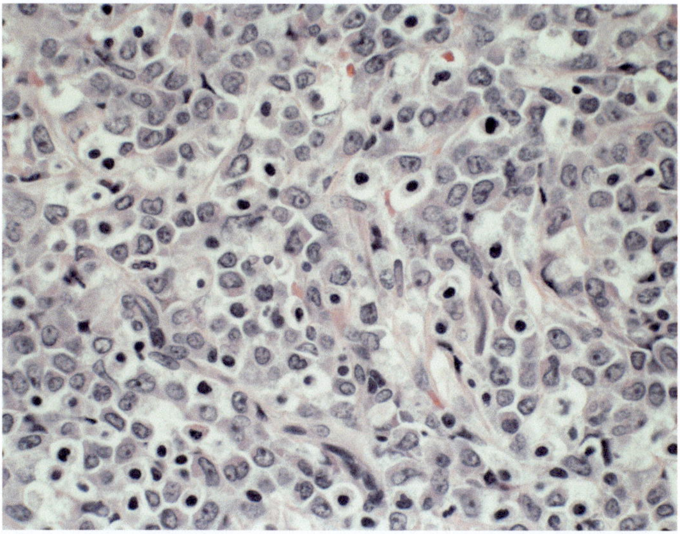

Myeloid sarcoma

Myeloid Proliferations Associated with Down Syndrome

Snapshot

- Newborn with Down syndrome and transient abnormal myelopoiesis
- Young child (<5 years) with Down syndrome and MDS/AML

Clinical Presentations

Transient Abnormal Myelopoiesis

- Newborn with thrombocytopenia and circulating megakaryoblasts
- Spontaneous resolution within 3 months
- 20–30% progress to AML within 3 years

Myeloid Leukemia Associated with Down Syndrome

- Young child (<5 *years*) with thrombocytopenia and MDS or acute megakaryoblastic leukemia

Morphology

Transient Abnormal Myelopoiesis

- Megakaryoblasts in blood and marrow
- Erythroid and megakaryocytic dysplasia

Myeloid Leukemia

- Includes both MDS and acute (megakaryoblastic) leukemia

Immunophenotype

- POSITIVE: CD41, CD42b, CD61, CD71, CD117, CD34 (TAM > AML)
- NEGATIVE: MPO, glycophorin A, CD14

Genetics

- *GATA1* mutations
- Trisomy 8
- Trisomy 21 (constitutional)

Differential Diagnosis

- *Conventional pediatric MDS/AML* (children >5 years of age with *GATA1*-negative disease)

Chapter 4
Mastocytosis

Cutaneous Mastocytosis

Snapshot

- Multifocal dense clusters/infiltrates of mast cells in the skin (dermis)

Clinical Features

- Commonly occurs in infants
- Pigmented macular or papular skin lesions
- Lesions may urticate when stroked (Darier's sign) or develop blistering
- No extracutaneous spread or systemic symptoms

Morphologic Features

- Compact clusters (≥ 15 cells each) or cohesive sheets of mature mast cells with round to ovoid, spindle-shaped, and/or metachromatic nuclei
- Predominantly involves the dermis, often in a periadnexal and perivascular distribution
- Limited epidermotropism

© Springer Nature Switzerland AG 2019

S. D. Hudnall et al., *Pocket Guide to Diagnostic Hematopathology*, https://doi.org/10.1007/978-3-030-10630-0_4

Immunophenotype

- POSITIVE: CD117 (*KIT*), mast cell tryptase, chymase, CD25 (variable)

Genetics

- *KIT* point mutations, including *D816V*

Variants

Urticaria Pigmentosa/Maculopapular Cutaneous Mastocytosis

- Disseminated red-brown macules or papules
- Mostly perivascular and periadnexal dermal aggregates

Diffuse Cutaneous Mastocytosis

- Band-like infiltrate in papillary and upper reticular dermis
- Skin thickened and often discolored

Mastocytoma of Skin

- Single nodular lesion of metachromatic mast cells with abundant cytoplasm in the dermis, may extend to subcutaneous tissue

Differential Diagnosis

- *Mast cell hyperplasia and mast cell activation* (mast cells aggregates are not compact. Lack CD25 expression; no *KIT* mutations)
- *Systemic mastocytosis* (extracutaneous involvement; systemic symptoms)

Systemic Mastocytosis

Snapshot

- Multifocal dense clusters/infiltrates of abnormal CD25+ mast cells in the marrow or other extracutaneous sites

Clinical Features

- Fever, weight loss, rash, abdominal pain, headache, hypotension, musculoskeletal symptoms, and organ failure
- Anemia, thrombocytopenia, neutropenia, eosinophilia, and elevated serum tryptase

Morphologic Features

- Compact clusters ($\geq$ 15 cells) or cohesive sheets of mast cells that may be associated with reticulin fibrosis or reactive polymorphic inflammation
- Variable cellular morphology (round with granular cytoplasm, spindled, bilobated to multilobate nuclei)
- May be accompanied by reticulin fibrosis and a reactive inflammatory infiltrate

Immunophenotype

- POSITIVE: CD117, mast cell tryptase, chymase, CD25, CD2 (+/−)

Genetics

- *KIT* point mutations, usually D816V

Variants[1]

Indolent Systemic Mastocytosis

- Low-level mast cell infiltration without end-organ damage

Smoldering Systemic Mastocytosis

- Marked mast cell infiltration, often with organomegaly, but no end-organ damage

---

[1] Note: Adapted from Tables 3.01, 3.02, 3.03 in Swerdlow SH; International Agency for Research on Cancer; World Health Organization; et al. WHO classification of tumours of haematopoietic and lymphoid tissues. Lyon: International Agency for Research on Cancer; 2017.

Systemic Mastocytosis with an Associated Hematologic Neoplasm

- Concomitant involvement by a myeloid neoplasm, non-Hodgkin lymphoma, or plasma cell neoplasm

Aggressive Systemic Mastocytosis

- Marked mast cell infiltration leading to end-organ damage

Mast Cell Leukemia

- Rare aggressive disease with >20% atypical mast cells in marrow aspirate and >10% of circulating leukocytes

Differential Diagnosis

- *Mast cell hyperplasia and mast cell activation* (mast cell aggregates are not well defined. CD25-negative; no *KIT* mutations)
- *Cutaneous mastocytosis* (aggregates/clusters of mast cells limited to the skin [dermis; no systemic symptoms])

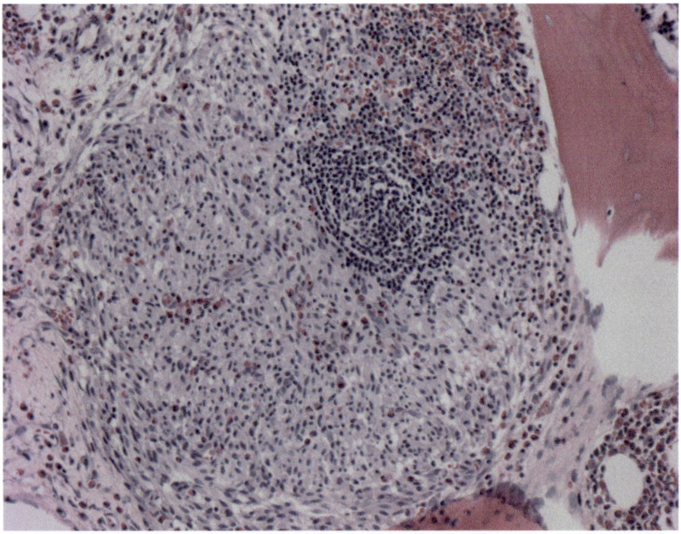

Systemic mastocytosis. Spindled mast cell aggregate with associated small lymphocytic aggregate (bone marrow)

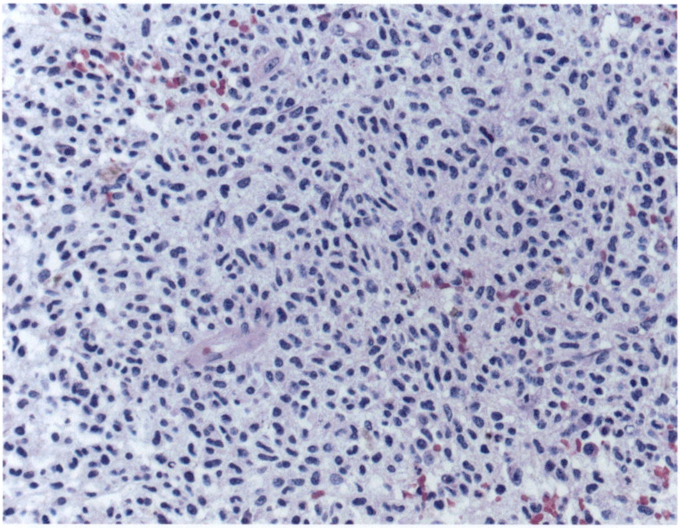

Sheets of spindled mast cells in marrow (mast cell leukemia)

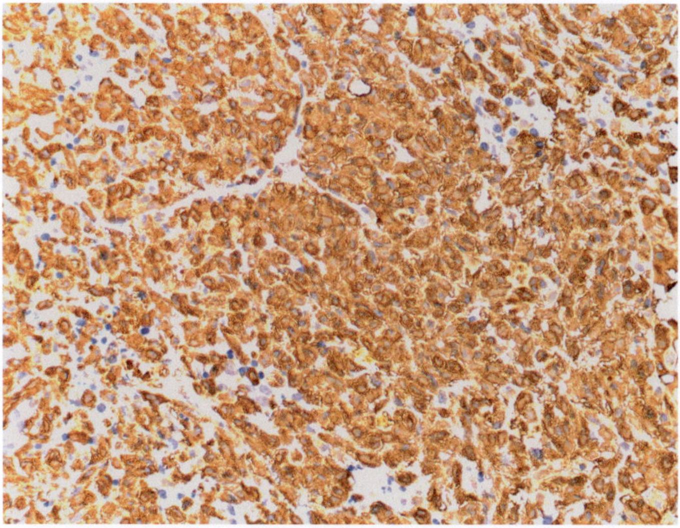

Sheets of mast cell tryptase-positive mast cells

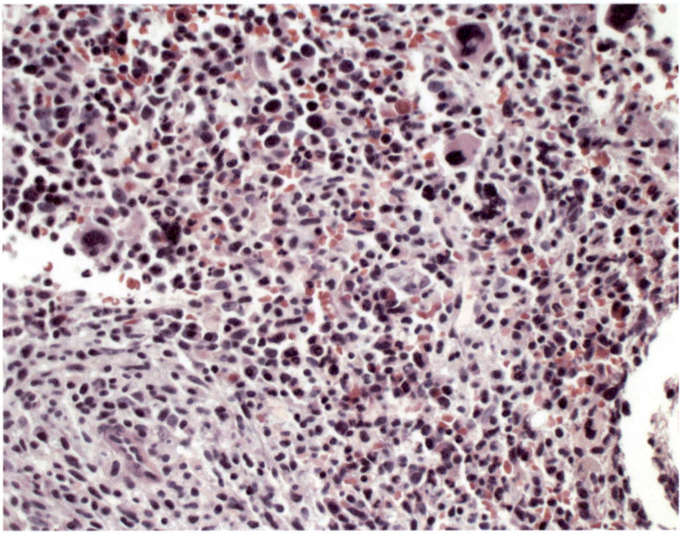

Systemic mastocytosis with an associated hematological neoplasm. Note the mast cell aggregate in lower left and myelodysplastic syndrome in upper right

Chapter 5
Blastic Plasmacytoid Dendritic Cell Neoplasm

Snapshot

- Monotonous infiltrate of blasts in dermis, commonly involving blood, marrow, nodes

Clinical Features

- Wide age range, most commonly in older males
- Sites include skin, blood, marrow, lymph nodes

Morphology

- Monomorphic infiltrate of medium-sized blasts in dermis, interfollicular infiltrate in nodes, interstitial infiltrate in marrow

Immunophenotype

- POSITIVE: CD4, CD56, CD123, and TCL1
- VARIABLY POSITIVE: CD68 and TdT
- NEGATIVE: CD3, CD20, CD34, CD117, lysozyme, MPO, NSE

© Springer Nature Switzerland AG 2019

S. D. Hudnall et al., *Pocket Guide to Diagnostic Hematopathology*, https://doi.org/10.1007/978-3-030-10630-0_5

Genetics

- Complex karyotypic defects (including 5q defects)

Differential Diagnosis

- *Acute leukemia of ambiguous lineage* (without classic BPDCN immunophenotype)
- *Myeloid*
- *NK lymphoblastic leukemia/lymphoma neoplasm-associated plasmacytoid dendritic cell infiltrate* (CD56–)

> **Caveats and Pearls**
> - May occur in association with acute myeloid leukemia

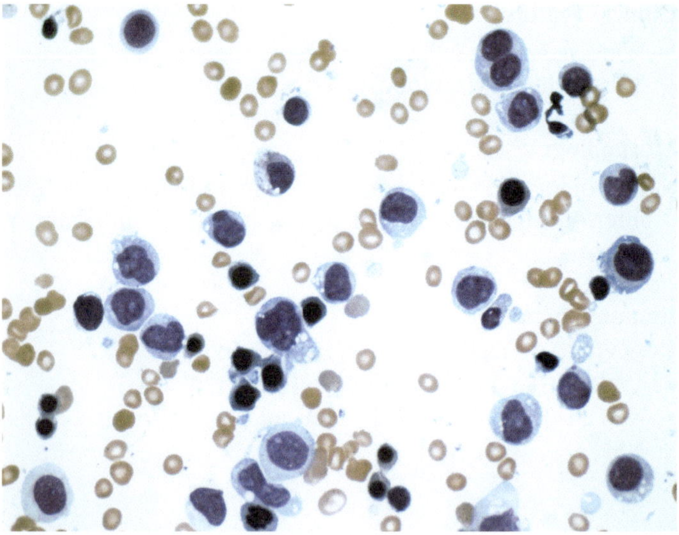

Blastic plasmacytoid dendritic cell neoplasm. Monoblast-like cells infiltrating the bone marrow

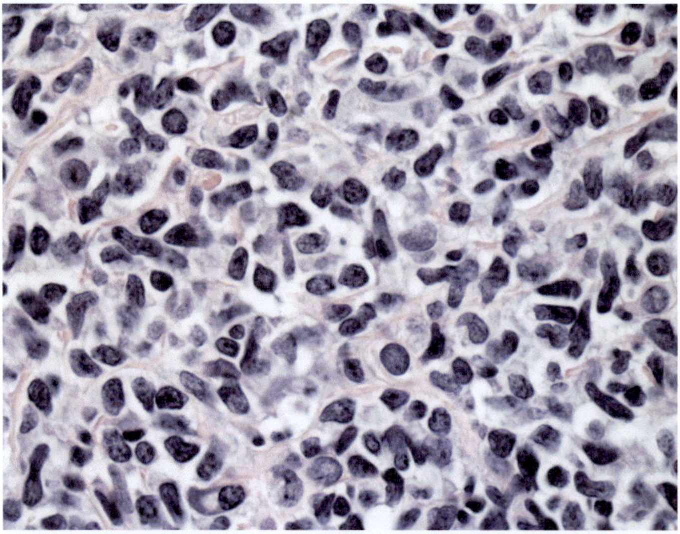

Blastic plasmacytoid dendritic cell neoplasm. Monoblast-like infiltrate in the bone marrow

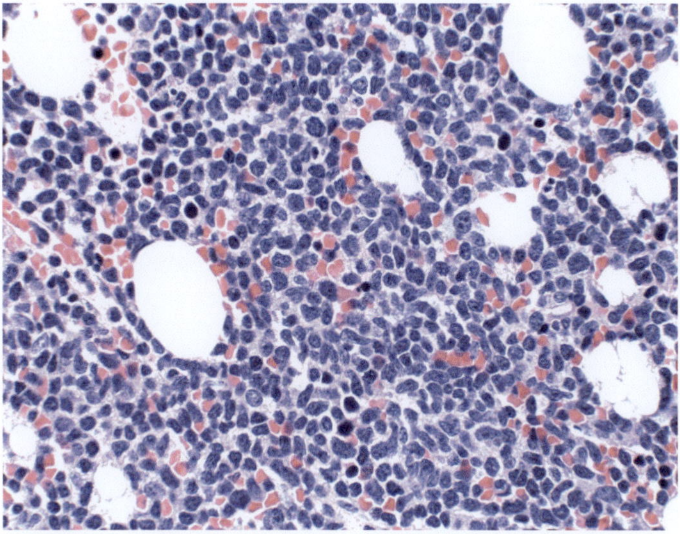

Blastic plasmacytoid dendritic cell neoplasm. Monoblast-like cells in peripheral blood

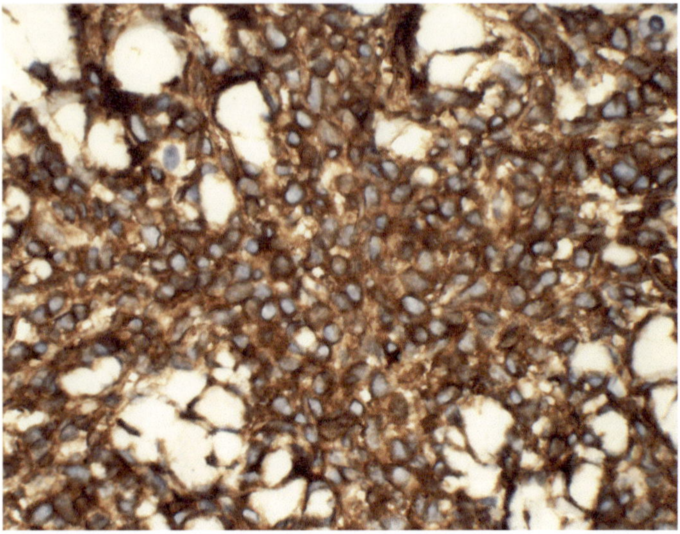

Blastic plasmacytoid dendritic cell neoplasm. Strong CD123 positivity

Chapter 6
Myeloid/Lymphoid Neoplasms with Eosinophilia and Rearrangement of *PDGFRA*, *PDGFRB*, *FGFR1*, or with *PCM1-JAK2*

Snapshot

- A chronic myeloproliferative neoplasm, lymphoid neoplasm, or acute myeloid leukemia, with associated eosinophilia and *PDGFRA*, *PDGFRB*, *FGFR1*, or *PCM1/JAK2* gene abnormality

Clinical Features

- Patients often present with fatigue or other symptoms due to eosinophilia (GI symptoms, respiratory symptoms, pruritus, etc.)
- Pulmonary and/or cardiac fibrosis
- Splenomegaly with or without hepatomegaly
- Mild elevation of serum tryptase

Immunophenotype

- Dependent on the type of morphology (myeloproliferative neoplasm, T- or B-cell lymphoblastic leukemia, acute myeloid leukemia)

© Springer Nature Switzerland AG 2019
S. D. Hudnall et al., *Pocket Guide to Diagnostic Hematopathology*, https://doi.org/10.1007/978-3-030-10630-0_6

Subtypes

- *Myeloid/lymphoid neoplasms with PDGFRA rearrangement* (most common type is a myeloproliferative neoplasm, morphologically similar to chronic eosinophilic leukemia, with *FIP1L1-PDGFRA* gene fusion; can be treated with imatinib)
- *Myeloid/lymphoid neoplasms with PDGFRB rearrangement* (generally presents as a myeloproliferative neoplasm with eosinophilia and sometimes neutrophilia or monocytosis; most common fusion is *ETV6-PDGFRB*; can be treated with imatinib)
- *Myeloid/lymphoid neoplasms with FGFR1 rearrangement* (can present as a myeloproliferative neoplasm with eosinophilia and sometimes neutrophilia or monocytosis, T- or B-lymphoblastic leukemia/lymphoma, mixed phenotype leukemia, or acute myeloid leukemia from MPN transformation)
- *Myeloid/lymphoid neoplasms with PCM1-JAK2* (provisional entity; can present as either chronic eosinophilic leukemia or primary myelofibrosis, or chronic myeloid leukemia. *BCR-ABL1*-negative, and rarely T- or B-lymphoblastic leukemia/lymphoma)

Differential Diagnosis[1]

- *Reactive eosinophilia (will not have a genetic rearrangement)*
- *Chronic myeloproliferative neoplasms (such as chronic eosinophilic leukemia; see diagnostic criteria for each)*
- *Transformation of a chronic myeloproliferative neoplasm into acute myeloid leukemia (will not have a genetic abnormality in PDFGRA, PDGFRB or FGFR1, or with PCM1-JAK2)*

---

[1] Note: Diagnostic criteria adapted from Tables 4.01, 4.02, and 4.03 from Swerdlow SH; International Agency for Research on Cancer; World Health Organization; et al. WHO classification of tumours of haematopoietic and lymphoid tissues. Lyon: International Agency for Research on Cancer; 2017.

- *T-lymphoblastic leukemia/lymphoma (will not have a genetic abnormality in PDFGRA, PDGFRB or FGFR1, or with PCM1-JAK2)*
- *B-lymphoblastic leukemia/lymphoma (will not have a genetic abnormality in PDFGRA, PDGFRB, or FGFR1, or with PCM1-JAK2)*
- *Systemic mastocytosis* (Mast cells are often spindled, have a *KIT D816V* mutation, aberrant CD25 expression with/without CD2)

Caveats and Pearls

- Tend to present with eosinophilia in peripheral blood
- May have increased mast cells in marrow, which can be spindled and express CD25 (and rarely CD2)

Chapter 7
Acute Leukemias of Ambiguous Lineage

Snapshot

- Acute leukemia with indeterminate or mixed lineage assignment (undifferentiated, mixed phenotype, ambiguous)
- Excludes all cases of AML with recurrent genetic abnormalities, AML with myelodysplasia-related changes, therapy-related AML, and CML in blast crisis

Lineage Assignment Criteria[1]

Myeloid

- MPO or any two of the following: NSE, CD11c, CD14, CD64, lysozyme

B-Lymphoid

- CD19 (strong) with CD10, CD79a, or cCD22
- CD19 (weak) with any two of the following: CD10, CD79a, cCD22

[1] Note: Adapted from Table 10.01 in Swerdlow SH; International Agency for Research on Cancer; World Health Organization; et al. WHO classification of tumours of haematopoietic and lymphoid tissues. Lyon: International Agency for Research on Cancer; 2017.

© Springer Nature Switzerland AG 2019
S. D. Hudnall et al., *Pocket Guide to Diagnostic Hematopathology*, https://doi.org/10.1007/978-3-030-10630-0_7

T-Lymphoid

- cCD3 (epsilon chain), or surface CD3

- *Acute undifferentiated leukemia*
  - Negative for MPO, NSE, cCD3, strong CD19, cCD22, and cCD79a
- *Mixed phenotype acute leukemia with BCR/ABL translocation t(9;22)*
  - p190 fusion transcript most common
  - Mixed B/myeloid phenotype most common
  - Must be distinguished from blast crisis of CML (especially if p210-positive)
- *Mixed phenotype acute leukemia with KMT2A (11q23) rearrangements*
  - Most common in infants and children
  - Mixed population of monoblasts and B-lymphoblasts
  - *Mixed phenotype acute leukemia, B/myeloid, NOS*
  - Monomorphic (lymphoblastic) or dimorphic (lymphoblastic and myeloblastic)
- *Mixed phenotype acute leukemia, T/myeloid, NOS*
  - Monomorphic (lymphoblastic) or dimorphic (lymphoblastic and myeloblastic)
- *Mixed phenotype acute leukemia, NOS*
  - Composed of both T- and B-lymphoblasts
- *Acute leukemia of ambiguous lineage, NOS*
  - Blasts with indefinite lineage assignment due to absence of lineage-specific phenotype (negative for MPO, CD3, strong CD19)
  - Aggressive NK cell leukemia
  - Positive for NK cell markers CD16 and CD56, T-lymphocyte markers (cCD3, CD2, CD5, CD7), and EBV, while negative for CD4 and TCR gene rearrangement

Chapter 8
Precursor Lymphoid Neoplasms

B-Lymphoblastic Leukemia/Lymphoma, NOS

Snapshot
- Numerous B-lymphoblasts in blood and marrow, or in extramedullary sites

Clinical Features

B-Lymphoblastic Lymphoma (B-LBL)
- Older children and adolescents, usually asymptomatic, with mass lesion
- Extramedullary disease (skin, soft tissue, bone, lymph nodes)

B-Acute Lymphoblastic Leukemia (B-ALL)
- Young children with peripheral blood cytopenia
- Marrow, blood, and extramedullary disease (CNS, testes, spleen, liver, lymph nodes)
- Increased incidence in Down syndrome

© Springer Nature Switzerland AG 2019

S. D. Hudnall et al., *Pocket Guide to Diagnostic Hematopathology*, https://doi.org/10.1007/978-3-030-10630-0_8

Morphology

- Diffuse infiltrate of small- to medium-sized blasts with scant pale cytoplasm, homogenous chromatin and nucleoli ranging from indistinct to prominent; azurophilic granules in some cases
- Diffuse or paracortical infiltrate in lymph nodes

Immunophenotype

- POSITIVE: CD10, CD19, cCD79a, cCD22, PAX5, TdT
- VARIABLE: CD20, CD34, myeloid markers (CD13, CD33, MPO [weak])

Cytochemical Stains

- MPO-negative; PAS-positive cytoplasmic granules (some cases)

Maturation Subtypes

- Progenitor B-ALL (CD19 and TdT-positive)
- Common B-ALL (CD10-positive)
- Precursor B-ALL (cytoplasmic mu heavy chain-positive)
- Transitional B-ALL (surface heavy chain-positive)

Differential Diagnosis

- *Hematogones* (small nonclonal CD10+ TdT+ CD19+ B-cell precursors, often seen post-therapy, range of B-cell maturation detected by flow cytometry)
- *Burkitt leukemia/lymphoma* (IHC-positive for CD20, BCL6, and MYC; IHC-negative for TdT and BCL2; positive for MYC-IGH rearrangement)

Caveats and Pearls

- Clonal TCR gene rearrangements are often seen

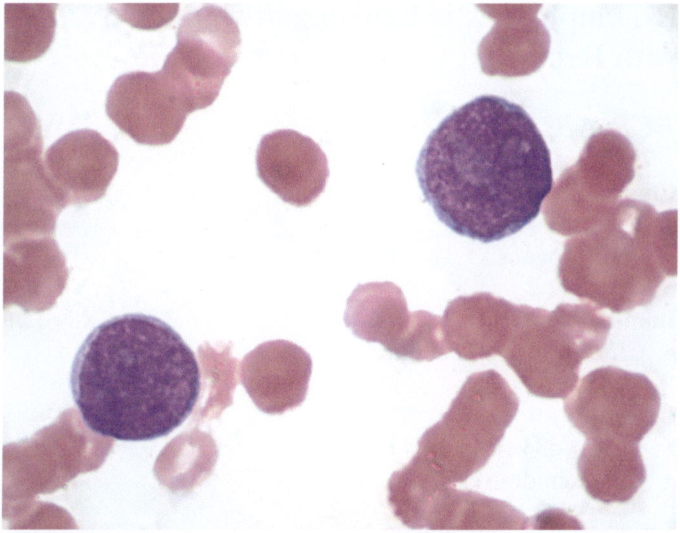

B-lymphoblastic leukemia/lymphoma, NOS. Circulating B-lymphoblasts in blood

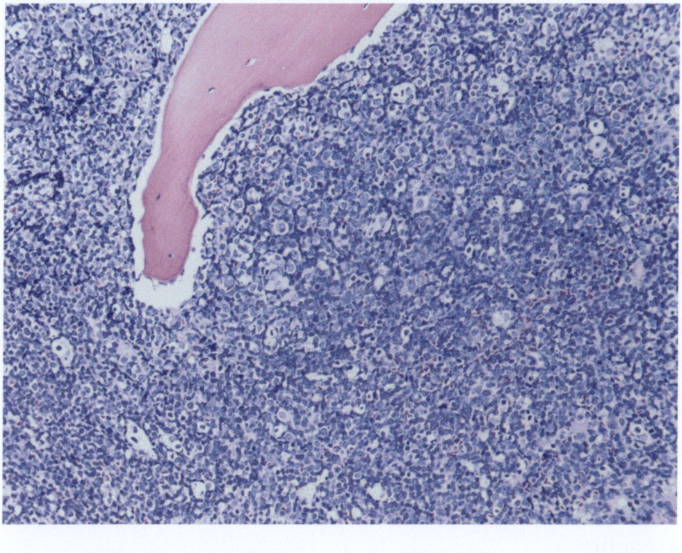

B-lymphoblastic leukemia/lymphoma, NOS. Marrow replacement by B-lymphoblastic infiltrate

B-Lymphoblastic Leukemia/Lymphoma with Recurrent Genetic Abnormalities

BCR-ABL1 Translocation

Clinical Features

- Adults > children
- Poor prognosis

Immunophenotype

- CD25-positive in adults

Genetics

- t(9;22)(q34.1;q11.2)
- p190 (children); p190 or p210 (adults)

KMT2A Rearrangement

Clinical Features

- Most common leukemia of infants
- Very high WBC counts, CNS involvement
  Poor prognosis

Immunophenotype

- CD15-positive, CD10-negative

Genetics

- t(v;11q23.3)

ETV6-RUNX1 Translocation

Clinical Features

- Children > adults
- Excellent prognosis

Genetics

- t(12;21)(p13.2;q22.1)

Hyperdiploidy

Clinical Features

- Common in children
- Excellent prognosis

Genetics

- >50 chromosomes

T(5;14) Rearrangement

Clinical Features

- Eosinophilia

Genetics

- t(5;14)(q31.1;q32.1)
- *IL3/IgH* rearrangement

T(1;19) Rearrangement

Immunophenotype

- Positive for cytoplasmic mu heavy chain

Genetics

- t(1;19)(q23;p13.3)
- *TCF3-PBX1* translocation

T-Lymphoblastic Leukemia/Lymphoma

Snapshot

- Cytoplasmic CD3-positive lymphoblastic infiltrate involving blood, marrow, and/or anterior mediastinum

Clinical Features

- Most common in adolescent males with high leukocyte count and/or anterior mediastinal mass

Morphology

- Diffuse, paracortical, or nodular infiltrate of small- to medium-sized lymphoblasts with scant cytoplasm and either condensed chromatin without distinct nucleoli or finely dispersed chromatin and distinct nucleoli

Immunophenotype

- POSITIVE: cCD3 (sometimes sCD3), TdT, CD34, CD1a, CD99, dual CD4/CD8 (common)
- Variable expression of myeloid antigens CD13 and CD33

Subtype

Early T-cell precursor lymphoblastic leukemia

- POSITIVE: cCD3 (rarely sCD3), CD7
- NEGATIVE: CD1a, CD8, MPO
- POSITIVE (1 or more): CD34, CD117, HLA-DR, CD11b, CD13, CD33, CD65

Genetics

- *TCR* gene translocations (14q11.2, 7q35, 7p14-15)
- del9p and *NOTCH* mutations in T-ALL

Differential Diagnosis

- *NK-lymphoblastic leukemia/lymphoma* (CD56+, CD2+, CD7+, cCD3+, B and myeloid markers-negative, germline TCR and IGH genes)

Caveats and Pearls

- T-LBL with eosinophilia and myeloid hyperplasia is associated with 8p11.2 rearrangement (*FGFR1* gene)

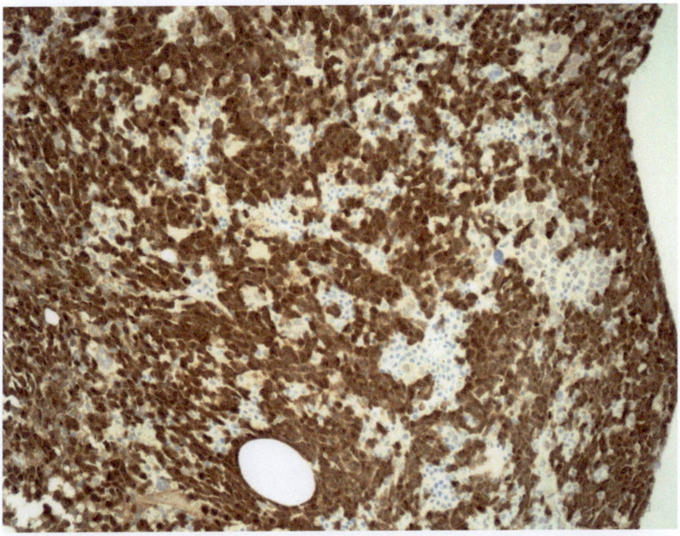

T-lymphoblastic leukemia/lymphoma. TdT-positive T-lymphoblastic infiltrate

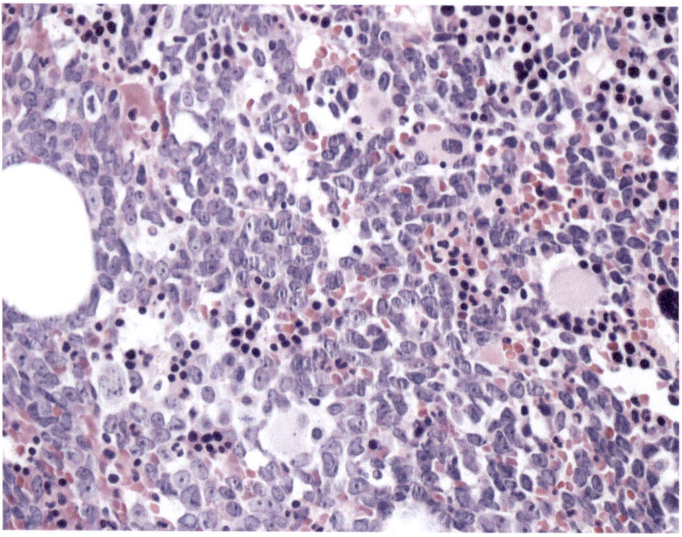

T-lymphoblastic leukemia/lymphoma. Close-up image of T-lymphoblastic leukemia in marrow—note the medium-large cells with immature chromatin and small basophilic nucleoli

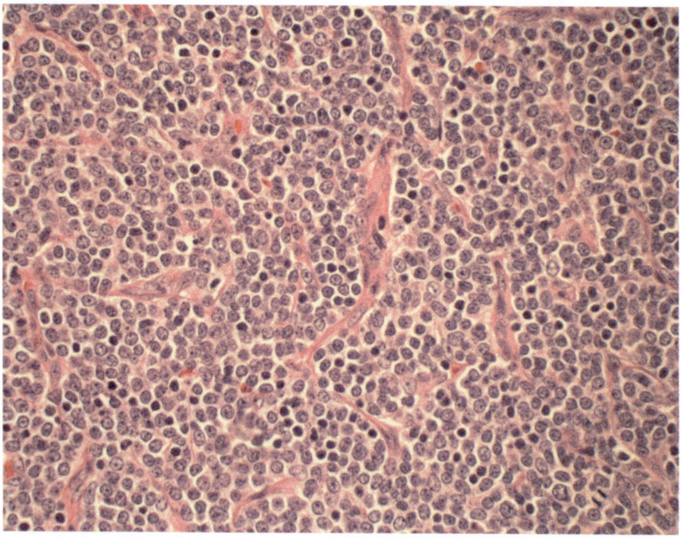

T-lymphoblastic leukemia/lymphoma. Monotonous T-lymphoblastic infiltrate in soft tissue

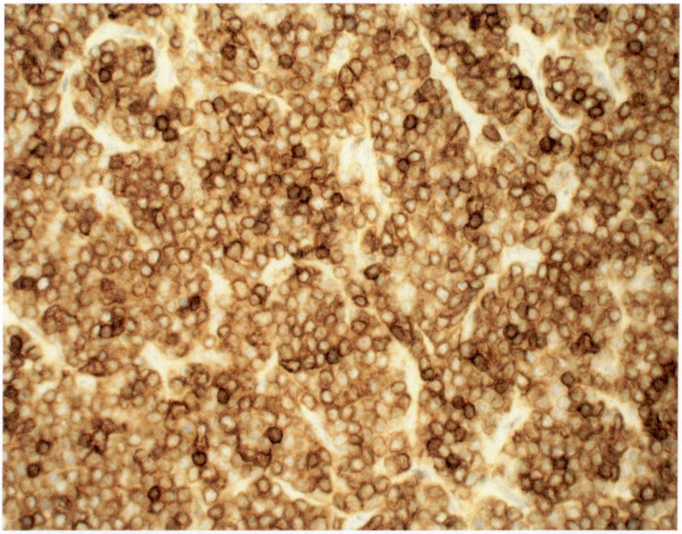

T-lymphoblastic leukemia/lymphoma. Cytoplasmic CD3-positive T-lymphoblasts

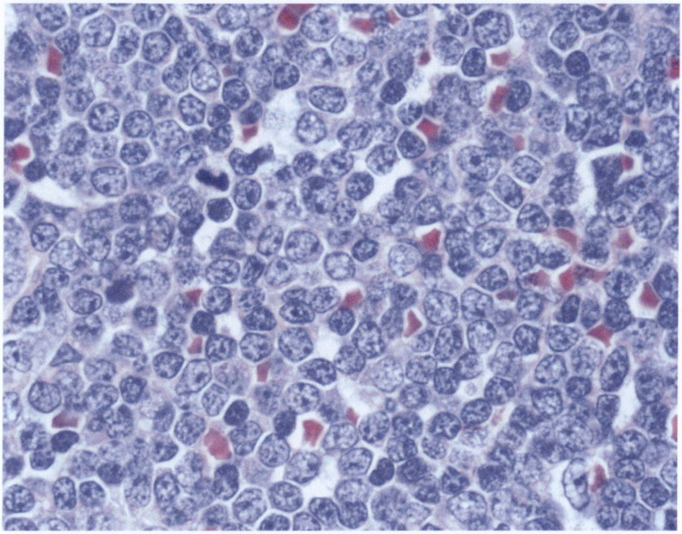

T-lymphoblastic leukemia/lymphoma. High power image of T-lymphoblastic infiltrate

NK-Lymphoblastic Leukemia/Lymphoma

Morphology

- Monotonous sheets of small-medium cells with finely dispersed chromatin, indistinct nucleoli, and sparse basophilic cytoplasm, with high proliferation rate

Immunophenotype

- POSITIVE: CD2, CD7, CD56, cytoplasmic CD3
- NEGATIVE: CD19, MPO, surface CD3

Genetics

- Germline TCR and IG genes

Differential Diagnosis

- *Blastic plasmacytoid dendritic cell neoplasm* (common skin involvement; positive for CD2AP, CD4, CD56, CD123, CD303, TCL1A, TCF4; negative for CD3, MPO, and lysozyme, CD68 [variable punctate positivity])
- *T-lymphoblastic leukemia/lymphoma* (surface CD3-positive, TCR rearrangement)

Chapter 9
Mature B-Cell Neoplasms

Chronic Lymphocytic Leukemia/Small Lymphocytic Lymphoma/Monoclonal B-Cell Lymphocytosis

Snapshot

- CD5+CD23+ = small lymphocytic infiltrate of blood and marrow (CLL), or diffuse small lymphocytic infiltrate of lymph nodes and extranodal sites (SLL), small serum M spike may be seen

SLL Morphology

- Effacement by a diffuse infiltrate of small mature lymphocytes with indistinct nucleoli, scattered large cells, vague proliferation centers, and low proliferative index

CLL Diagnosis

- >5000 clonal CD5+ B-cells per microliter blood (requirement may be relaxed if cytopenias or symptoms present)

Immunophenotype

- POSITIVE: CD5 (dim), CD20 (dim), CD23, LEF1
- NEGATIVE: CD10, cyclin D1, SOX11
- Atypical cases may be CD5 and/or CD23-negative

© Springer Nature Switzerland AG 2019

S. D. Hudnall et al., *Pocket Guide to Diagnostic Hematopathology*, https://doi.org/10.1007/978-3-030-10630-0_9

Cytogenetics

- Del(6q), del(13q), del(11q), del(17p); trisomy 12

Prognosis

- *Unfavorable*: Prominent proliferation centers, high proliferative index, CD38/ZAP70 positivity, germline IGHV, del(6q), del(11q), del(17p)
- *Favorable*: Isolated del(13q), mutated IGHV

Progression

- High-grade diffuse large B-cell lymphoma (Richter syndrome) or rarely Classic Hodgkin lymphoma

Differential Diagnosis

- *Monoclonal B-cell lymphocytosis* (<5000 clonal B-cells/microliter blood for ≥3 months), low count MBL with ≤500 clonal B-cells per microliter blood, high count MBL with >500 and <5000 clonal B-cells per microliter blood, and non-CLL type (CD5-) MBL that may be related to splenic marginal zone lymphoma
- *B-prolymphocytic leukemia* (marked lymphocytosis with >55% prolymphocytes)
- *Mantle cell lymphoma* [CD5+ CD23−, LEF1−, cyclin D1+ and/or SOX11+, t(11;14)+]
- *Marginal zone lymphoma* (CD5−, CD43+, admixed plasma cells)
- *Lymphoplasmacytic lymphoma* (CD5−, clonal plasma cells, IgM paraprotein, MYD88 mutation)

Caveats and Pearls

Asymptomatic nonprogressive SLL may represent a tissue-based form of MBL—minimal lymphadenopathy without proliferation centers

Isolated EBV+ classic RS cells in SLL—must differentiate from transformation to *Hodgkin lymphoma*

- Monoclonal B cell lymphocytosis - an asymptomatic CLL-related condition with low-level clonal B-cell lymphocytosis (<5000 clonal B-cells per microliter blood)—three variants (low count, high count, non-CLL type)
- *Low count MBL* (≤500 clonal B-cells per microliter blood)
- *High count MBL* (>500 – <5000 clonal B-cells per microliter blood)—a clinically significant distinction
- *Non-CLL type MBL* (CD5 negative)—may be related to splenic marginal zone lymphoma

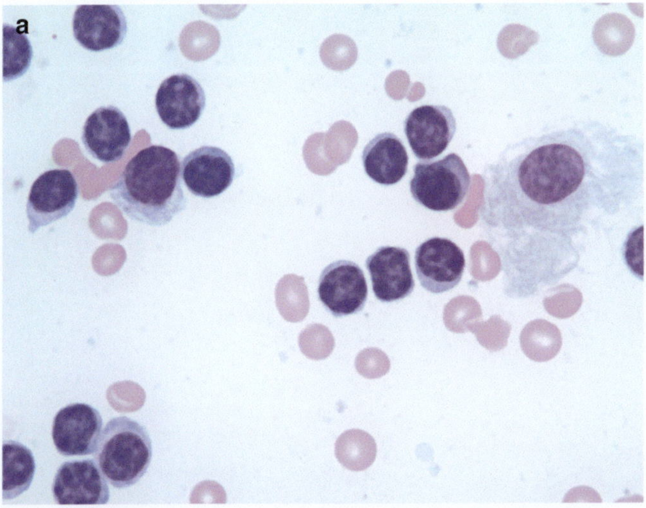

Chronic lymphocytic leukemia (CLL). Small lymphocytic leukemia (SLL). (**a**) CLL with small mature lymphocytes in peripheral blood; (**b**) CLL with sheets of small mature lymphocytes in marrow aspirate; (**c**) SLL with diffuse infiltrate of small mature lymphocytes with a central vaguely defined proliferation center; (**d**) SLL with lymphoid aggregate in marrow; (**e**) SLL with scattered paraimmunoblasts; (**f**) CLL with prolymphocytes in blood smear; (**g**) SLL with Richter transformation

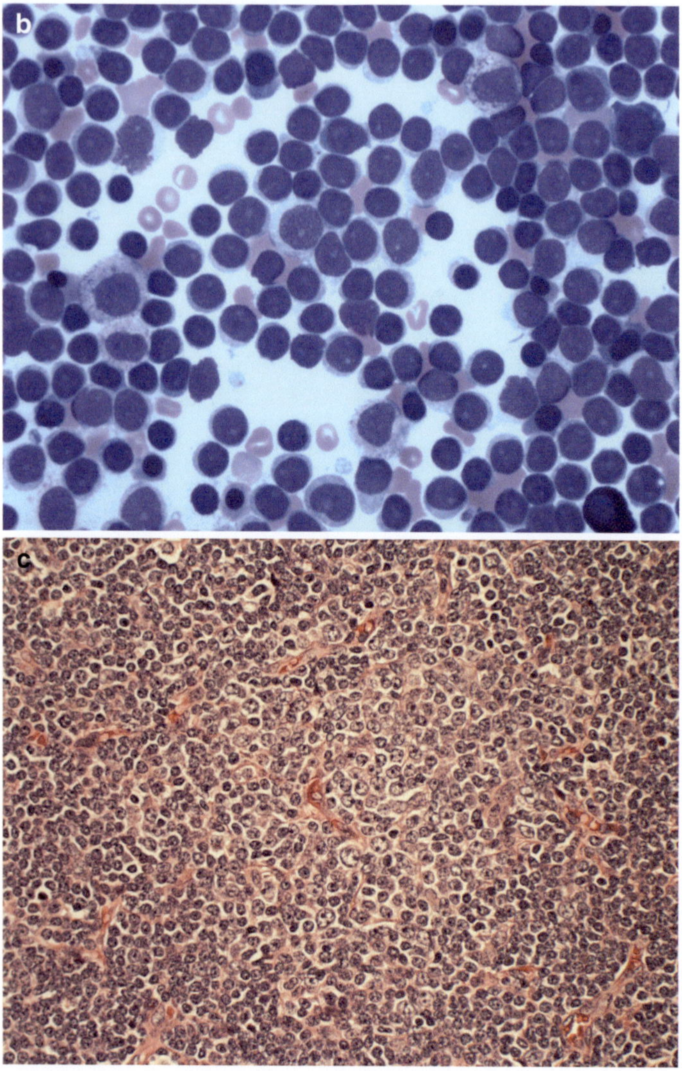

(continued)

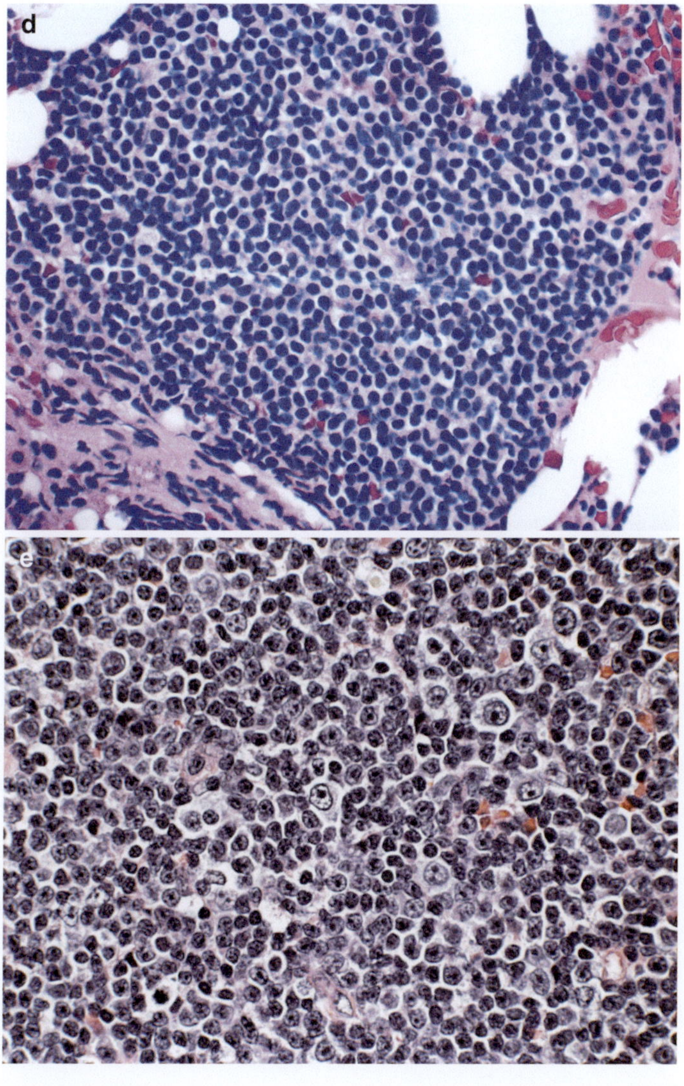

(continued)

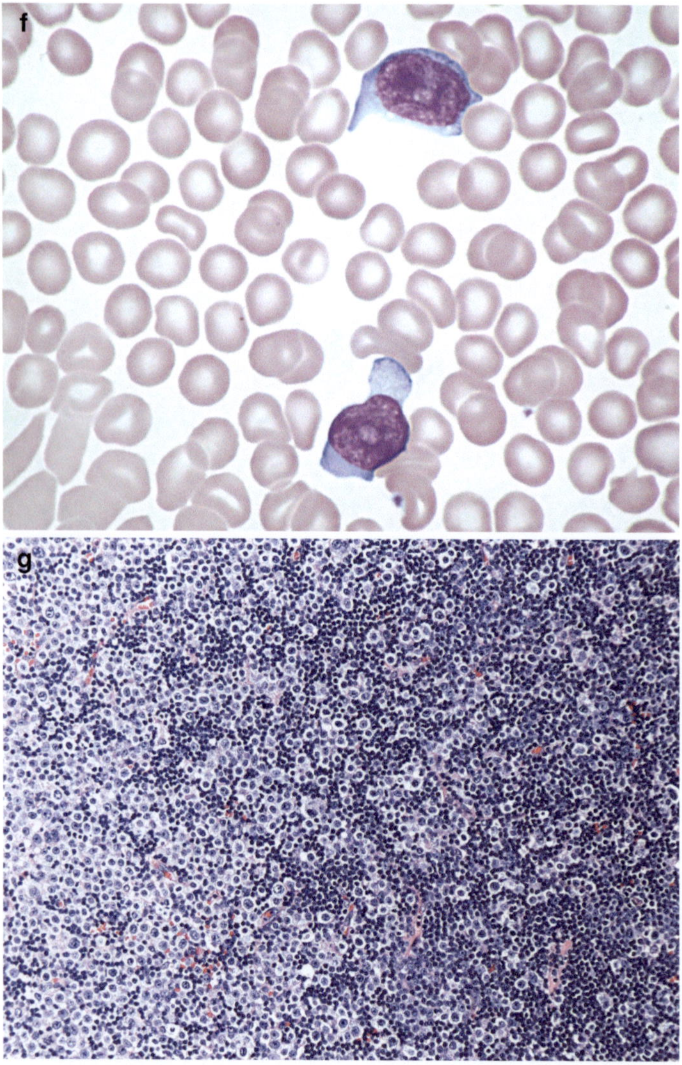

(continued)

B-Cell Prolymphocytic Leukemia

Snapshot

- Marked peripheral lymphocytosis with predominance of abnormal medium-sized lymphoid cells with prominent central nucleoli

Clinical Features

- Elderly adult with fever, weakness, weight loss, marked leukocytosis, and splenomegaly; minimal-absent lymphadenopathy

Morphology

- Medium-sized lymphoid cells with round nuclei and prominent central nucleoli, representing the majority of circulating cells

Immunophenotype

- POSITIVE: CD20, CD79a
- USUALLY NEGATIVE: CD5, CD23

Genetics

- Complex karyotypes, del(17p), del(13q14)

Differential Diagnosis

- *Mantle cell lymphoma, blastoid leukemic variant* (cyclin D1+, t[11;14]+)
- Spleen involvement may resemble *splenic marginal zone lymphoma*
- Node involvement may resemble *CLL/SLL with increased prolymphocytes* (proliferation centers)

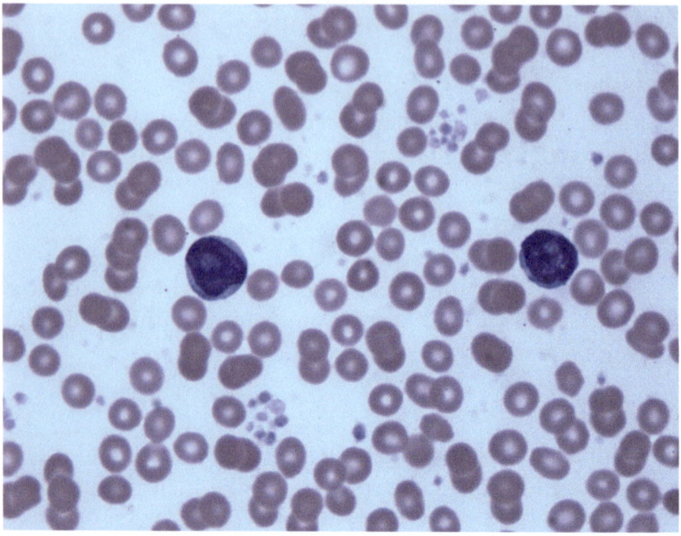

B-cell prolymphocytic leukemia with medium-large lymphoid cells with prominent central nucleoli in blood smear

Splenic Marginal Zone B-Cell Lymphoma

Snapshot

- Spleen with white pulp expansion and effacement by monocytoid B-cells, with extension into red pulp

Clinical Features

- Older adults with splenomegaly; autoimmune anemia (some cases); autoimmune thrombocytopenia (some cases); villous lymphocytes on blood smear
- Peripheral lymphadenopathy and extranodal disease are uncommon

Morphology

- Circulating villous lymphocytes in blood
- White pulp infiltrated and expanded by B-lymphocytes with abundant pale cytoplasm (monocytoid B-cells), leading to germinal center and mantle zone effacement, and marginal zone expansion; involvement of red pulp
- Splenic hilar nodes and marrow involved
- Nodular marrow infiltrate with intrasinusoidal involvement

Immunophenotype

- POSITIVE: CD20, CD79a
- NEGATIVE: CD5 (−/+), CD10, CD23, CD43, CD103, BCL6, LEF1, cyclin D1, annexin A1

Cytogenetics

- NEGATIVE: t(14;18), t(11;14), t(1;14), t(11;18)

Differential Diagnosis

- *CLL/SLL* (CD5+, CD23+, LEF1+)
- *Mantle cell lymphoma* (CD5+, cyclin D1/SOX11+, t[11;14])
- *Hairy cell leukemia* (splenic red pulp expansion, atretic white pulp, nodular marrow infiltrate, CD25+, CD103+, annexinA1+)
- *Follicular lymphoma* (CD10+, BCL6+, t[14;18]
- *Lymphoplasmacytic lymphoma* (CD5 and LEF1-negative, IgM spike, *MYD88 L265P* mutation)

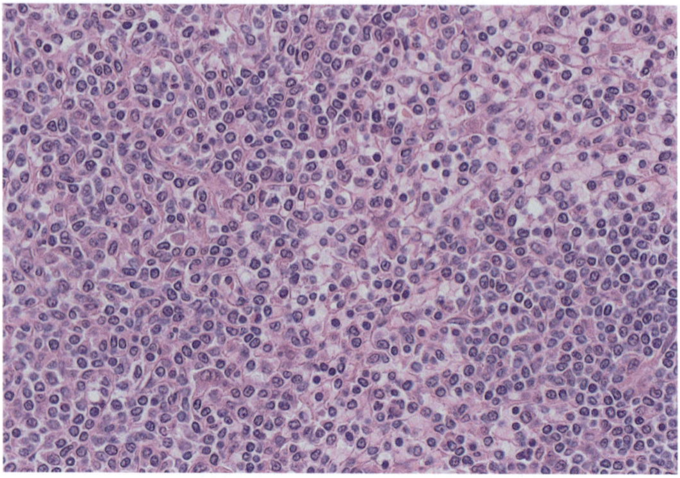

Splenic marginal zone lymphoma with monocytoid B-cells

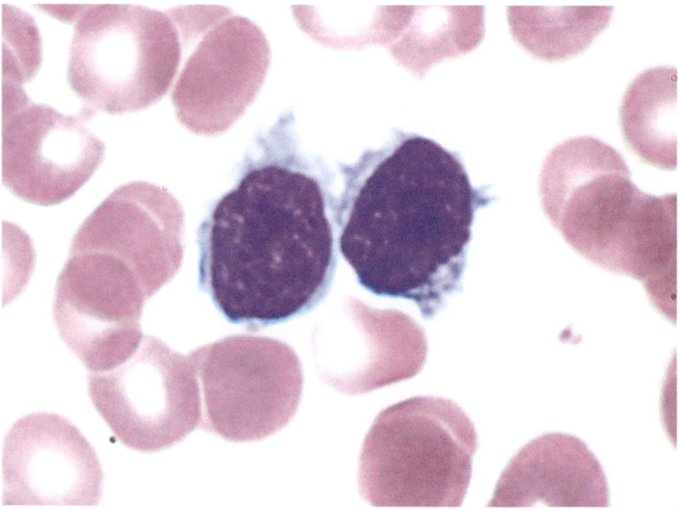

Splenic marginal zone lymphoma. Medium-sized lymphocytes with polar villi in peripheral blood

Hairy Cell Leukemia

Snapshot

- Adult male with splenomegaly and pancytopenia
- Interstitial marrow infiltrate of widely spaced small B-cells with abundant clear cytoplasm (fried eggs), diffuse reticulin fibrosis, and circulating small cells with hairy cytoplasmic projections

Clinical Features

- Middle-aged to elderly males>females; fever, weakness, fatigue, pancytopenia, monocytopenia, splenomegaly; hepatomegaly; recurrent infections

Morphology

- Small cells with oval to bean-shaped nuclei, indistinct nucleoli, abundant pale cytoplasm, and hairy circumferential cytoplasmic projections (seen only on smears)
- Interstitial marrow infiltrate of small cells with diffuse reticulin fibrosis
- Splenic red pulp infiltrate with atrophic white pulp
- Sinusoidal infiltrate in liver

Cytochemical Stains

- Tartrate-resistant acid phosphatase (TRAP) positive

Immunophenotype

- POSITIVE: CD20 (bright), DBA.44 (CD72), CD11c, CD25, CD103, TRAP, annexin A1, BRAF, cyclin D1 (weak); usually negative for CD5 and CD10

Genetics

- *BRAF V600E* mutation (most negative cases carry *MAP2K1* mutations)

Differential Diagnosis

- *Hairy cell leukemia variant* (leukocytosis, villous lymphocytes, negative for CD25, CD103, tartrate-resistant acid phosphatase [TRAP] [IHC], and annexin A1; *BRAF* mutation negative, many positive for *MAP2K1* mutations)

> **Caveats and Pearls**
> - Myeloid cells are annexin A1-positive—careful evaluation of marrow biopsy is required to avoid false-positive interpretation

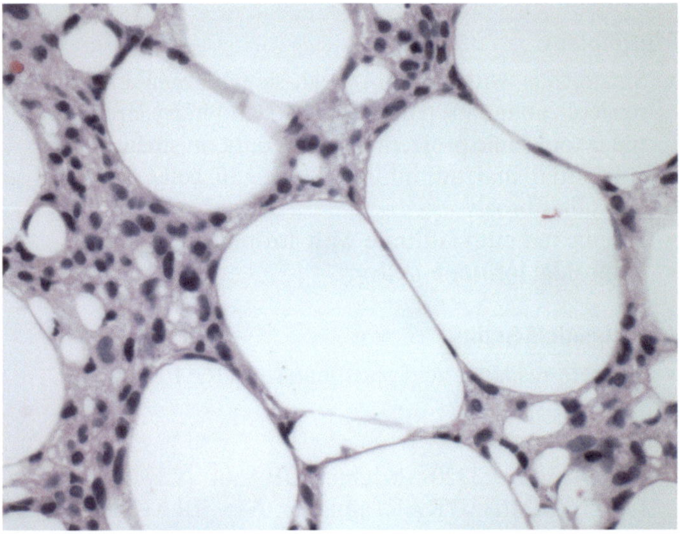

Hairy cell leukemia with subtle interstitial small lymphocytic infiltrate in marrow

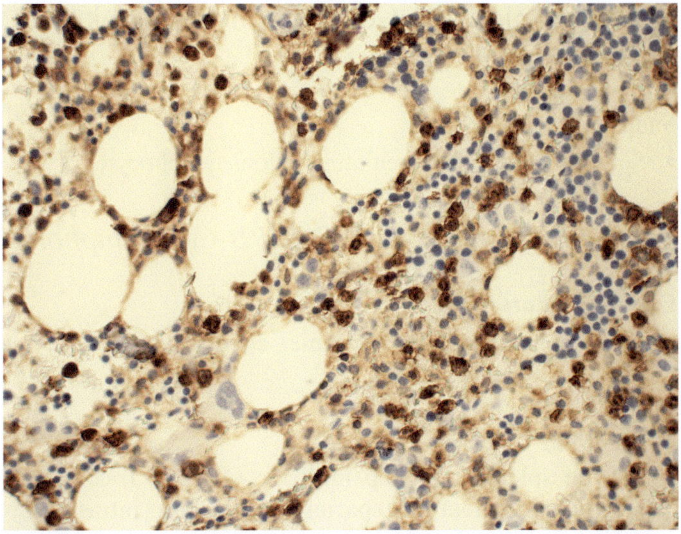

Hairy cell leukemia. Annexin A1-positive hairy cells in marrow (IHC)

Primary Splenic B-Cell Lymphoma/Leukemia (Nonmarginal)

Snapshot

- Splenomegaly with circulating villous lymphocytes

Splenic Diffuse Red Pulp Small B-Cell Lymphoma

Clinical Features

- Leukopenia, thrombocytopenia, circulating villous lymphocytes, splenomegaly

Morphology

- Diffuse splenic red pulp infiltrate of small B-cells with mostly mature features; sparing of white pulp; intrasinusoidal marrow involvement

Immunophenotype

- POSITIVE: CD20, DBA.44 (CD72)
- NEGATIVE: CD5, CD10, CD11c, CD25, CD103, CD123, IgD, annexin A1, TRAP

Genetics

- Often positive for *CCND3* mutations, infrequent *BRAF* mutations

Hairy Cell Leukemia Variant

Clinical Features

- Leukocytosis, circulating villous lymphocytes with prominent central nucleoli, splenomegaly

Morphology

- Diffuse splenic red pulp infiltrate of small B-cells with prominent nucleoli (prolymphocytic); atretic white pulp; intrasinusoidal marrow involvement

Immunophenotype

- POSITIVE: CD20, DBA.44 (CD72), CD11c, CD103
- NEGATIVE: CD5, CD10, CD25, CD123, IgD, TRAP, annexin A1

Genetics

- Negative for *BRAF V600E* mutation, may be positive for *MAP2K1* mutations

Differential Diagnosis

- *Hairy cell leukemia* (positive for TRAP, CD25, CD123, annexin A1, and *BRAF V600E* mutation)
- *Splenic marginal zone lymphoma* (infiltration of white pulp by small-large lymphocytes with abundant pale cytoplasm; nodular marrow infiltrates; CD103-negative)

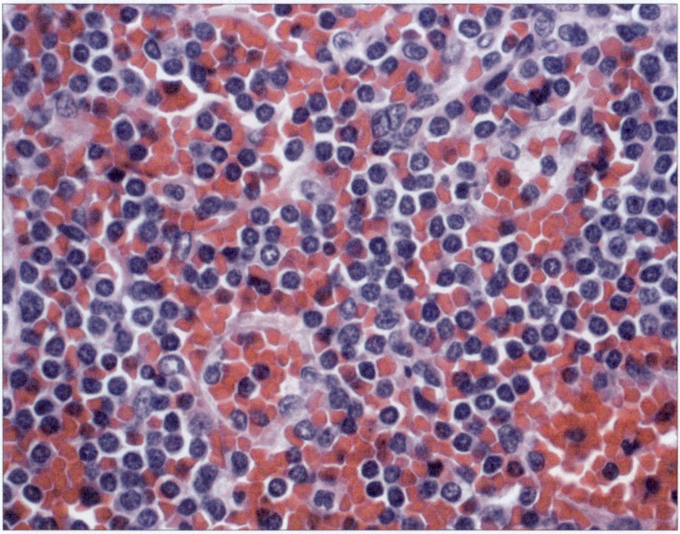

Primary splenic B-cell lymphoma/leukemia, hairy cell variant (splenic red pulp)

Lymphoplasmacytic Lymphoma

Snapshot

- Lymphoplasmacytic infiltrate in marrow, lymph nodes, and/or spleen

Clinical Features

- Older adults with weakness, fatigue, anemia, hyperviscosity, cryoglobulinemia, autoimmune manifestations, and IgM gammopathy (Waldenstrom macroglobulinemia)
- Lymphadenopathy and/or hepatosplenomegaly in some cases
- Uncommonly preceded by cryoglobulinemia or IgM MGUS

Morphology

Marrow

- Admixture of small lymphocytes, plasma cells, and plasmacytoid lymphocytes
- Dutcher bodies and increased mast cells may be seen

Lymph node and spleen

- Generally monotonous lymphoplasmacytic infiltrate with variable growth pattern (diffuse to follicular, sometimes with partial effacement)
- Splenic red pulp infiltrate

Immunophenotype

- POSITIVE: CD20 (B-cells), CD138 (plasma cells), cytoplasmic IgM (most common)
- NEGATIVE: CD5, CD10, CD103

Genetics

- *MYD88 L265P* mutation (90%)

Differential Diagnosis

- *IgM MGUS* (asymptomatic, <10% marrow involvement, *MYD88* mutation +/−)

- *Marginal zone B-cell lymphoma* (larger cells with abundant pale cytoplasm, marginal zone pattern with follicular colonization, *MYD88* mutation negative)
- *Plasma cell neoplasm with lymphoplasmacytic features* (incomplete "CRAB" features, cyclin D1+ plasma cells, no clonal B-cells)

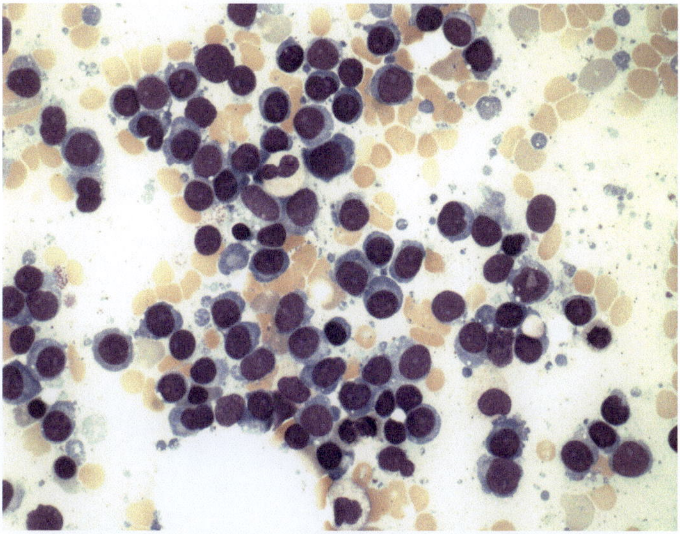

Lymphoplasmacytic lymphoma with admixed plasmacytoid lymphocytes and plasma cells in marrow aspirate

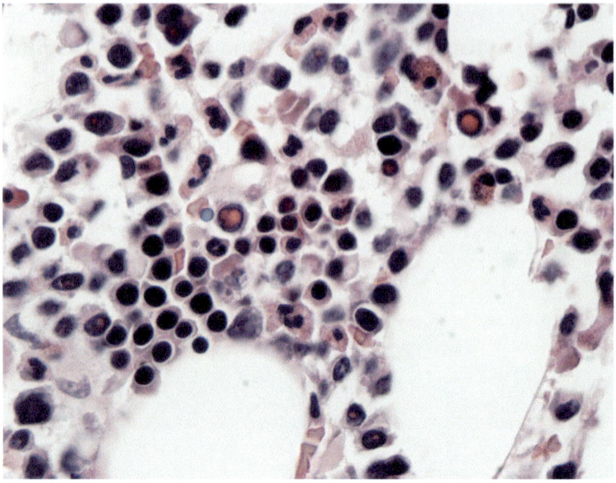

Lymphoplasmacytic lymphoma. Prominent intranuclear inclusions (Dutcher bodies) in lymphoplasmacytic cells

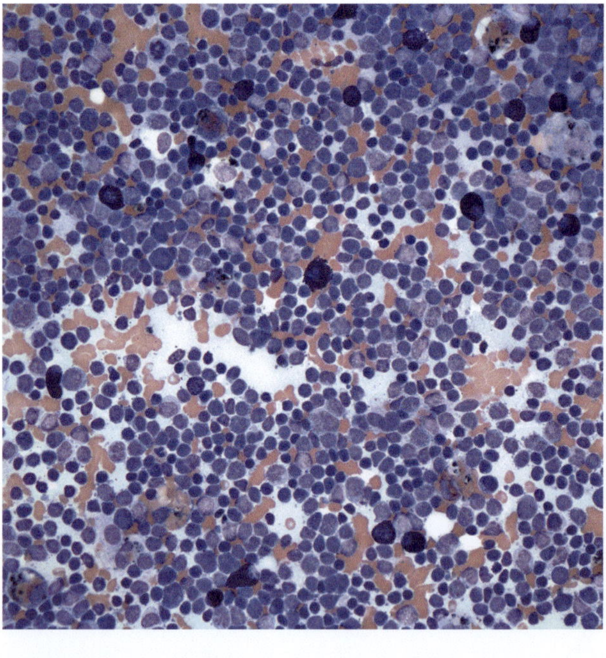

Lymphoplasmacytic infiltrate in marrow aspirate with scattered deeply basophilic mast cells

IgM Monoclonal Gammopathy of Undetermined Significance (IgM MGUS)

Snapshot

- Asymptomatic older adults with low-level monoclonal IgM serum paraprotein (<3gdL)

Morphology

- Inconspicuous marrow infiltrate of clonal IgM-positive lymphoplasmacytic B-cells (<10%)

Immunophenotype

- CD20-positive B-cells
- CD138/IgM-positive CD56-negative plasma cells

Genetics

- *MYD88 L265P* mutation (50%), *CXCR4* mutation

Differential Diagnosis

- *Lymphoplasmacytic lymphoma* (symptomatic disease, conspicuous marrow infiltrate, *MYD88* mutation nearly always present)
- *IgM-related disorder* (symptomatic IgM gammopathy with LPL-like symptoms of peripheral neuropathy, cryoglobulinemia, or cold agglutinin disease)

Non-IgM Monoclonal Gammopathy of Undetermined Significance

Snapshot

- Asymptomatic condition of older adults with a small amount of monoclonal paraprotein (IGH or light chain) in serum and/or urine

Clinical Features

- Absence of myeloma-related symptoms and light chain amyloidosis
- Reduced normal immunoglobulin (–/+)
- Low rate of progression to myeloma

Lab Features

- Serum M protein <30 g/L
- Light chain MGUS—clonal light chain urinary excretion <500 mg/24 hours

Morphology

- <10% clonal plasma cells in marrow

Abnormal Plasma Cell Immunophenotype

- CD19-CD56 +/–

Caveats and Pearls

- In some cases, the kappa/lambda ratio in marrow may fall within the normal range

Plasma Cell Myeloma

Snapshot

- Clonal plasma cell tumor in marrow, most often with M spike and disease-related symptoms

Clinical Features

- Typically, older adults with myeloma-related symptoms, including hypercalcemia, renal failure, anemia, lytic bone lesions, amyloidosis, hyperviscosity, hyperuricemia, and recurrent infections

Clinical Variants

Symptomatic Myeloma

- Monoclonal paraprotein (IgG, IgA, and light chain) in serum or urine (no minimum)
- Monoclonal plasma cells in marrow (no minimum)
- Myeloma-related symptoms

Asymptomatic (Smoldering) Myeloma

- M protein in serum or urine (>3 g/dL)
- Monoclonal plasma cells in marrow (10–60%)
- No myeloma-related symptoms

Nonsecretory Myeloma

- No secreted M protein detected (cytoplasmic only, nonproducer)
- Myeloma-related symptoms

Plasma Cell Leukemia

- Defined as increased clonal plasma cells in blood (either >20% of leukocytes or absolute count >2000/μL)
- Mostly primary (no antecedent myeloma)
- Often CD20-positive, CD56-negative

Morphology

- Plasma cells with variable morphology, including mature, plasmablastic, pleomorphic, spindle, and lymphoplasmacytic forms

Immunophenotype

- POSITIVE: CD138, CD38, kappa or lambda (unless nonproducer)
- VARIABLY POSITIVE: CD56, CD117, CD79a, cyclin D1 (lymphoplasmacytic)
- NEGATIVE: CD45, CD19, CD20 (most cases)

Genetics

- t(4;14), t(14;16), t(14;20), del(17p13), del(13)

Differential Diagnosis

- *Lymphoplasmacytic lymphoma* (*MYD88* mutation)
- *Reactive polyclonal plasmacytosis* (infection [syphilis, tuberculosis], chronic inflammation [rheumatoid arthritis])
- *Plasma cell–rich MALT lymphoma* (particularly thyroid, admixed CD20-positive B-cells)

Caveats and Pearls

- Tumor plasma cells are rarely CD138-negative (CD38-positive)
- Plasma cells are often difficult to identify on H&E-stained marrow sections and underrepresented on smears and by flow cytometry, requiring CD138 IHC for accurate counting
- Kappa/lambda in situ hybridization (ISH) is useful in cases with high IHC background staining
- Absence of detectable light chain expression may be indicative of *nonproducer myeloma*; staining for IgG, IgA, and IgM is recommended to rule out *heavy chain disease*

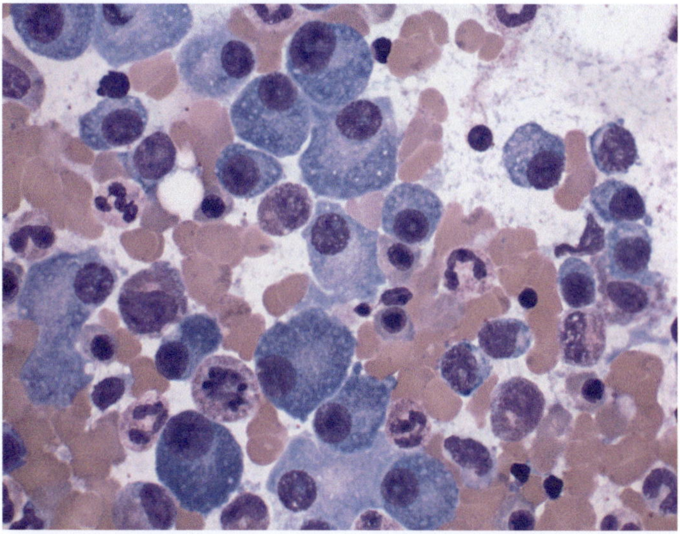

Plasma cell myeloma. Numerous abnormal plasma cells in marrow aspirate

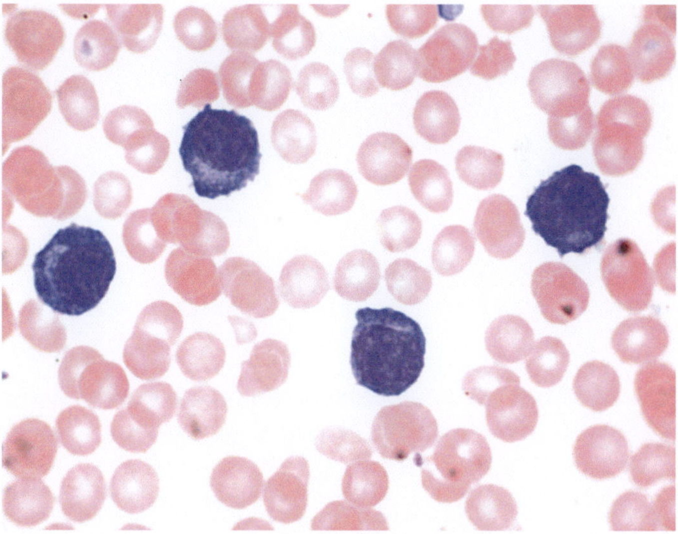

Plasma cell leukemia. Numerous circulating plasma cells

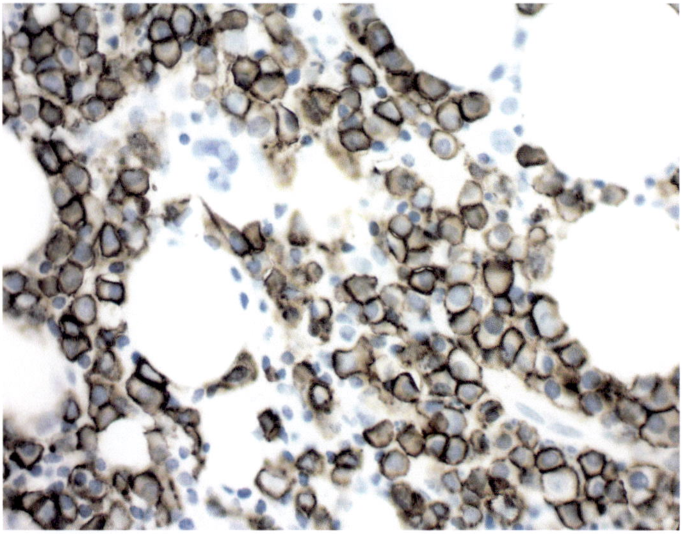

Plasma cell myeloma. Numerous CD138-positive plasma cells in myeloma (IHC)

Plasmacytoma

Snapshot

- Monotonous sheet of clonal plasma cells (may be anaplastic or plasmablastic) in an extramedullary site, with no myeloma-related findings (M spike +/−)

Variants

Solitary Plasmacytoma of Bone (SBP)

- Single lesion (vertebral, ribs, skull, pelvis)
- Localized bone pain, pathologic fracture
- M protein +/−

Extraosseous Plasmacytoma (EP)

- Upper respiratory tract mass with nasal symptoms
- Other sites include GI tract, lymph node, skin, CNS
- M protein −/+

Immunophenotype

- POSITIVE: CD138 (CD38), kappa or lambda, CD56
- NEGATIVE: CD19, CD20, CD45

Differential Diagnosis

- *Plasma cell myeloma* (marrow disease, usually with myeloma-related findings [hypercalcemia, renal failure, anemia, lytic bone lesions])
- *Plasmacytic hyperplasia* (polyclonal plasma cells without atypia)
- *Plasma cell–rich MALT lymphoma* (admixed clonal B-cells; thyroid common site)
- *Lymphoplasmacytic lymphoma* (admixed clonal B-cells, typically IgM+)
- *Plasmablastic lymphoma* (CD45+ CD20+ plasmablasts, often EBV+)

Caveats and Pearls

- Admixed clonal B-cells favor marginal zone lymphoma
- Mu heavy chain expression favors lyphoplasmacytic lymphoma
- If >1 bone lesion, myeloma is favored over solitary plasmacytoma of bone
- CD56 expression may be negative to weak in extraosseous plasmacytoma

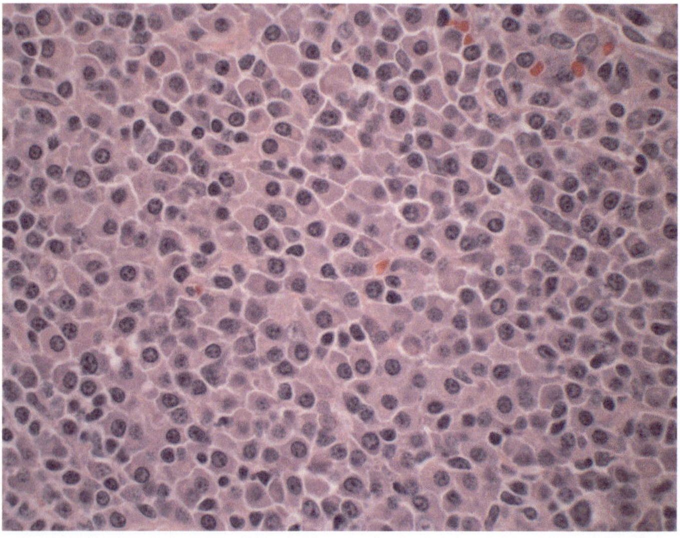

Extraosseous plasmacytoma. Sheets of plasma cells in soft tissue

Monoclonal Immunoglobulin Deposition Diseases

Snapshot

- Deposition of pink amorphous material in small vessels leading to a wide range of symptoms, with underlying MGUS, myeloma, or lymphoplasmacytic lymphoma

Clinical Presentations

Amyloidosis

- Organomegaly, purpura, peripheral neuropathy, carpal tunnel syndrome, heart failure, nephrotic syndrome, bone pain

Monoclonal Light/Heavy Chain Deposition Disease

- Nephrotic syndrome, renal failure

Morphology (Marrow)

- Ranges from mild increase in plasma cells (most commonly) to overt myeloma or lymphoplasmacytic lymphoma

Immunophenotype

- Monoclonal CD138/CD38-positive plasma cells

Variants

Primary Amyloidosis

- Underlying diagnosis of MGUS, myeloma, or lymphoplasmacytic lymphoma, almost always with an M protein
- Involvement of numerous sites
- Congo Red positive material in vessel walls, basement membranes, interstitium

Light/Heavy Chain Deposition Disease (LCDD/HCDD)

- Most often associated with myeloma or MGUS, with M spike
- Renal presentation most common (nephrotic syndrome, renal failure)
- Pink amorphous Congo Red negative material

Caveats and Pearls

- AL amyloid usually composed of lambda protein
- LCDD material usually composed of kappa protein

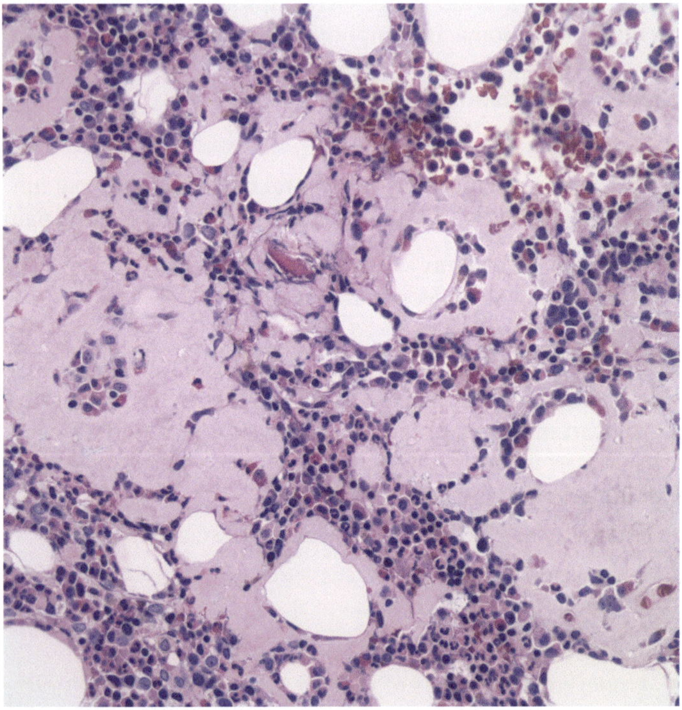

Primary amyloidosis. Amyloid deposition in bone marrow

Plasma Cell Neoplasms with Paraneoplastic Syndromes

Plasma Cell Neoplasms with POEMS Syndrome

POEMS Syndrome

- Acronym for polyneuropathy, organomegaly (liver, spleen), endocrinopathy (hypogonadal, thyroid), monoclonal gammopathy, and skin changes (hyperpigmentation, hypertrichosis)
- Mandatory criteria are polyneuropathy and clonal plasma cell disorder
- Other findings include increased vascular endothelial growth factor (VEGF) and thrombocytosis

Morphology

- Osteosclerotic plasmacytoma (thickened trabecular bone with paratrabecular fibrosis and spindle-shaped plasma cells, usually lambda-restricted)
- Often associated with nodal Castleman disease, plasma cell variant

Plasma Cell Neoplasms with TEMPI Syndrome

TEMPI Syndrome

- Acronym for telangiectasia, erythrocytosis with high erythropoietin, monoclonal gammopathy, perinephric fluid collection, and intrapulmonary shunting
- Hypercellular erythroid predominant marrow with <10% clonal plasma cells; M spike

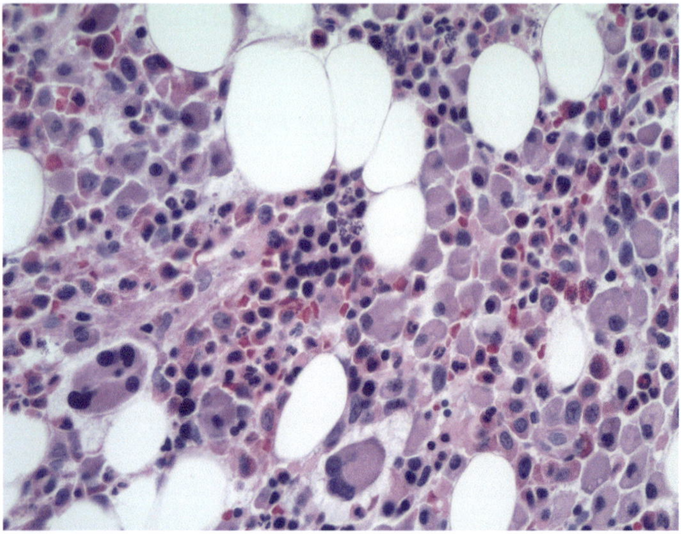

Plasma cell neoplasm in POEMS syndrome. Marrow with numerous abnormal plasma cells

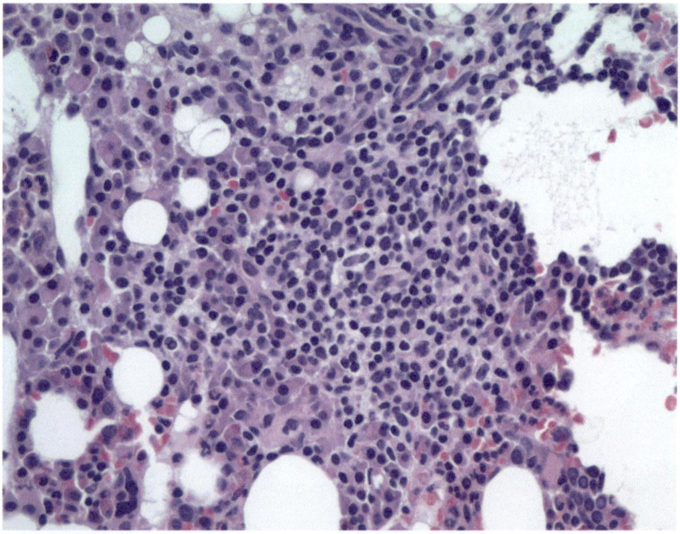

Plasma cell neoplasm in POEMS syndrome. Marrow with lymphoid aggregate surrounded by abnormal plasma cells

Extranodal Marginal Zone Lymphoma of Mucosa-Associated Lymphoid Tissue (Malt Lymphoma)

Snapshot

- Diffuse polymorphic lymphoid infiltrate in mucosal sites often with monocytoid B-cells, plasma cells, and lympho-epithelial lesions

Clinical Features

- Mucosal sites (GI tract [stomach, small bowel], salivary glands, thyroid, conjunctiva, breast, lung, skin)
- Often arises in setting of chronic infection (stomach—*Helicobacter pylori*, skin—*Borrelia burgdorferi*, intestine—*Campylobacter jejuni*, conjunctiva—*Chlamydia psittaci*) or chronic inflammation (salivary glands—Sjogren syndrome [salivary glands], Hashimoto thyroiditis [thyroid])
- Small monoclonal paraprotein sometimes detected

Morphology

- Extrafollicular lymphoid infiltrate, often with follicular colonization
- Small-intermediate-sized B-cells, often monocytoid
- Lymphoepithelial lesions seen (prominent in GI tract)
- Admixed plasma cells and large lymphocytes (thyroid cases often plasma cell–rich)

Immunophenotype

- POSITIVE: CD20, CD43, in some cases light chain restriction (kappa/lambda IHC)
- NEGATIVE: CD5, CD10, BCL6, cyclin D1

Genetics

- Translocations involving *MALT1*, *BCL10*, and *FOXP1* genes [t(11;18), t(1;14), t(14;18), t(3;14)]; trisomy 3; trisomy 18

Variant

Immunoproliferative Small Intestinal Disease (IPSID)

- Middle East and South Africa; associated with malabsorption; IgA+ plasma cells with no light chain expression (*IgA heavy chain disease*)

Differential Diagnosis

- *Reactive lymphoid hyperplasia* (polyclonal kappa/lambda)
- *Small lymphocytic lymphoma* (CD5+ CD23+, rare-absent plasma cells)
- *Mantle zone lymphoma* (monotonous CD5+ cyclin D1+ infiltrate)
- *Plasmacytoma* (no clonal B-cells)
- *Follicular lymphoma* (CD10+ centrocytes/centroblasts)
- *DLBCL* (sheets of large B-cells without FDC networks)

Caveats and Pearls

- CD21/CD23 IHC is useful for highlighting disrupted follicular dendritic cell (FDC) networks in follicular colonization
- Small endoscopic biopsies may be insufficient for diagnosis—detection of clonal IgH by *polymerase chain reaction* (PCR) may be required
- MALT lymphoma may undergo transformation to *diffuse large B-cell lymphoma*
- Sheets of large cells is best classified as *diffuse large B-cell lymphoma*
- The term *high-grade MALT lymphoma* should not be used

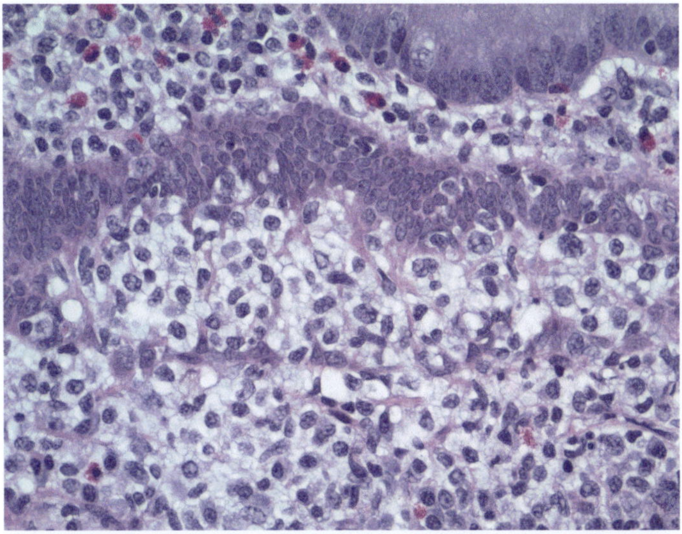

Gastric MALT lymphoma with lymphoid infiltrate within gastric gland (lymphoepithelial lesion)

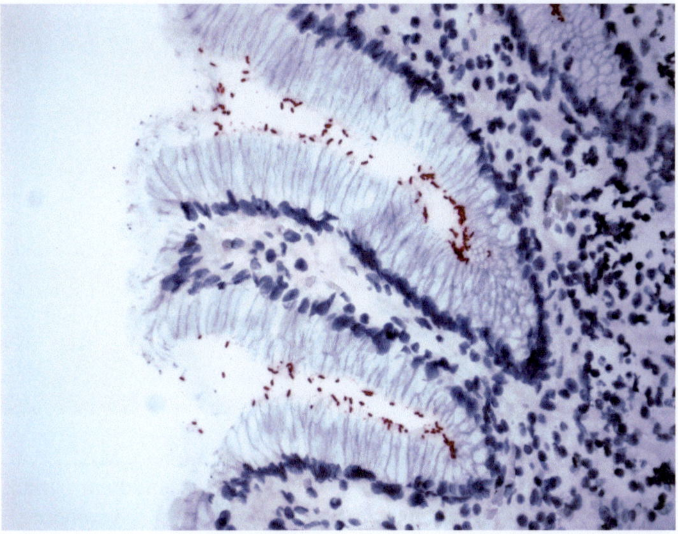

MALT lymphoma. *Helicobacter pylori* (red IHC) on gastric mucosa

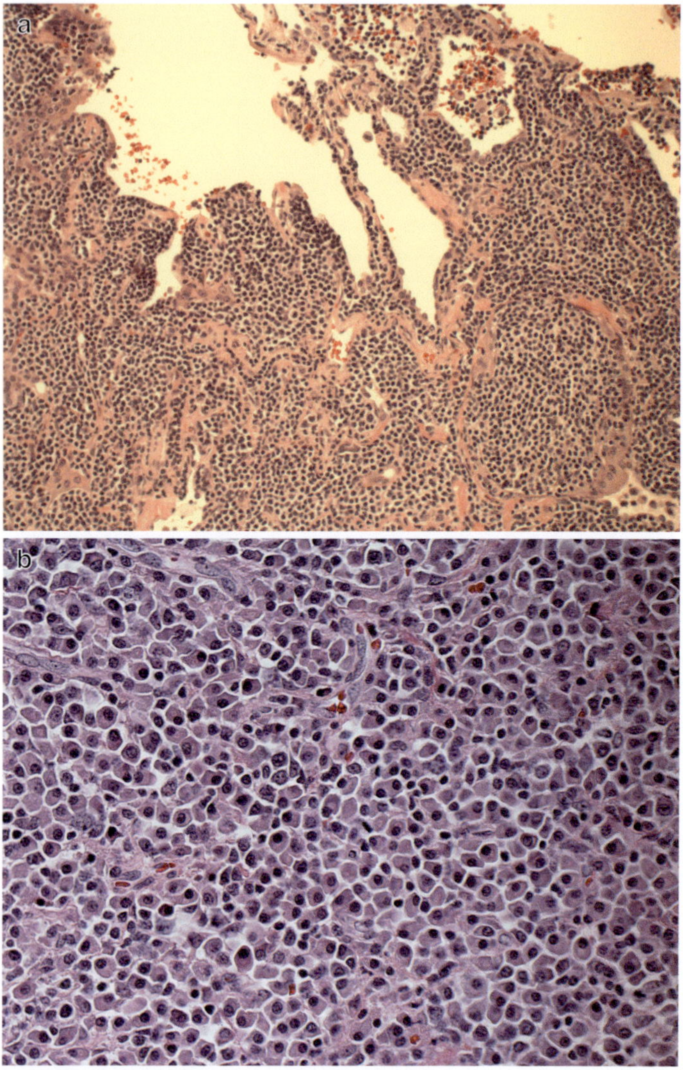

(**a**) Extensive small lymphocytic infiltrate in pulmonary MALT lymphoma; (**b**) plasma cell–rich MALT lymphoma; (**c**) nodular periadnexal lymphoid infiltrate in primary cutaneous MALT lymphoma

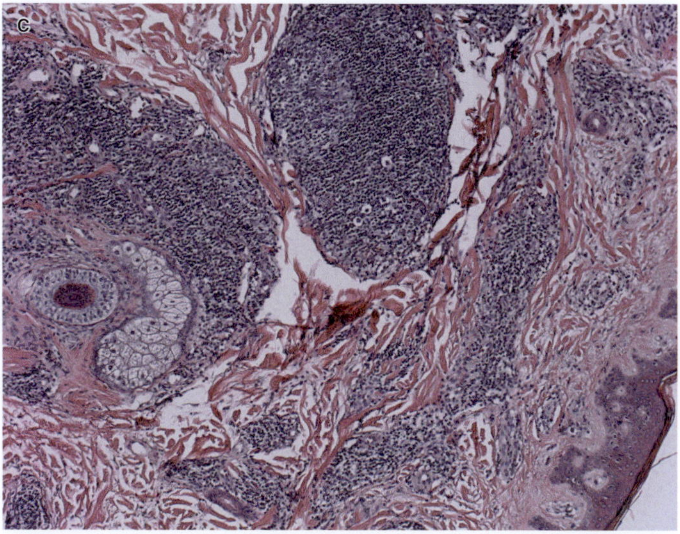

(continued)

Nodal Marginal Zone Lymphoma

Snapshot

- Asymptomatic lymphadenopathy with partial effacement by a vaguely nodular infiltrate of monocytoid B-cells and plasma cells (adult form) or by progressively transformed germinal centers (pediatric form)

Clinical Features

- *Adult Form*: Older adults with asymptomatic peripheral lymphadenopathy (and no evidence of extranodal disease)
- *Pediatric Form*: Male predominance with asymptomatic enlargement of peripheral nodes, most often head and neck

Morphology

- Perifollicular infiltrate of small- to medium-sized lymphoid cells with abundant pale cytoplasm (monocytoid B-cells), variable admixture of plasma cells; partial effacement of reactive follicles (with follicular colonization)
- In pediatric form, the infiltrate often contains enlarged progressively transformed germinal centers

Immunophenotype

- Admixture of CD20+ B-cells and CD138+ plasma cells, light chain (kappa/lambda) restriction; B-cells typically negative for CD5, CD10, CD23, *BCL6*; and cyclin D1; CD43 expression is variable

Genetics

- Absence of extranodal MALT lymphoma translocations

Differential Diagnosis

- *Extranodal MALT lymphoma* (nodal disease may represent spread from an extranodal site [e.g., thyroid, salivary gland])

- *Atypical marginal zone hyperplasia (pediatric)* (CD43 is an unreliable marker in this setting, immunoglobulin gene rearrangement analysis is required)

Caveats and Pearls
- In rare cases, the marginal zone B-cells are large and pleomorphic
- If infiltrate appears diffuse, inapparent primary follicles may be detected by detection of CD21/CD23+ FDC
- In worrisome adult cases without detectable light chain restriction, CD43 expression may be helpful in diagnosis of B-cell lymphoma

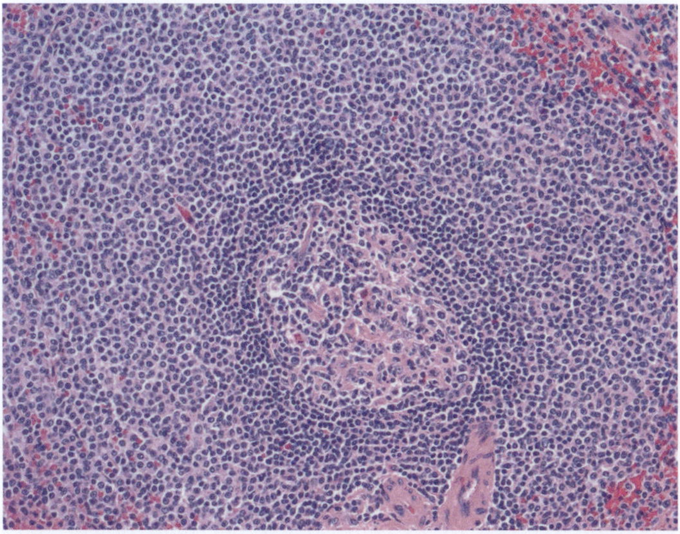

Nodal marginal zone lymphoma, marginal zone pattern. Note the aberrant expansion of marginal zone in lymph node

Follicular Lymphoma

Snapshot

- Effacement by multiple enlarged haphazardly arranged follicles with loss of polarity and indistinct mantle zones

Clinical Features

- Adults with asymptomatic lymphadenopathy, splenomegaly and marrow involvement (common); can be extranodal
- Distinctive pediatric, primary cutaneous, testicular, and duodenal forms—all indolent

Morphology

- Abnormal follicles—back-to-back, attenuated mantle zone, no polarity, decreased tingible-body macrophages
- Variable number of small centrocytes and large centroblasts (see grading)
- Low mitotic rate (most cases)
- Significant interfollicular expansion sometimes seen
- Tight paratrabecular aggregates in marrow

Immunophenotype

- POSITIVE: CD20, CD10, BCL6, BCL2 (unless high-grade), CD21/CD23/CD35 (to highlight FDC networks)
- NEGATIVE: CD5, CD43, cyclin D1

Genetics

- *BCL2* translocation [t(14;18)]

Grading

- Grade 1/2 (up to 15 centroblasts per high power field [/HPF])
- Grade 3a (>15 centroblasts/HPF)
- Grade 3b (centroblasts only)

Subtypes and Variants

Pediatric-Type Follicular Lymphoma

- Localized indolent disease with large irregular follicles often with blast-like germinal center B-cells, often grade 3 and *BCL2*-negative

Duodenal-Type Follicular Lymphoma

- Features may overlap in situ follicular neoplasia and MALT lymphoma, FDC often restricted to follicle periphery, t(14;18)-positive, indolent process

Primary Cutaneous Follicle Center Lymphoma

- Adults with localized lesions of head or trunk, dermal disease, follicular and diffuse growth patterns; FDC meshworks may be absent in diffuse variant, variable CD10, and *BCL2* expression; if CD10 and *BCL2* expression is strong, consider secondary involvement by a nodal primary, t(14;18) often absent

Testicular Follicular Lymphoma

- Children>adults, often grade 3A, t(14;18)-negative, good prognosis

Diffuse Follicular Lymphoma Variant

- Inguinal mass, diffuse pattern with small *BCL2* neg/wk + follicles, CD10 and CD23-positive, t(14;18)-negative, 1p36 deletion

In Situ Follicular Neoplasia

- Normal-appearing follicles with strong positivity for CD10 and BCL2; t(14;18)-positive, indolent process

Differential Diagnosis

- *Reactive follicular hyperplasia* (BCL2-negative germinal center B-cells)
- *Mantle cell lymphoma, mantle zone pattern* (CD5+ cyclin D1/SOX11+)

- *Marginal zone lymphoma with follicular colonization* [CD43+ monocytoid B-cells, absence of t(14;18)]
- *Diffuse large B-cell lymphoma* (absent centrocytes, absent FDC networks; may arise from follicular lymphoma)

Caveats and Pearls

- Cases with sheets of centroblasts (absent CD21/CD23+ FDC networks) are best classified as *diffuse large B-cell lymphoma*
- Some high-grade FL cases are negative for CD10 and/or BCL2
- Some healthy persons carry small numbers of germinal center B-cells with t(14;18) *BCL2* translocation—avoid overdiagnosis
- Beware normal BCL2+ primary follicles
- In grading, do not confuse FDC with centroblasts
- In rare cases of *pediatric follicular hyperplasia*, clonal CD10+ B-cells are detected by flow cytometry
- FDC in FL may be CD21 or CD23-negative

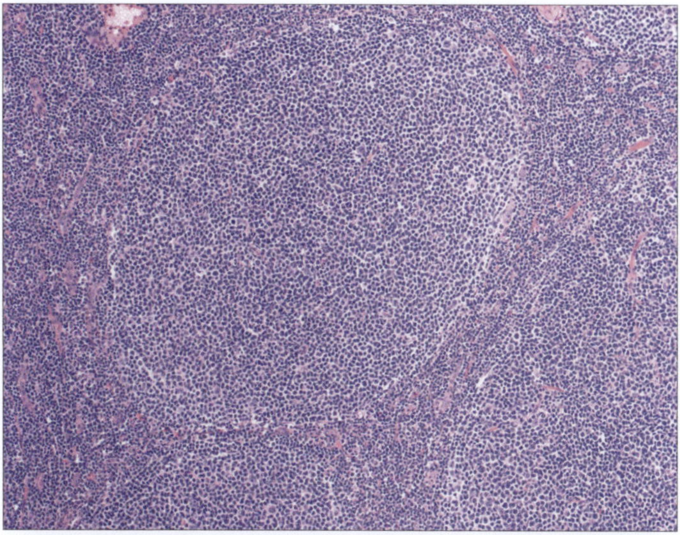

Low-grade follicular lymphoma with abnormal lymphoid follicles

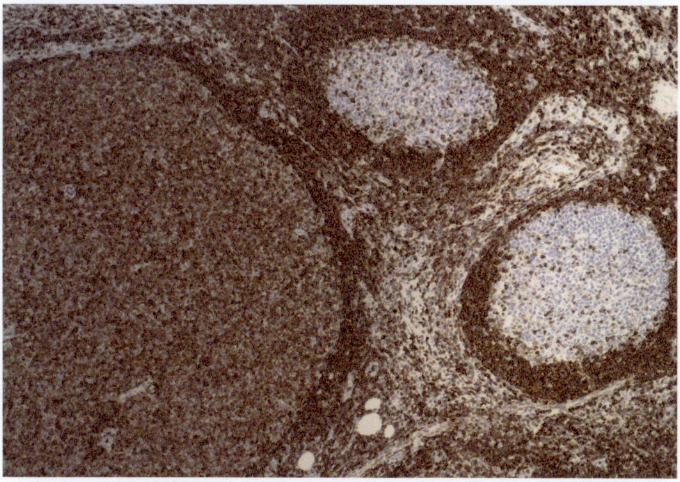

Low-grade follicular lymphoma with a single enlarged follicle with BCL2-positive germinal center B-cells on left and two benign BCL2 negative follicles on right. Note the BCL2 positivity of the mantle zones

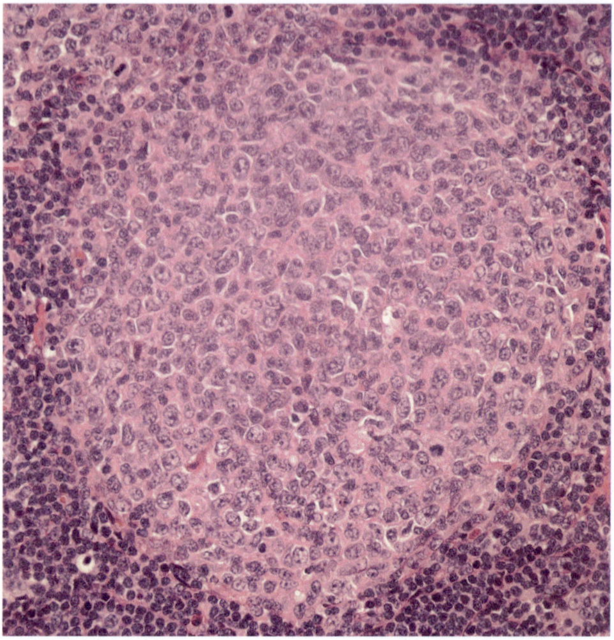

Neoplastic follicle composed entirely of large centroblasts (follicular lymphoma, grade 3B)

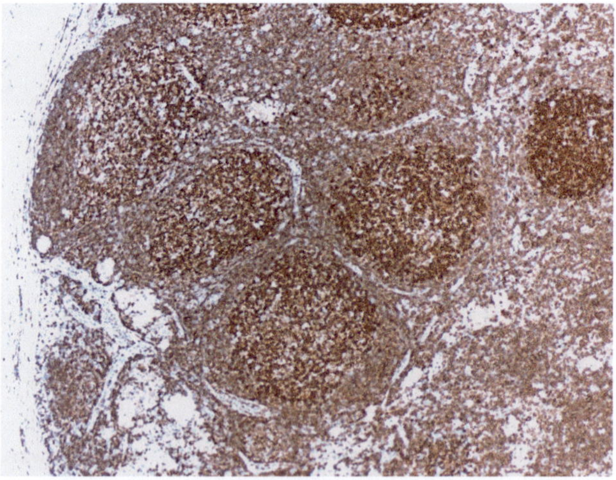

Normal-appearing follicles with BLC2-positive germinal centers (in situ follicular neoplasia)

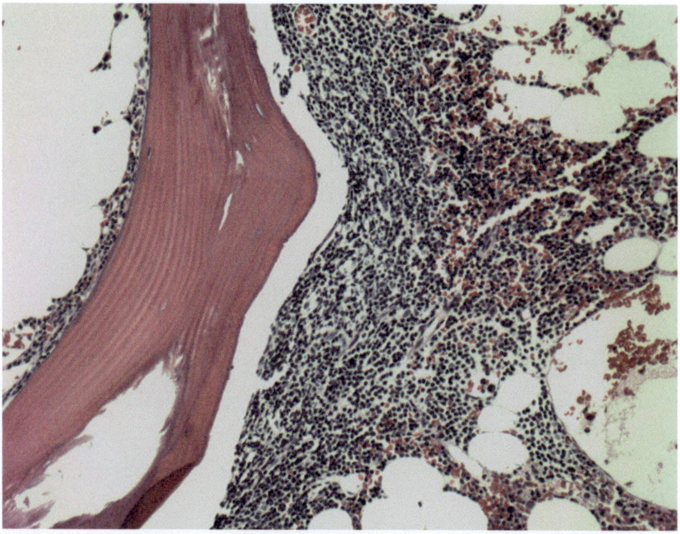

Tight paratrabecular lymphoid infiltrate in marrow involvement by follicular lymphoma

Large B-Cell Lymphoma with *IRF4* Rearrangement

Snapshot

- Large B-cell lymphoma with follicular or diffuse pattern, often limited to Waldeyer's ring and/or cervical nodes

Clinical Features

- Children and young adults with limited stage disease

Morphology

- Follicular (grade 3B), diffuse large B-cell lymphoma rearrangement

Immunophenotype

- Strong positive *MUM1*, usually *BCL6*-positive, CD10 and *BCL2*-positive in 50%, sometimes CD5-positive, high Ki-67 proliferative index

Genetics

- *Ig/IRF4* rearrangement (most cases), *BCL6* rearrangement (some cases), no *BCL2* rearrangement

Differential Diagnosis

- *Follicular lymphoma* (MUM1-negative, t[14;18]-positive)
- *Diffuse large B-cell lymphoma* (older adults, higher stage, *IRF1* rearrangement negative)
- *MUM1+ follicular lymphoma* (older adults, seen with DLBCL)

Primary Cutaneous Follicle Center Lymphoma

Snapshot

- Skin lesions, usually scalp, forehead, or trunk, composed of a follicular to diffuse infiltrate of *BCL6*-positive small to large centrocytes

Morphology

- Follicles typically lack polarization and tingible-body macrophages, with attenuated mantle zones
- Diffuse form composed of large centrocytes, may be multilobate or spindle-shaped

Immunophenotype

- POSITIVE: CD20, BCL6, BCL2 (variable), CD10 (variable), CD21/CD35 FDC (follicular pattern)

Genetics

- *BCL2* rearrangement t(14;18) in some cases

Caveats and Pearls

- If BCL2 and CD10 are strongly and uniformly positive, consider secondary involvement by a nodal primary

Mantle Cell Lymphoma

Snapshot

- Monotonous infiltrate of atypical small-medium-sized lymphocytes with irregular nuclear contour

Sites of Involvement

- Lymph node, spleen, marrow, blood, Waldeyer's ring, GI tract
- Multiple lymphomatous polyposis (intestine)
- Leukemic non-nodal disease (often small cell variant)

Morphology

- Effacement by a small lymphocytic infiltrate (nodular or diffuse)
- Small-medium in size with irregular nuclear contours
- Monomorphic without large cells or proliferation centers

Immunophenotype

- POSITIVE: CD5, CD20 (strong), BCL2, cyclin D1 and/or SOX11
- NEGATIVE: CD10, CD23, BCL6

Genetics

- *Cyclin D1* translocation into heavy chain locus [t(11;14)(q13;q32)]
- Rare variant translocations of 11q13 (*cyclin D1*) into light chain loci
- *Cyclin D1*-negative MCL harbor alternate *cyclin D2* or *cyclin D3* translocations

Prognostic Factors

- ADVERSE: High mitotic rate (>10 mitotic figures or >40% Ki-67+), blastoid or pleomorphic variant
- FAVORABLE: Small cell variant, in situ mantle cell neoplasia

Variants

Blastoid

- Small-intermediate cells with immature (salt and pepper) chromatin, indistinct nucleoli, and high mitotic index

Pleomorphic

- Intermediate-large pleomorphic cells with variably prominent nucleoli
- *Small cell* (small round cells with dense heterochromatin resembling SLL)
- *Marginal zone-like* (foci of medium-sized cells with abundant pale cytoplasm [monocytoid])

In Situ Mantle Cell Neoplasia

- Cyclin D1+ cells confined to the inner mantle zone of follicles—to be distinguished from mantle zone pattern of MCL!

Leukemic Non-nodal Mantle Cell Lymphoma

- *SOX1*-negative; blood, marrow, and spleen; frequently indolent, may be small cell variant, aggressive if secondary mutations present

Differential Diagnosis

- *Small lymphocytic lymphoma* (typically CD20 dim, CD23+, cyclin D1/*SOX11*−)
  Marginal zone lymphoma (CD5−, cyclin D1−)
- *Lymphoblastic lymphoma* (vs. blastoid variant) (CD5−, cyclin D1−, TdT+)
- *DLBCL* (vs. pleomorphic variant) (cyclin D1−, *SOX11*−)

Caveats and Pearls

- Some cases are CD5−, CD23+, cyclin D1−(SOX11+)
- Scattered epithelioid histiocytes and hyalinized vessels often seen
- Plasma cells are usually rare and polyclonal
- Marked lymphocytosis may mimic *B-prolymphocytic leukemia*
- In situ *mantle cell neoplasia* is characterized by cyclin D1+ cells confined to the inner mantle zone, while in MCL with a mantle zone growth pattern cyclin D1+ cells populate the entire mantle zone

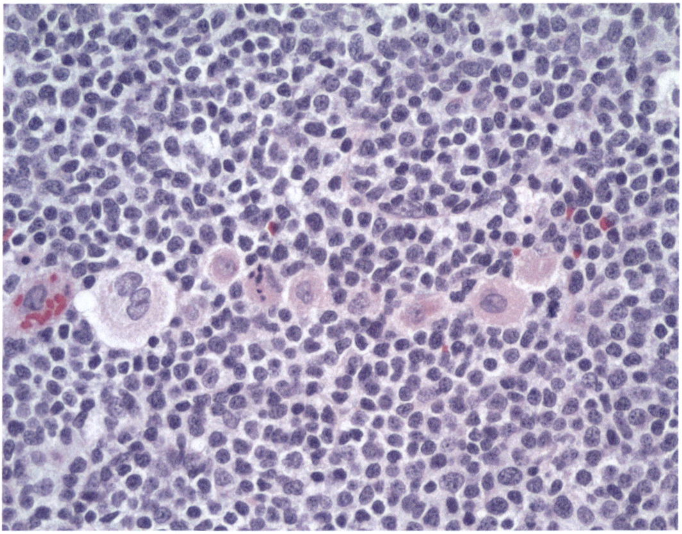

Mantle cell lymphoma with monotonous population of small-medium lymphocytes with immature chromatin and scattered epithelioid histiocytes with eosinophilic cytoplasm

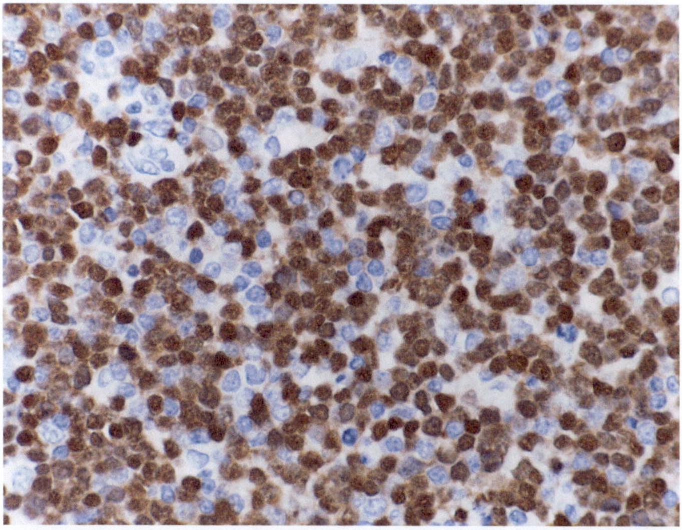

Mantle cell lymphoma. Cyclin D1 (BCL1)-positive lymphoid infiltrate

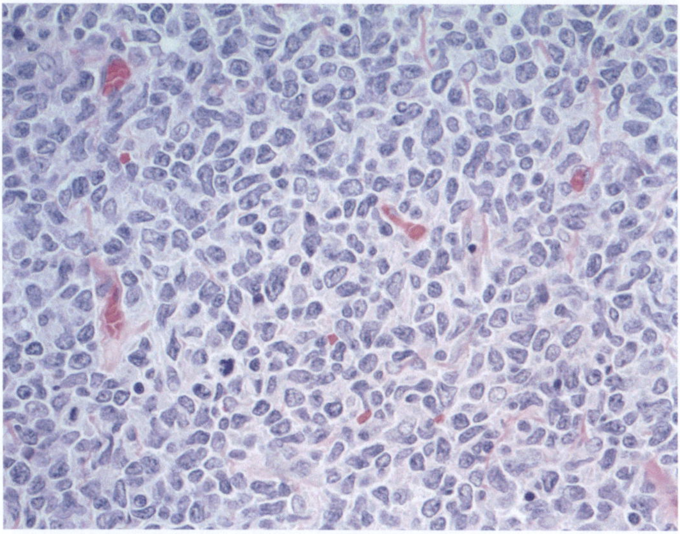

Mantle cell lymphoma. Pleomorphic variant

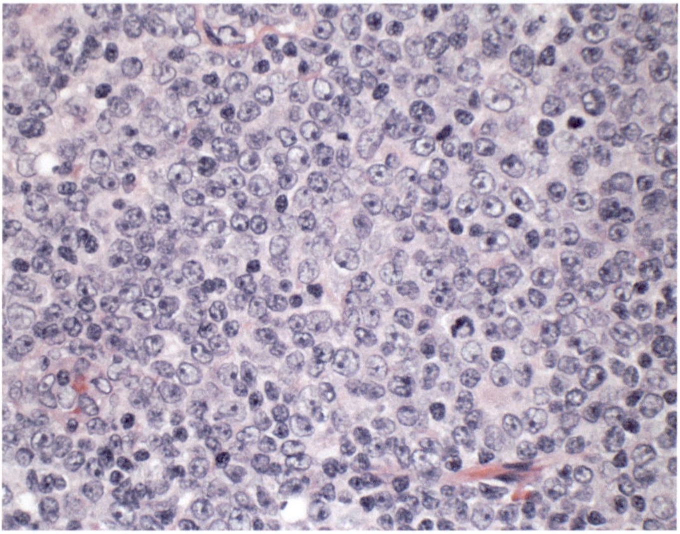

Mantle cell lymphoma. Blastoid variant

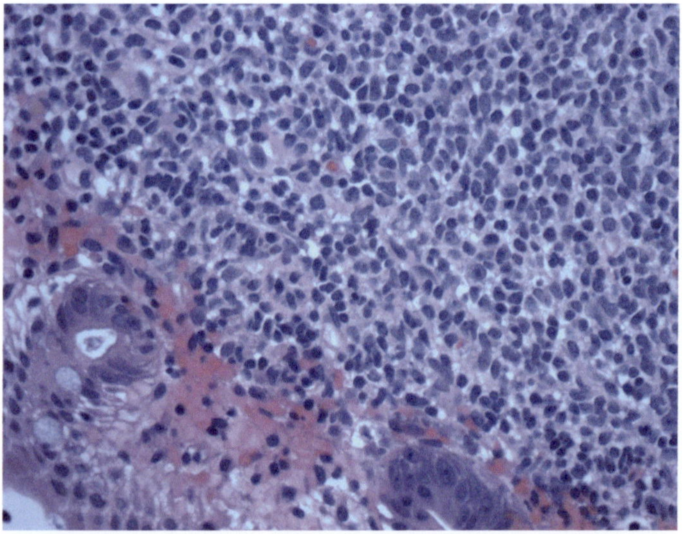

Lymphomatous polyposis (intestinal mantle cell lymphoma)

Diffuse Large B-Cell Lymphoma (DLBCL), NOS

Snapshot

- Diffuse infiltrate of medium to large B-cells with centroblastic, immunoblastic, or anaplastic morphology

Clinical Features

- Most often, older adults with nodal and/or extranodal disease (GI tract most common)
- May represent progression from low-grade lymphoma

Immunophenotype

- Suggested panel (pan-B-cell markers [CD20, CD79a, PAX5], subset classifier markers [CD10, BCL6, MUM1], FDC marker [CD21], prognostic markers [BCL2, Ki-67, c-MYC, ALK1, EBER])
- High proliferative rate (Ki-67 [40–95%])

Prognostic Subtypes

- *Germinal center (GC) type*: (CD10+ or CD10– BCL6+ MUM1–) (30% positivity threshold)
- *Activated B-cell (ABC) type*: (CD10– BCL6– MUM1+/–)
- Adverse features include double-expresser phenotype[1] (>40% MYC and >50% BCL2), *MYC* translocation, *BCL2* translocation, EBV positivity, and large cell morphology in marrow

DLBCL Variants

EBV+ DLBCL

- Commonly extranodal, usually ABC type, often polymorphous with scattered large immunoblasts and Hodgkin/RS-like cells, poor prognosis in elderly, excellent prognosis in younger adults

---

[1] Note: If double or triple rearrangements present, classify as *high-grade B-cell lymphoma with double/triple hit*

Primary Cutaneous DLBCL, Leg Type

- Elderly females, dermal tumors usually of lower legs, dissemination common, usually ABC type

DLBCL Associated with Chronic Inflammation

- Elderly males, extranodal mass (chronically inflamed pleura, bone, joints, periarticular area), usually EBV+

Fibrin-Associated DLBCL

- Incidental finding, large EBV+ B-cells found singly or in small aggregates within fibrinous material in pseudocysts, hematomas, cardiac thrombus

Primary DLBCL of the CNS

- Parenchymal disease with perivascular infiltrates, prominent necrosis, absence of immunodeficiency, dissemination rare, CD10-negative (if positive, search for non-CNS primary), EBV-negative (if positive, search for immunodeficiency)

Differential Diagnosis

- *High-grade B-cell lymphoma* (admixed medium and large cells; numerous phagocytic histiocytes [starry sky]; >90% Ki-67+; *c-MYC*, *BCL2*, *BCL6* rearrangements)
- *Burkitt lymphoma* (monotonous medium-size cells, numerous phagocytic histiocytes [starry sky], *BCL2* –/+, Ig-*MYC* translocation, no *BCL2* or *BCL6* rearrangement)
- ALK+ *large B-cell lymphoma* (CD20-negative, ALK-positive)
- *Follicular lymphoma, grade 3B* (centroblastic infiltrate in a nodular growth pattern with intact CD21/CD23+ FDC networks)
- *Classic Hodgkin lymphoma* (CD45– CD30+ CD15+/– PAX5 wk + fascin+ classic RS cells)
- *Seminoma* (PLAP-positive, CD45/CD20-negative)

Caveats and Pearls

- Diffuse sheets devoid of intact CD21+ FDC meshworks
- Focal involvement of follicles may be seen
- In small biopsies, distinction between high-grade follicular lymphoma and DLBCL may be difficult

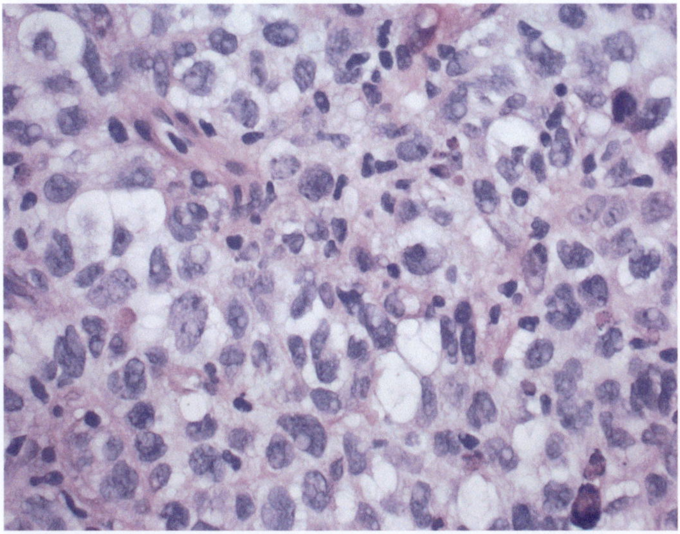

Diffuse large B-cell lymphoma. Centroblastic variant

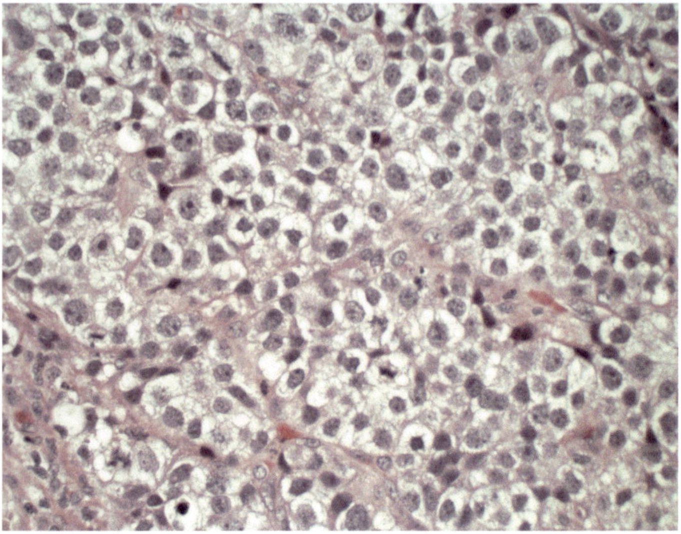

Diffuse large B-cell lymphoma. Clear cell variant

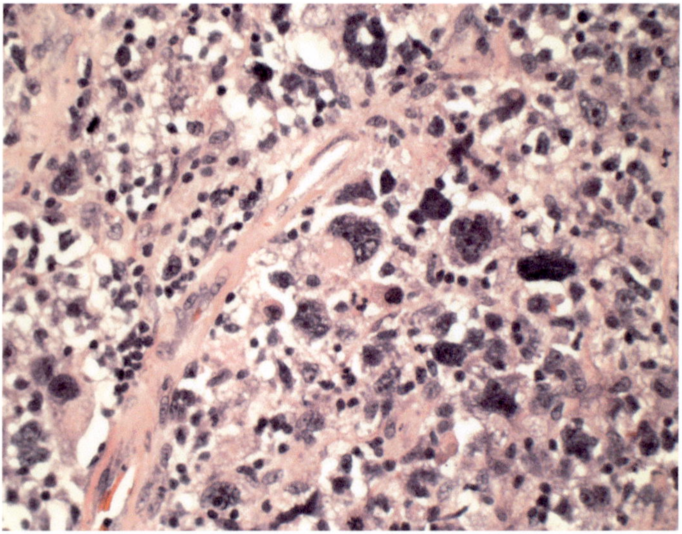

Diffuse large B-cell lymphoma. Anaplastic variant

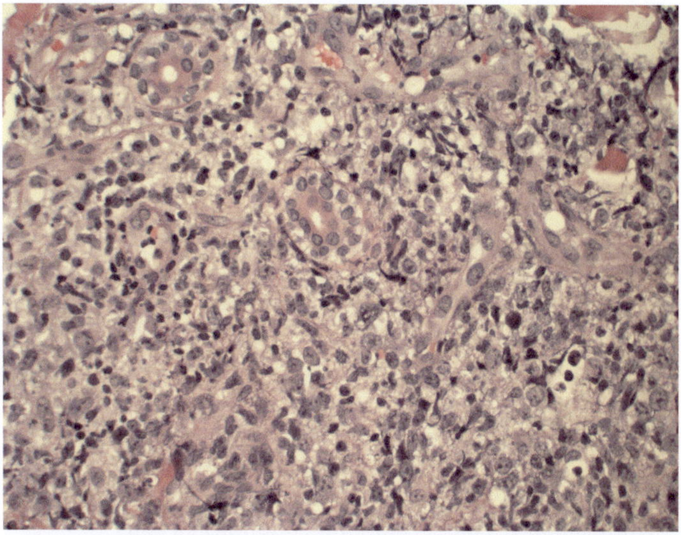

Primary cutaneous diffuse large B-cell lymphoma, leg type

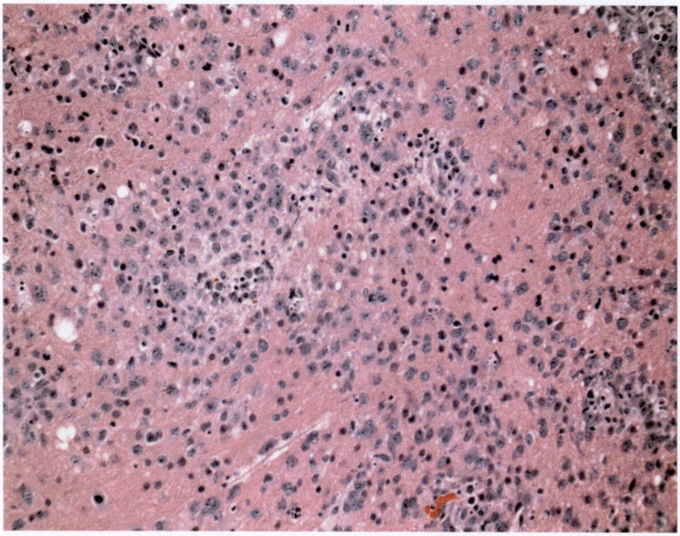

Primary CNS lymphoma (cerebrum)

T-Cell/Histiocyte-Rich Large B-Cell Lymphoma

Snapshot

- Diffuse T-cell/histiocyte-rich infiltrate with scattered large EBV-negative B-cells

Clinical Features

- Middle-aged males >females with fever, malaise, lymphadenopathy, hepatosplenomegaly

Morphology

- Diffuse infiltrate of small mature T-cells, histiocytes (non-epithelioid), and scattered large clonal B-cells
- No residual BCL6+ follicles or CD21+ FDC networks
- Rare small B-cells, eosinophils, and plasma cells
- No classic RS cells
- EBV-negative large cells

Immunophenotype

- CD4+ small T-cells
- CD68+ histiocytes
- CD20+ BCL6+ EBV- large B-cells

Differential Diagnosis

- *Nodular lymphocyte predominant Hodgkin lymphoma* (nodular infiltrate, B-cell-rich nodules, EMA+ LP cells; rare diffuse variant with T-cell-rich background)
- *Angioimmunoblastic T-cell lymphoma* (clonal PD1/CD10+ T-cells, EBV+ large B-cells)

Caveats and Pearls

- Some cases may be histiocyte-poor

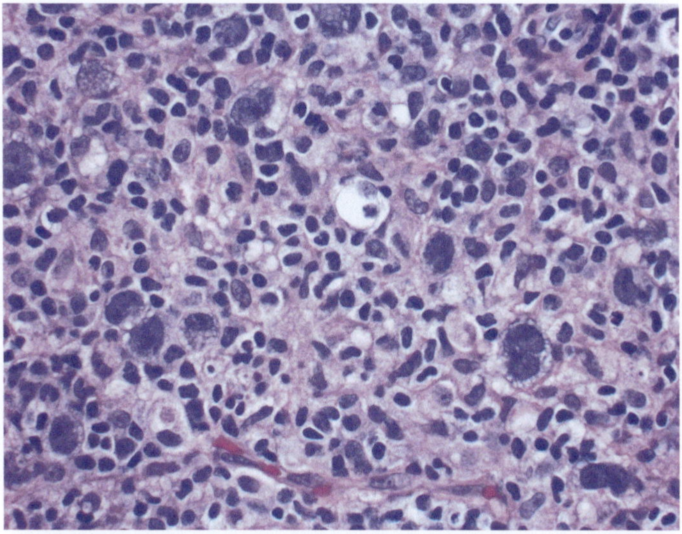

T-cell-rich large B-cell lymphoma. Note the scattered large cells and numerous background small lymphocytes

EBV-Positive Mucocutaneous Ulcer

Snapshot

- Ulcerated mucosal lesion with underlying polymorphous EBV-positive lymphoid infiltrate

Clinical Features

- Older adults with iatrogenic or age-related immunodeficiency
- Sites include oral cavity, skin, or GI tract

Morphology

- Ulcerated mucosa with polymorphous infiltrate with scattered large EBV+ immunoblasts or RS-like cells and numerous small CD8+ T-cells

Immunophenotype (Large Cells)

- POSITIVE: CD20, PAX5, OCT2, MUM1, CD30, EBV (EBER)
- NEGATIVE: CD10, BCL6

Genetics

- Clonal immunoglobulin gene rearrangement not detected (most cases)

Differential Diagnosis

- *EBV+ DLBCL* (nodal disease, clonal B-cells)
- *EBV+ Classic Hodgkin lymphoma* (nodal disease, classic RS cell phenotype)

Lymphomatoid Granulomatosis

Snapshot

- Extranodal polymorphic angiocentric lymphoid infiltrate with EBV+ B-cells

Clinical Features

- Adult males (most common) with evidence of immunodeficiency
- Fever, malaise, weight loss
- Other site-specific presentations (lung, CNS, kidney, skin)
- Lung symptoms (cough, dyspnea, chest pain)
- Lesions are usually bilateral

Morphology

- Polymorphic angiocentric lymphoid infiltrate composed of variable numbers of small T-cells, histiocytes, plasma cells, and scattered clonal EBV+ B-cells; variable necrosis; granulomas are uncommon

Immunophenotype

- Numerous small CD3+ CD4+ T-cells
- Scattered large CD20+ EBER+ B-cells

Grading

Based upon the relative number of large, often pleomorphic EBER+ B-cells:

- Grade 1 (rare-absent EBV+ B-cells)
- Grade 2 (few large EBV+ B-cells)
- Grade 3 (many large EBV+ B-cells

Differential Diagnosis

- *Diffuse large B-cell lymphoma* (sheets of large B-cells)
- *Extranodal NK/T-cell lymphoma* (abnormal sCD3−/CD56+ EBV+ NK/T-cells)
- *Classic Hodgkin lymphoma* (CD30 + CD15 + CD45− RS cells)

Caveats and Pearls

- Some large RS-like B-cells may be CD30+ but CD45-positive, CD15-negative
- Cases with large confluent sheets of EBV+ B-cells are best classified as DLBCL
- Leukocytes are rare
- Granulomas are uncommon

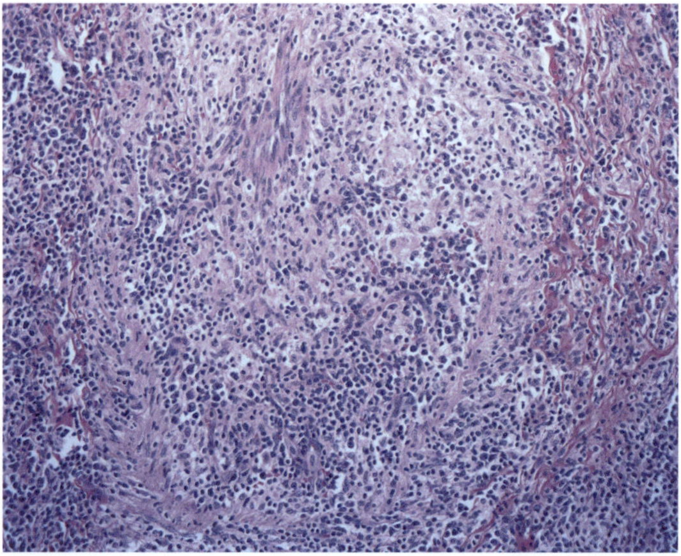

Lymphomatoid granulomatosis with angiocentric/angiodestructive infiltrate of lung

Primary Mediastinal (Thymic) Large B-Cell Lymphoma

Snapshot

- Anterior mediastinal mass composed of large B-cells with abundant cytoplasm and delicate interstitial fibrosis

Clinical Features

- Young adults (females>males), frequently with local extension to lung, pleura, or pericardium
- Rare involvement of lymph nodes and marrow
- May progress to extranodal sites

Morphology

- Sheets or nests of centroblast-like large cells, sometimes pleomorphic and multilobate, with varying degrees of delicate interstitial fibrosis

Immunophenotype

- POSITIVE: CD20, CD30 (weak variable), MUM1, CD23, MAL, PDL1, nuclear REL, c-MYC (variable)
- NEGATIVE: Immunoglobulin (common) and EBV

Genetics

- Multiple defects (9p24, 16p13 common)
- *BCL2*, *BCL6*, *MYC* rearrangements rarely

Differential Diagnosis

- *DLBCL* (nodal involvement common)
- *Classic Hodgkin lymphoma* (admixed inflammatory cells, dense sclerosis [in NSHL], RS cells with prominent nucleoli, CD30+ [strong, uniform], CD20 −/+, CD45−)
- *B-cell lymphoma unclassifiable with features intermediate between DLBCL and HL* (IHC expression of both B-cell and HL markers)

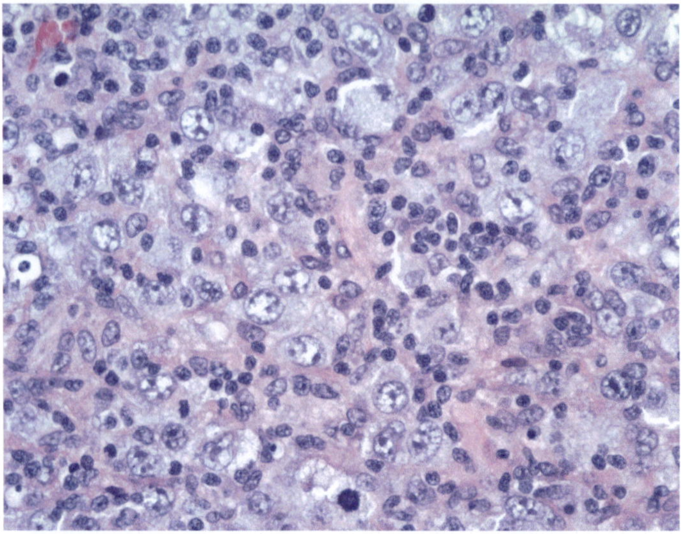

Primary mediastinal large B-cell lymphoma (PMLBCL)

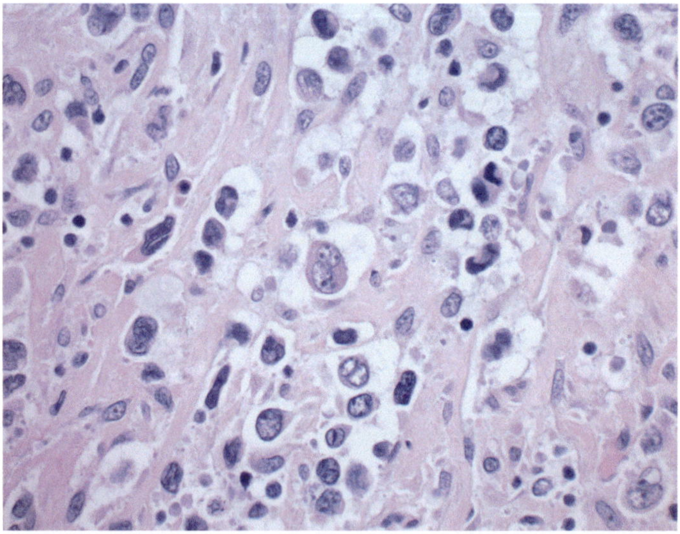

Primary mediastinal large B-cell lymphoma (PMLBCL) with fibrosis

Intravascular Large B-Cell Lymphoma

Snapshot

- Older adults with fever and intravascular collections of large B-cells in extranodal sites

Clinical Subtypes

- *Western type*: Site-specific symptoms (neurologic or cutaneous)
- *Asian type*: Systemic symptoms (hepatosplenomegaly, pancytopenia with hemophagocytosis)

Morphology

- Collections of large centroblastic or immunoblastic lymphoid cells within the lumen of small-medium-sized blood vessels, often capillaries; intrasinusoidal infiltrates in liver, spleen, and marrow; limited extravascular extension may be seen

Immunophenotype

- POSITIVE: pan-B-cell markers (CD20, CD79a, PAX5), MUM1 (if CD10+)
- VARIABLE: CD5−/+, CD10−/+

Differential Diagnosis

- *NK/T-cell lymphoma, intravascular variant* (CD2+, CD56+, EBV+)
- *Anaplastic large cell lymphoma, ALK-negative* (positive for CD30, and one or more pan-T-cell markers [most cases])

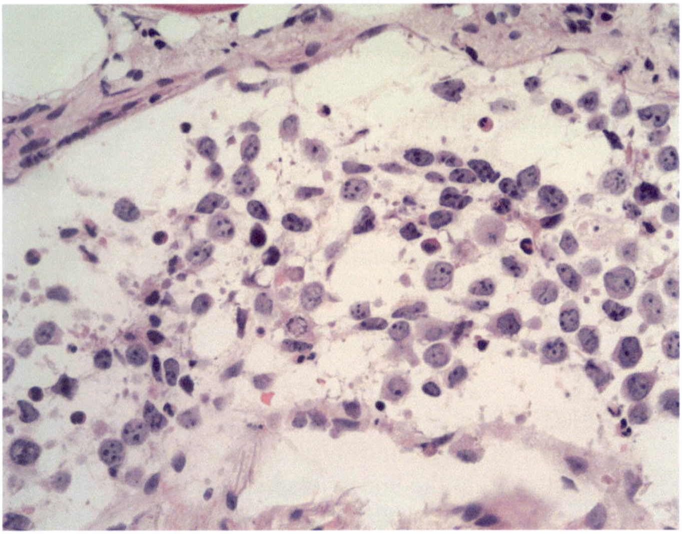

Intravascular large B-cell lymphoma

ALK-Positive Large B-Cell Lymphoma

Snapshot

- Diffuse cohesive immunoblastic infiltrate often with sinusoidal growth pattern

Clinical Features

- Young adult males (most common) with involvement of lymph nodes or mediastinum

Morphology

- Large cells with prominent central nucleoli, some with plasmablastic features

Immunophenotype

- POSITIVE: ALK1, CD138, MUM1, EMA, IgA>>IgG
- USUALLY NEGATIVE: Pan-B-cell markers and CD30
- EBV/HHV8-negative

Genetics

- *ALK1* translocation [t(2;7), t(2;x), rarely t(2;5)]

Differential Diagnosis

- *Plasmablastic lymphoma* (ALK-*negative*, EBV-positive)
- *ALK1+ anaplastic large cell lymphoma* (pan-T-cell markers and CD30-positive, pan-B-cell markers negative)

Caveats and Pearls

- With IgH-*MYC* translocation, consider plasmablastic lymphoma
- Some cases may be cytokeratin-positive

Plasmablastic Lymphoma

Snapshot

- Sheets of large CD138+ plasmablasts in a mucosal site

Clinical Features

- Seen in patients with immunodeficiency (HIV, aging-related, iatrogenic [post-transplant, autoimmune disease])
- Mucosal sites common, especially oral cavity

Morphology

- Sheets of large plasmablasts with abundant amphophilic cytoplasm and prominent central nucleoli, variable degree of plasmacytic differentiation; large anaplastic multinucleated cells sometimes seen

Immunophenotype

- POSITIVE: CD38, CD138, EBV+/−, MUM1, EMA, CD30, Ki-67 (>90%), MYC+/−
- NEGATIVE: CD45, CD20, PAX5, CD79a, ALK1, CD56 −/+

Genetics

- *MYC* translocation (50%), complex karyotype

Differential Diagnosis

- *Anaplastic or plasmablastic myeloma* (myeloma-related symptoms, marrow involvement, EBV-negative, CD56-positive)
- *Diffuse large B-cell lymphoma* (positive pan-B-cell markers, negative CD38/CD138, proliferative rate < 90%)
- *ALK-positive large B-cell lymphoma* (ALK+, EBV−, sinusoidal growth pattern)
- *Plasmablastic transformation of myeloma* (prior history of plasma cell neoplasm)

Caveats and Pearls

- If strongly positive for pan-B-cell markers, best classified as *DLBCL, NOS*
- If CD56-positive, rule out *myeloma*
- If prior history of plasma cell neoplasm, classify as *plasmablastic transformation of myeloma*
- If myeloma-related features are present, consider a diagnosis of *plasmablastic neoplasm (plasmablastic lymphoma/anaplastic myeloma)*

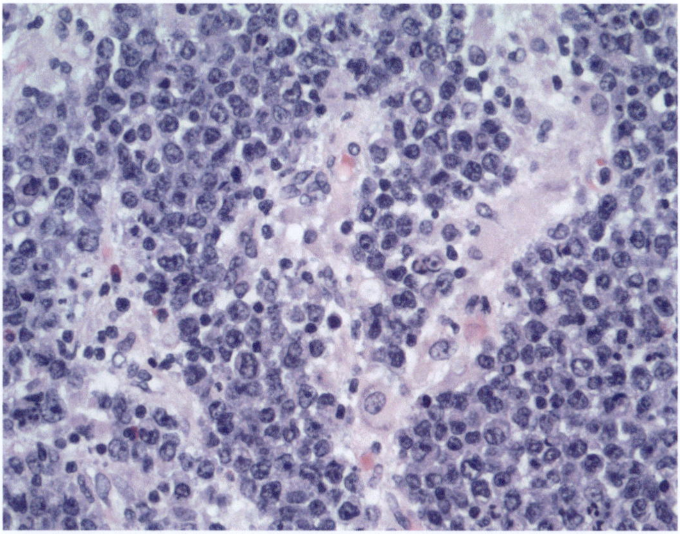

Plasmablastic lymphoma

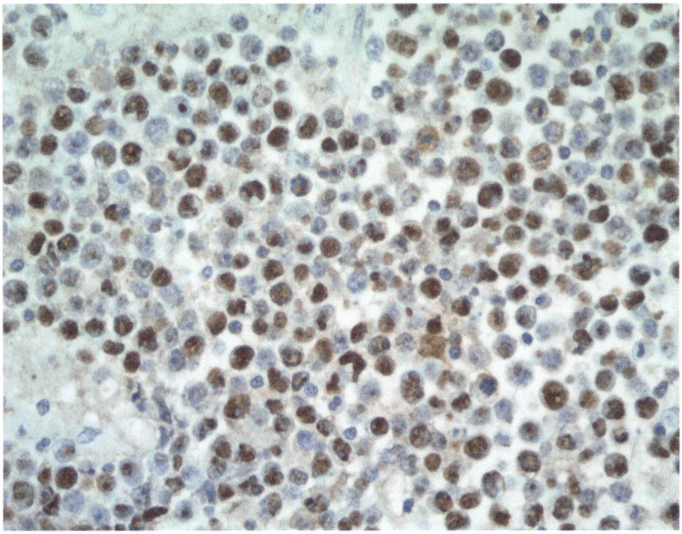

Plasmablastic lymphoma with EBV positivity (EBER ISH)

Primary Effusion Lymphoma

Snapshot

- Malignant effusion (or rarely extracavitary mass) of large pleomorphic HHV8/EBV-positive B-cell-derived lymphoid cells with null phenotype

Clinical Features

Three clinical settings:

1. HIV+ patients with severe immunodeficiency
2. Solid organ transplant recipients
3. Elderly HIV persons from the human herpesvirus-8 (HHV8)-endemic Mediterranean region

Rare presentation as an extracavitary mass (extranodal sites, lymph nodes)

Morphology

- Large pleomorphic cells with immunoblastic, plasmablastic, or anaplastic features

Immunophenotype

- POSITIVE: CD45, CD138/CD38, CD30, EMA, HHV8 LANA1, EBV EBER1 (most cases)
- NEGATIVE: Pan-B-cell markers (CD20, CD79a)

Differential Diagnosis

- *Diffuse large B-cell lymphoma* (positive for pan-B-cell markers, HHV8-negative)
- *Plasmablastic lymphoma* (extranodal sites, CD79a-positive [most cases], HHV8-negative)

Caveats and Pearls

- May occur with Kaposi sarcoma or multicentric Castleman disease

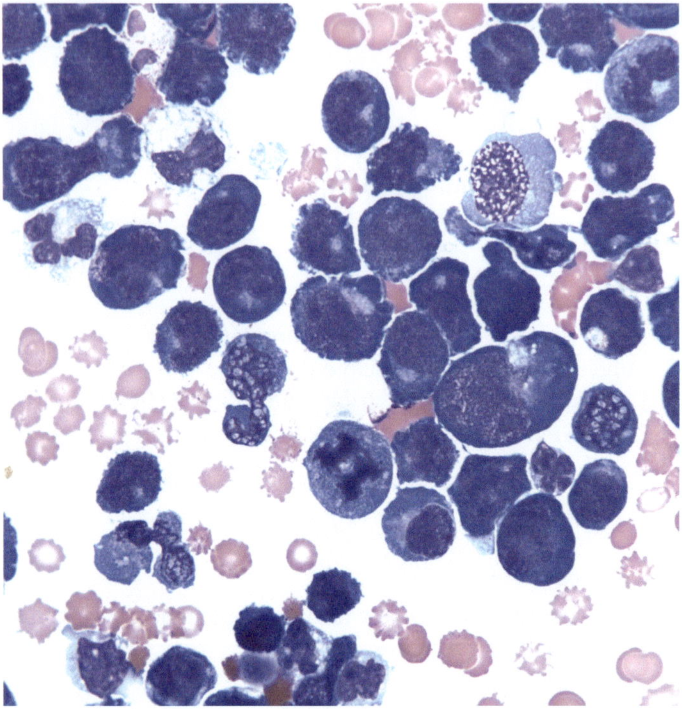

Primary effusion lymphoma (pleural fluid)

HHV8-Associated Lymphoproliferative Disorders

Primary Effusion Lymphoma (see separate entry)

HHV8+ Multicentric Castleman Disease

Snapshot

- Lymphoid follicle involution with HHV8+ plasmablasts in mantle zones and interfollicular areas and numerous interfollicular plasma cells

Clinical Features

- Constitutional symptoms (fever, night sweats, weight loss); lymphadenopathy; splenomegaly in immunosuppressed patients

Immunohistochemistry

- POSITIVE: IgM lambda (polyclonal), CD20 variable, CD38, IgA-positive plasma cells
- NEGATIVE: PAX5, CD138

HHV8+ Diffuse Large B-Cell Lymphoma, NOS

Snapshot

- Diffuse sheets of HHV8+ plasmablasts in lymph nodes and spleen

Clinical Features

- Progressive lymphadenopathy and splenomegaly, usually arising in setting of HHV8+ multicentric Castleman disease

Immunohistochemistry

- Clonal IgM lambda-positive plasmablasts, variably positive for CD20 and CD38, negative for CD79a and CD138

Differential Diagnosis

- *Plasmablastic lymphoma* (HHV8-negative, EBV-positive)
- *Extracavitary primary effusion lymphoma* (EBV-positive)

HHV8+ Germinotropic Lymphoproliferative Disorder

Snapshot

- Plasmablastic infiltration of lymph node germinal centers and atrophic Castleman-like follicles

Clinical Features

- Localized lymphadenopathy in otherwise healthy HIV-negative individuals

Immunohistochemistry

- POSITIVE: HHV8 (LANA), EBV (EBER ISH), monotypic kappa or lambda in some cases
- NEGATIVE: CD20, CD138

Genetics

- Polyclonal or oligoclonal immunoglobulin gene rearrangements

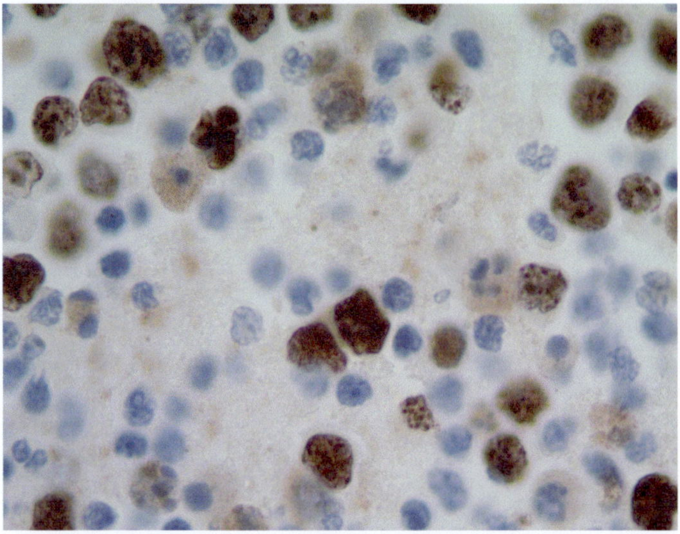

HHV-8-positive large cells in PEL (LANA1 IHC)

Burkitt Lymphoma

Snapshot

- Highly proliferative lymphoid neoplasm composed of monomorphic sheets of immature medium-sized B-cells with numerous admixed starry-sky pattern histiocytes

Clinical Features

- *Endemic disease*—Jaw/facial bone tumors in children from malaria-endemic regions (Africa, New Guinea)
- *Sporadic disease*—Ileocecal tumor (most common site) in young adults; lymph node tumors in older adults
- *Immunodeficiency-related disease*—Lymph node disease (most common site), most often in HIV+ adults

Morphology

- Diffuse monomorphic sheets of medium-sized immature B-cells with oval nuclei, several small basophilic nucleoli, and basophilic cytoplasm with small lipid-laden vacuoles best seen on smears or touch preps
- Prominent apoptosis and starry-sky pattern histiocytes
- Very high Ki-67 proliferative index (95–100%)
- Rarely, tumor cells may exhibit plasmacytoid or pleomorphic features ('atypical BL')

Immunophenotype

- CD10, CD20, and BCL6-positive; BCL2-negative/weak, TdT-negative

Virology

- EBV positivity (detected best by EBER ISH) ranges from 100% in endemic disease to approximately 30% in sporadic and immunodeficiency-related disease

Genetics

- *c-MYC* rearrangements with immunoglobulin loci [t(8;14), t(2;8), t(8;22)]

- Absence of *BCL2* or *BCL6* translocation
- *TCF3* or *ID3* mutations in most (70%) sporadic and immunodeficiency-related cases, and many (40%) endemic cases; *cyclin D3* mutations in 30%

Differential Diagnosis

- *Burkitt-like lymphoma with 11q aberration* (provisional entity)—More cellular pleomorphism, lower c-MYC expression by IHC, negative for *c-MYC* rearrangement, *11q* abnormalities, more complex karyotype
- *B-lymphoblastic leukemia/lymphoma*—TdT-positive; negative for surface Ig, EBV, and *c-MYC* rearrangements

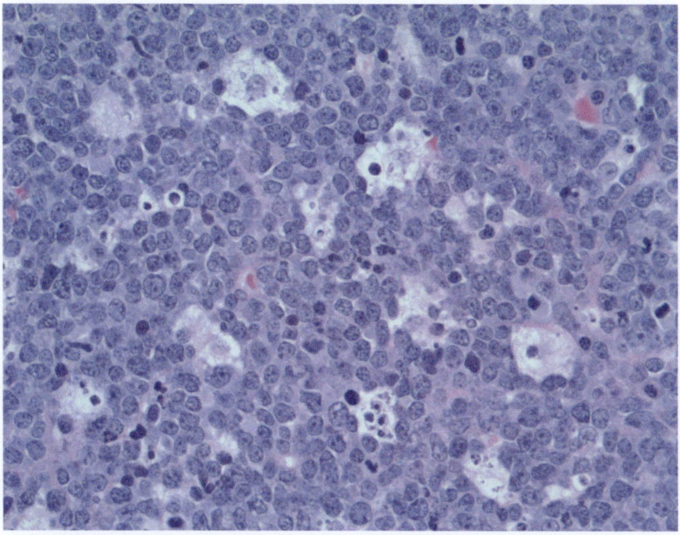

Burkitt lymphoma with admixed starry-sky histiocytes

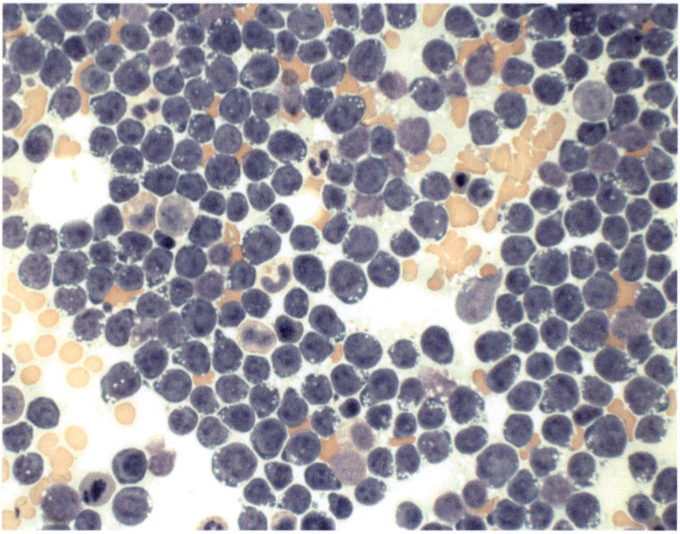

Burkitt lymphoma, marrow aspirate smear. Note the cytoplasmic vacuoles

Burkitt-Like Lymphoma with 11q Aberration

Snapshot

- Infiltrate of medium-large Burkitt-like cells with high mitotic index, 11q abnormalities, and absence of *c-MYC* translocation

Morphology

- Medium-large lymphoid cells with high proliferative index (>95%) and starry-sky pattern

Immunophenotype

- POSITIVE: CD20, PAX5, CD10, BCL6, MYC (variable), CD16/CD56+/−
- NEGATIVE: BCL2, EBV

Genetics

- *11q23* (gain) or *11q24* (loss); complex karyotype; no *MYC-IG* rearrangements

Differential Diagnosis

- *Burkitt lymphoma* (*MYC-IG* translocation, EBV+/−, CD38 high, CD45 weak)

High-Grade B-Cell Lymphoma with *MYC* and *BCL2* and/or *BCL6* Rearrangement

Snapshot

- High-grade diffuse B-cell lymphoma with variable cytologic features and *MYC* rearrangement plus *BCL2* and/or *BCL6* rearrangement

Morphology

- Diffuse infiltrate of medium to large cells with variable morphologic features resembling DLBCL, BL, intermediate DLBCL/BL, or lymphoblastic lymphoma
- Highly variable proliferative rate (may range from <30% [DLBCL-like] to >80% [BL-like])

Immunophenotype

- POSITIVE: CD20, CD10, BCL6, BCL2, and MYC (most cases)
- NEGATIVE: TdT, cyclin D1, and MUM1 (most cases)

Genetics

- Double hit (*MYC* and *BCL2* rearrangement, or *MYC* and *BCL6* rearrangement)
  Triple hit (*MYC*, *BCL2*, and *BCL6* rearrangement)
- Complex karyotypes are common

Differential Diagnosis

- *Burkitt lymphoma* (monomorphic infiltrate of medium-sized CD10+ BCL2-cells, very high proliferative rate [>90%], *MYC* rearrangement only with immunoglobulin gene partner, no *BCL2* or *BCL6* rearrangement, simple karyotype)
- *Diffuse large B-cell lymphoma* (sheets of large often pleomorphic cells, *BCL2*, *BCL6*, or *MYC* rearrangement may be seen, but no double or triple hit)
- *B-lymphoblastic leukemia/lymphoma* (small-medium-sized lymphoblasts, positive for TdT, cCD79a, cCD22)

- *Blastoid variant of mantle cell lymphoma* (small-medium-sized with lymphoblast-like features, CD5 and cyclin D1/SOX11-positive, CD10 and BCL6-negative)

Caveats and Pearls

- Gains and amplifications of *MYC*, *BCL2*, and/or *BCL6* genes *do not meet diagnostic criteria*

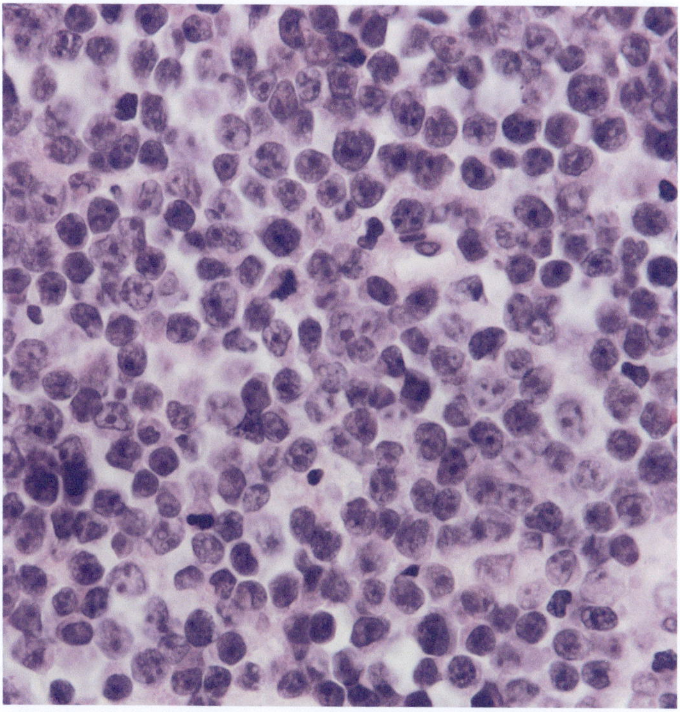

High-grade B-cell lymphoma with double hit (c-*MYC* and *BCL2* translocations)

High-Grade B-Cell Lymphoma, NOS

Snapshot

- Blastoid or Burkitt-like lymphoid infiltrate without double or triple hit (*MYC*, *BCL2*, *BCL6*)

Morphology

- Diffuse infiltrate of B-cells with variable morphology (Burkitt-like, centroblast-like, blastoid) and variable proliferative index

Immunophenotype

- POSITIVE: CD20, BCL6, CD10 (variable), MYC (variable)
- NEGATIVE: MUM1, TdT, cyclin D1, SOX11

Genetics

- Isolated *MYC* or *BCL2* rearrangement may be seen

Differential Diagnosis

- *DLBCL* (large cell infiltrate [centroblasts or immunoblasts])
- *Burkitt lymphoma* (monomorphic infiltrate, strong MYC expression, *MYC-IG* translocation, starry sky, very high proliferative index)
- *Blastoid variant of mantle cell lymphoma* (positive for CD5 and cyclin D1 or SOX11)

B-Cell Lymphoma, Unclassifiable, with Features Intermediate Between DLBCL and Classic Hodgkin Lymphoma

Snapshot

- Pleomorphic large cell infiltrate with morphologic and immunophenotypic features that overlap primary mediastinal large B-cell lymphoma (PMBL) and nodular sclerosis Hodgkin lymphoma (NSHL)

Clinical Features

- Young adult males with anterior mediastinal mass (most common)
- Supraclavicular nodes, lung, liver, spleen, marrow

Morphology

- Confluent sheets of pleomorphic large cells with diffuse fibrosis, sparse inflammatory infiltrate, bland neutrophil-poor necrosis

Immunophenotype

- POSITIVE: B-cell markers (CD45, CD20, CD79a, OCT2, BOB1) and classic RS-cell markers (CD15+/–, CD30, PAX5 [weak])
- NEGATIVE: EBV (most cases)

Genetics

- Clonal immunoglobulin heavy chain rearrangement

Differential Diagnosis

- *Classic Hodgkin lymphoma* (prominent inflammatory background, usually negative for CD45, CD20, OCT2; weak positive for PAX5, fascin positive)
- *Primary mediastinal large B-cell lymphoma* (no RS cells, CD23 positive)

Caveats and Pearls

- If EBV-positive, consider EBV+ DLBCL
- In PMBL-like cases, a CD20– CD15+ phenotype favors gray zone lymphoma
- In HL-like cases, a CD20++ PAX5++ CD15– phenotype favors gray zone lymphoma

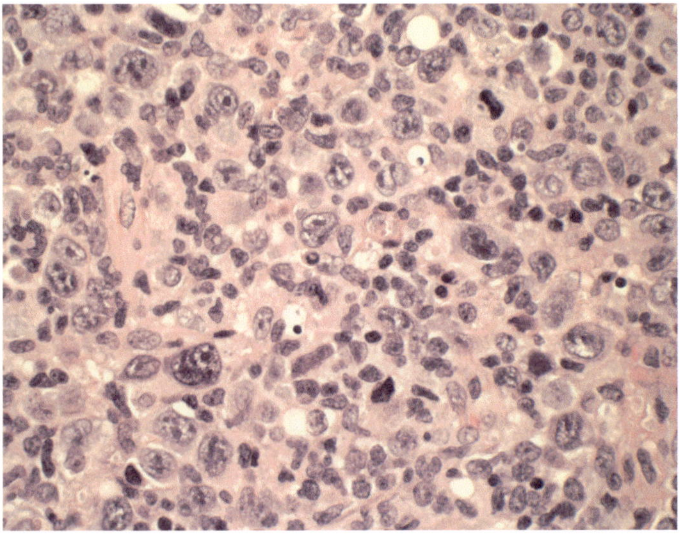

B-cell lymphoma, unclassifiable, with features of DLBCL and classic Hodgkin lymphoma

Chapter 10
Immunodeficiency-Associated Lymphoproliferative Disorders

Lymphoproliferative Disorders Associated with Primary Immune Disorders

Ataxia Telangiectasia

- Ataxia, telangiectasia, chronic lung infections
- LPD types—B-cell lymphoma (DLBCL, BL), T-cell lymphoma (PTCL), CHL, and nonleukemic clonal T-cell proliferations

Autoimmune Lymphoproliferative Syndrome

- Hepatosplenomegaly, lymphadenopathy, autoimmune cytopenia
- Double negative (CD4– CD8–) T-cells in blood, nodes, and spleen
- Follicular hyperplasia and progressive transformation of germinal centers
- LPD types—Hodgkin lymphoma (NLPHL and CHL), B-cell lymphoma (DLBCL, BL), and T-cell LPD (T-PLL, T-ALL)

Common Variable Immunodeficiency

- Nodal and extranodal lymphoid infiltrates (often polyclonal) with follicular and/or paracortical hyperplasia; nodular lymphoid hyperplasia of GI tract

© Springer Nature Switzerland AG 2019
S. D. Hudnall et al., *Pocket Guide to Diagnostic Hematopathology*, https://doi.org/10.1007/978-3-030-10630-0_10

- LPD types—EBV+ DLBCL, EBV+ CHL, low-grade BCL (SLL, LPL, MALT lymphoma), PTCL

Hyper-IgM Syndrome
- Absence of lymph node germinal centers
- IgM+/IgD+ B-cells in blood
- Proliferation of nonclonal IgM+ plasma cells in extranodal sites
- LPD types—EBV+ DLBCL, EBV+ CHL, T-LGL

Nijmegen Breakage Syndrome
- LPD types—DLBCL, PTCL, T-ALL/LBL, CHL

Severe Combined Immunodeficiency and X-Linked LPD
- LPD types—EBV+ DLBCL, EBV+ BL, fatal infectious mononucleosis with hemophagocytic syndrome

Wiskott-Aldrich Syndrome
- Microthrombocytopenia, eczema, and recurrent infections
- LPD types—EBV+ DLBCL, EBV+ CHL, lymphomatoid granulomatosis

HIV-Associated Lymphomas

Snapshot

- Variety of lymphomas (primarily aggressive B-cell lymphomas and classic Hodgkin lymphoma) seen in HIV+ persons, often EBV+, and often with extranodal disease (GI tract, CNS, liver, marrow)

Burkitt Lymphoma

- Often presents in GI tract
- Plasmacytoid features
- 30–50% EBV+

DLBCL

- Primary CNS lymphoma
- HHV-8+ DLBCL, NOS (EBV−)
- Overall 30% EBV+

Plasmablastic Lymphoma

- Oral cavity, jaw, other extranodal sites
- 60–70% EBV+ (EBER+ LMP1−)

Hodgkin Lymphoma

- 50% are NSHL type
- 80–100% EBV+ RS cells

Primary Effusion Lymphoma

- HHV-8+ EBV+/−
- Pan-B-cell antigens not expressed
- CD38/CD138-positive

Post-Transplant Lymphoproliferative Disorders (PTLD)

Snapshot

- Wide variety of frequently EBV-positive lymphoid lesions in the immune-compromised post-transplant setting that range from polyclonal B-cell and plasma cell hyperplasia to monoclonal B-cell and T-/NK-cell lymphoma and Hodgkin lymphoma

Plasmacytic Hyperplasia

- Polyclonal plasma cell–rich interfollicular infiltrate with variable EBV positivity

Infectious Mononucleosis

- Polyclonal interfollicular to diffuse EBV+ infiltrate of small lymphocytes, plasma cells, immunoblasts, and RS-like cells (CD45+ CD20+ CD15−)

Florid Follicular Hyperplasia

- Multiple enlarged secondary follicles with variable EBV positivity

Polymorphic PTLD

- Effacing/destructive lesion composed of B-cells (small- and medium-sized), T-cells (may be numerous), plasma cells, immunoblasts, and RS-like cells (CD45+ CD20+ CD15−)
- Most often positive for EBV and clonal immunoglobulin rearrangement
- *CAVEAT*: EBV+ mucocutaneous ulcer is not classified as PTLD

Monomorphic PTLD

Monomorphic B-Cell LPD

- Clonal B-cell or plasmacytic infiltrate meeting criteria for diffuse large B-cell lymphoma (most common), Burkitt

lymphoma, plasmacytoma, or, rarely, myeloma with variable EBV positivity
- NOTE: Category includes post-transplant EBV+ MALT lymphoma of skin and subcutaneous tissues

Monomorphic T-/NK-Cell LPD
- Neoplastic T-cell infiltrate meeting criteria for PTCL, NOS, hepatosplenic TCL, or other T- and NK-cell neoplasms (including T-LGL leukemia)
- Commonly extranodal

Classic Hodgkin Lymphoma LPD
- Typical classic Hodgkin lymphoma histology and immunophenotype
- Usually EBV+ mixed cellularity subtype

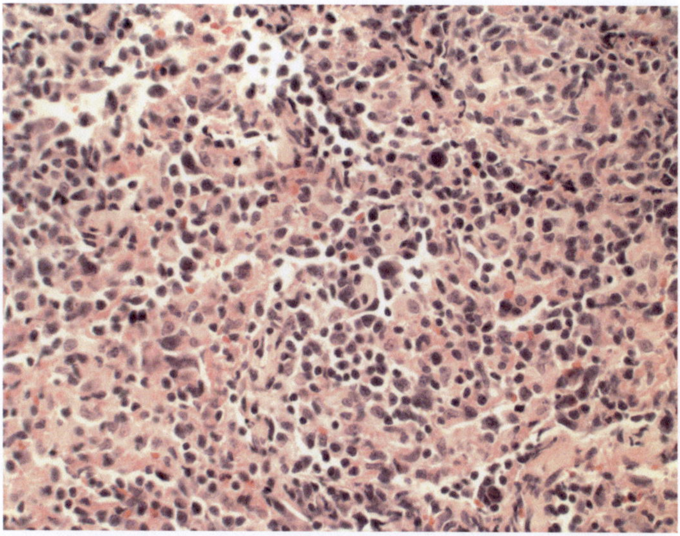

Post-transplant lymphoproliferative disorder (PTLD) of the lung

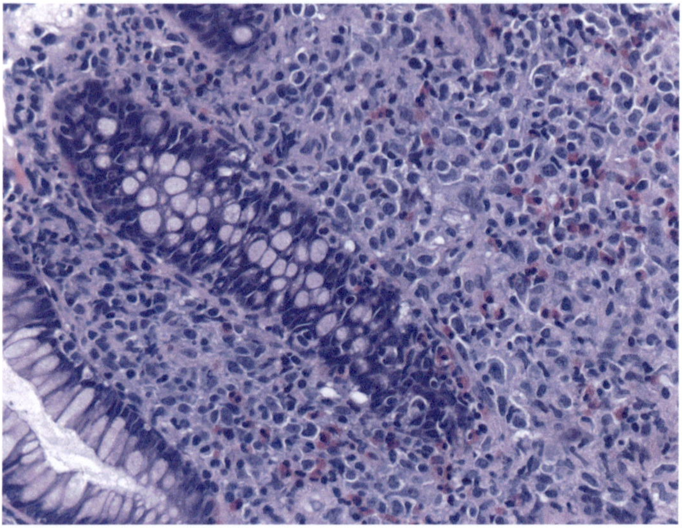

Post-transplant lymphoproliferative disorder (PTLD) of the gastro-intestinal tract

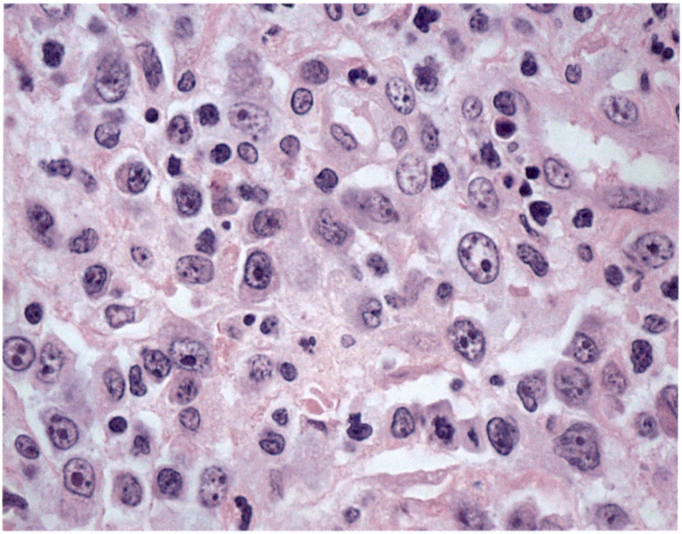

Polymorphic post-transplant lymphoproliferative disorder (PTLD)

Other Iatrogenic Immunodeficiency-Associated Lymphoproliferative Disorders

Snapshot

- Wide variety of lymphoproliferative disorders (LPD) arising in the setting of prolonged iatrogenic immunosuppression for autoimmune disease

Types of LPD

- DLBCL, classic Hodgkin lymphoma, HL-like B-cell LPD, polymorphic PTLD-like lesions, T-/NKT-cell lymphoma, follicular lymphoma, and other B-cell lymphomas
- EBV most often positive in HL, HL-like B-LPD, and polymorphic LPD, and less often positive in DLBCL and other B-cell lymphomas
- Often extranodal (except HL)

Autoimmune Diseases

- Rheumatoid arthritis
- Inflammatory bowel disease
- Psoriasis
- Psoriatic arthritis
- Systemic lupus erythematosus

Implicated Drugs

- Methotrexate
- TNF inhibitors
- Thiopurines

Specific Clinical Scenarios

- Rheumatoid arthritis treated with methotrexate (DLBCL, HL, T-cell lymphoma, polymorphic LPD)
- Crohn's disease treated with thiopurine +/− TNF inhibitor (hepatosplenic T-cell lymphoma)

Clinical Outcome

- Regression seen in some cases following drug withdrawal (excluding TNF inhibitors), particularly in HL, HL-like B-cell LPD, and polymorphic LPD

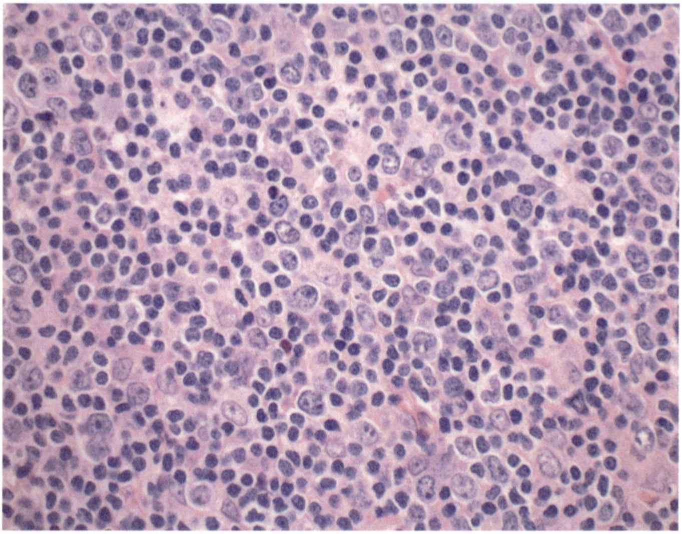

Methotrexate-associated polymorphic lymphoproliferative disorder

Chapter 11
Mature T- and NK-Cell Neoplasms

T-Cell Prolymphocytic Leukemia (T-PLL)

Snapshot

- Marked increase in blood of small- to medium-sized prolymphocytes with ovoid-irregular nuclei and with prominent central nucleoli, often with cytoplasmic blebbing

Clinical Features

- Rare aggressive neoplasm of adults >30 years
- Marked leukocytosis (WBC often >100 K/μL), anemia, and thrombocytopenia
- Hepatosplenomegaly, lymphadenopathy, rash, effusions

Morphology

- Monotonous infiltrate of small-medium prolymphocytes with ovoid-irregular nuclei, prominent central nucleoli, and basophilic cytoplasm, often with protrusions
- Morphologic variant—cerebriform nuclear contour
- Can involve lymph nodes, splenic red pulp, liver, and dermis (with epidermal sparing)

Immunophenotype

- POSITIVE: CD2, CD3 (weak surface), CD5, CD7, TCL1
- Variable CD4/CD8 expression: (CD4+/CD8−, CD4+/CD8+, or CD4−/CD8+)

© Springer Nature Switzerland AG 2019
S. D. Hudnall et al., *Pocket Guide to Diagnostic Hematopathology*, https://doi.org/10.1007/978-3-030-10630-0_11

Genetics

- Chromosome 14—inv(14)(q11q32) (80%), t(14;14)(q11;q32), t(X;14)(q28;q11)
- Chromosome 8—trisomy 8q (70–80%), gain of *MYC*

Differential Diagnosis

- *Peripheral T-cell lymphoma, NOS* (WBC count is not markedly elevated; lacks prolymphocytic morphology [prominent central nucleolus, cytoplasmic blebs]; pan-T-cell antigen loss is common (CD2, CD5, CD7); no expression of TCL1)
- *B-cell prolymphocytic leukemia* (may be morphologically similar, but easily distinguished by expression of pan-B-cell antigens

Caveats and Pearls

- Distinctive morphology is best evaluated by peripheral blood smear
- The dual CD4+/CD8+ immunophenotype is unique
- No pan-T antigen loss
- TCL1 positivity is unique

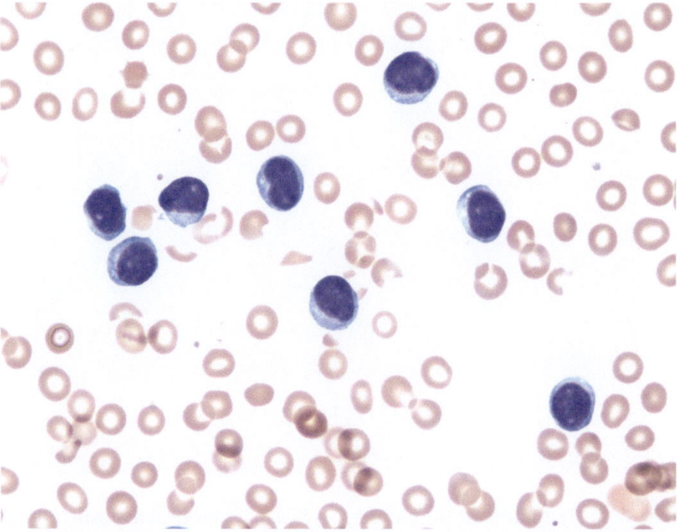

T-cell prolymphocytic leukemia (T-PLL). Abnormal prolymphocytes in blood smear

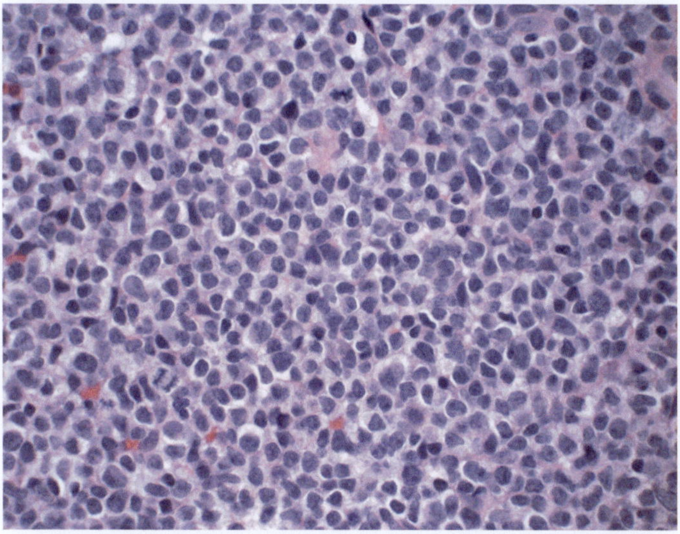

T-cell prolymphocytic leukemia (T-PLL). Diffuse monomorphic infiltrate in prolymphocytes

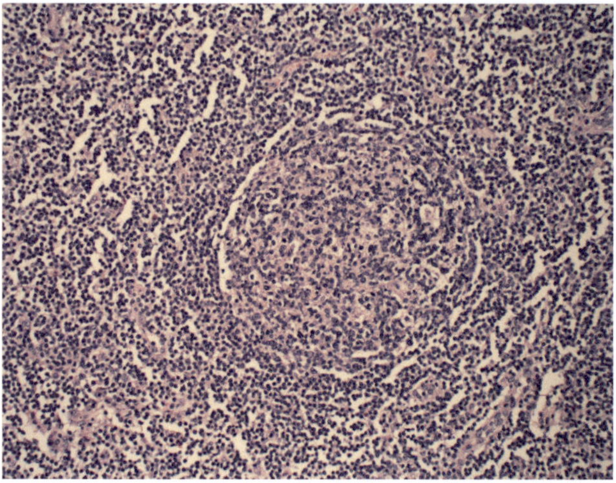

T-cell prolymphocytic leukemia (T-PLL). Paracortical infiltrate of prolymphocytes with sparing of follicle (lymph node)

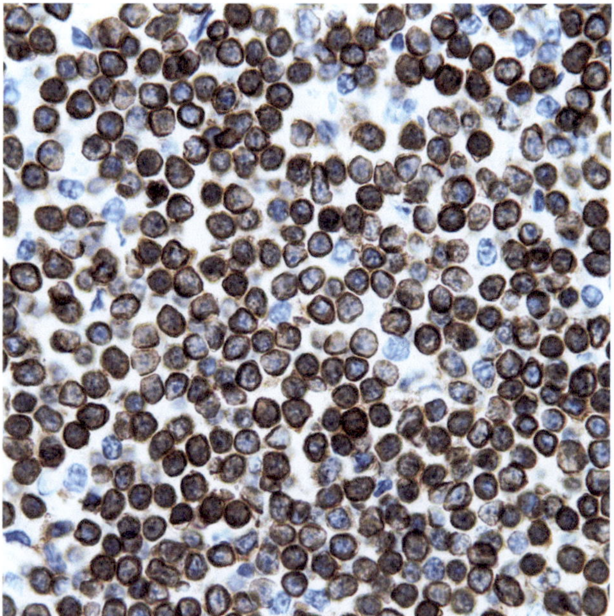

T-cell prolymphocytic leukemia (T-PLL). Cytoplasmic CD3 positivity

T-Cell Large Granular Lymphocytic Leukemia (T-LGLL)

Snapshot

- Persistent increase in blood of clonal medium-large CD57-positiveT-lymphocytes with abundant granular cytoplasm (LGL)

Clinical Features

- Persistent (>6 months) absolute lymphocytosis (often >2 K/μL)
- Involves blood, marrow, and spleen
- Neutropenia and anemia often present
- Hypergammaglobulinemia, autoantibodies (ANA, RF) often present
- Associated with autoimmune conditions, especially rheumatoid arthritis

Morphology

- Medium-large lymphoid cells with round to irregular nuclei with inconspicuous nucleoli, and abundant pale cytoplasm with variably prominent granules
- Sinusoidal infiltration of bone marrow and spleen

Immunophenotype

- POSITIVE: CD2, CD3, CD8, CD16, CD57, TCRαβ, TIA1, granzyme B, KIR (incomplete expression)
- NEGATIVE/WEAK POSITIVE: CD5, CD7, CD56
- UNCOMMON PHENOTYPES: CD4+/−, CD8−, TCRγδ+

Genetics

- Clonal TCR-positive

Differential Diagnosis

- *Reactive T-LGL population* (nonclonal; may have identifiable cause [e.g., infection, malignancy]; resolves with treatment of primary condition; no splenomegaly)
- *Hepatosplenic T-cell lymphoma* (lacks cytoplasmic granules; marked splenomegaly, usually with hepatomegaly; uniform expression of all three KIR antigens [CD158a, CD158b, CD158e]
- *Chronic lymphoproliferative disorder of NK-cells* (morphologically similar, can be distinguished by flow cytometry [surface CD3–]; no TCR rearrangement)

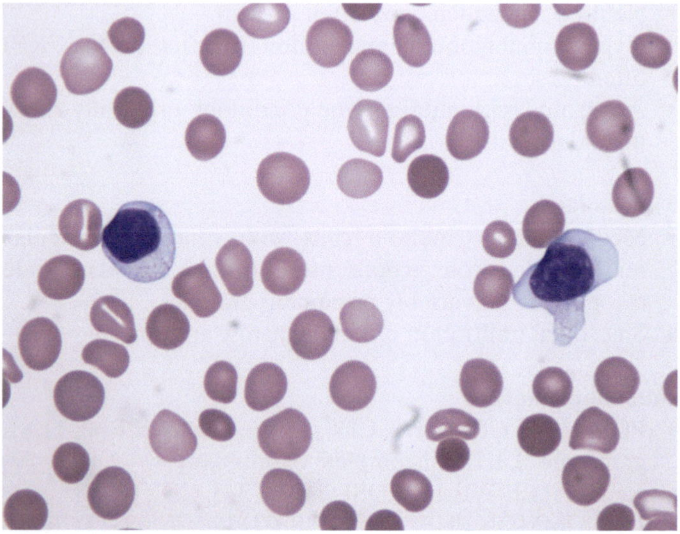

T-cell large granular lymphocytic leukemia (T-LGLL). Large granular lymphocytes in blood smear

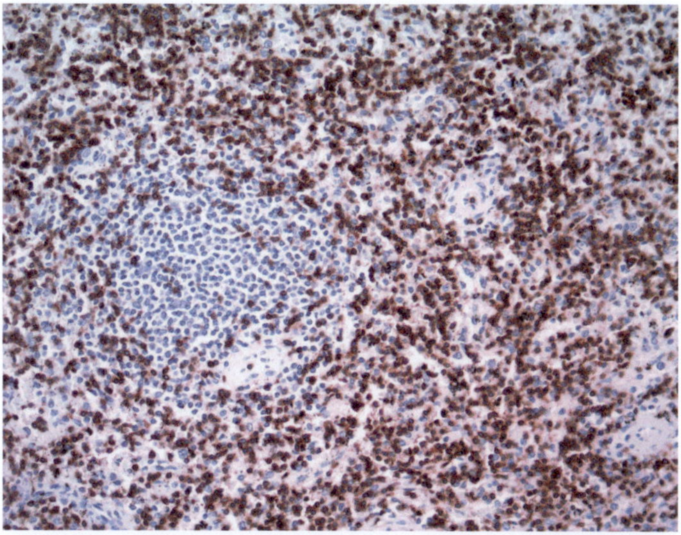

T-cell large granular lymphocytic leukemia (T-LGLL). CD8-positive T-cell infiltrate in splenic red pulp with sparing of white pulp

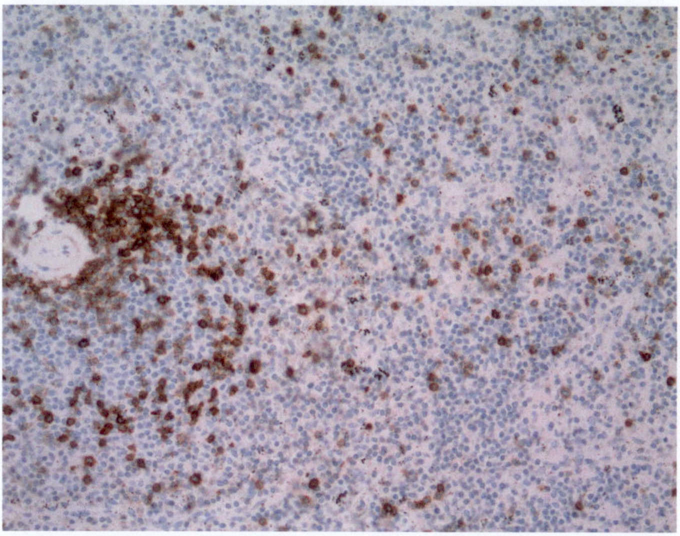

T-cell large granular lymphocytic leukemia (T-LGLL). Aberrant CD5-negativity of the splenic T-cell infiltrate

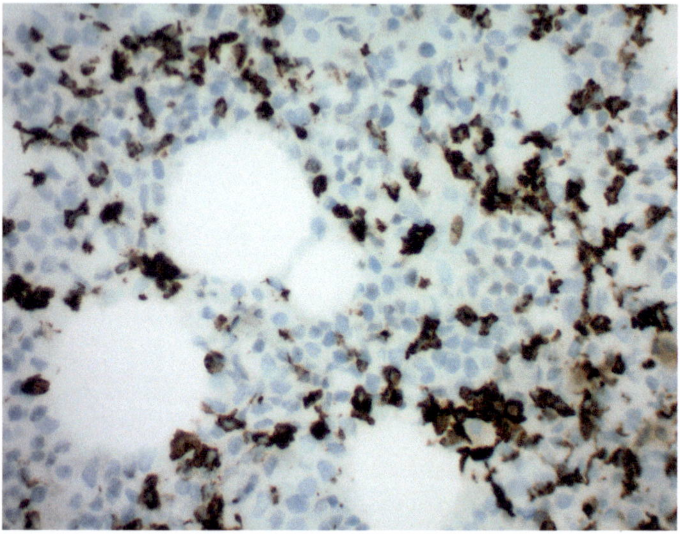

T-cell large granular lymphocytic leukemia (T-LGLL). CD57-positive T-cell infiltrate in marrow

Chronic Lymphoproliferative Disorder of NK-Cells

Snapshot

- Persistent increase (>6 months) of large granular NK-cells in peripheral blood with moderate-abundant granular cytoplasm

Clinical Features

- Primarily involves blood, bone marrow, liver, and spleen (moderate splenomegaly)
- Absolute lymphocyte count (often >2 K/μL)
- Neutropenia (<1.8 K/μL) and/or anemia (<10 g/dL) are common

Morphologic Features

- Increased circulating LGLs with round to mildly irregular nuclei, moderate to abundant pale cytoplasm, and variably prominent granules
- Sinusoidal infiltrates in bone marrow and spleen

Immunophenotype

- POSITIVE: cytoplasmic CD3ε, CD2, CD8, CD16, CD94, cytotoxic molecules
- Variable: CD2, CD7, CD56, CD57
- NEGATIVE: surface CD3, CD5, EBV (EBER)
- Restricted or absent expression of KIR antigens (CD158a, CD158b, CD158e)

Differential Diagnosis

- *Reactive NK-cell lymphocytosis* (may have identifiable cause [e.g., infection, malignancy] with resolution after treatment of primary condition; no splenomegaly)
- *Aggressive NK-cell leukemia; extranodal NK-/T-cell lymphoma* (aggressive clinical course; frequently EBV-positive)
- *T-cell large granular lymphocytic leukemia* (morphologically similar but can be distinguished by flow cytometry [notably surface CD3+]; positive for T-cell receptor gene rearrangement)

Aggressive NK-Cell Leukemia

Snapshot

- Peripheral blood and tissue involvement by medium-large lymphoid cells with variable morphology ranging from LGL to immature or pleomorphic lymphoid cells

Clinical Features

- Young adults; more common in Asian populations
- Involves peripheral blood, bone marrow, liver, and spleen
- Symptoms include pancytopenia, coagulopathy, hepatosplenomegaly, effusions
- May progress to hemophagocytic syndrome and multiorgan failure

Morphologic Features

- Circulating leukemic cells with variable morphology (including LGL-like, immature forms, immunoblastic, and pleomorphic forms)
- Dense diffuse infiltrates, often with necrosis and angioinvasion/destruction

Immunophenotype

- POSITIVE: cytoplasmic CD3ε, CD2, CD16 (+/−), CD56, cytotoxic molecules (perforin, granzyme B, TIA-1), EBER
- NEGATIVE: surface CD3, CD5, CD7 (−/+), CD57 (−/+)

Genetics

- TCR locus in germline configuration del7p, del17p, +1q

Differential Diagnosis

- *Chronic lymphoproliferative disorder of NK-cells* (indolent clinical course; EBV-negative)
- *Extranodal NK-/T-cell lymphoma* (involves upper aerodigestive tract, particularly nasal cavity)
- *Systemic EBV-positive T-cell lymphoma* (affects children and adolescents; NK-cell markers [CD16, CD56] not expressed; positive for T-cell receptor gene rearrangement)

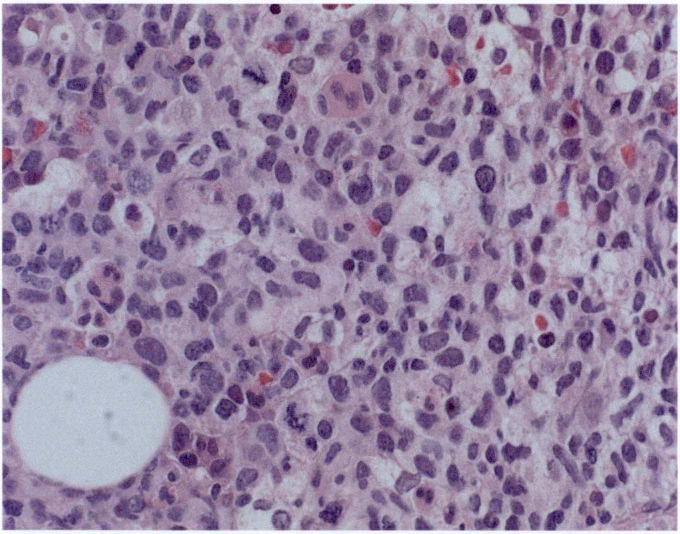

Aggressive NK-cell leukemic infiltrate with nuclear pleomorphism and abundant cytoplasm

EBV-Positive T-Cell and NK-Cell Lymphoproliferative Diseases of Childhood

Snapshot

- Proliferation of EBV-positive T-cells or NK-cells, usually in children from Asia, Central America, and South America

Systemic EBV-Positive T-Cell Lymphoma of Childhood

- Develops following acute primary EBV infection
- Clonal proliferation of small EBV-positive T-cells (usually CD8+) in liver, spleen, bone marrow, lymph nodes, and other locations
- Frequently complicated by fever, pancytopenia, hepatosplenomegaly, liver failure, and hemophagocytic syndrome

Chronic Active EBV Infection of T- and NK-Cell Type, Systemic Form

- Variable clinical presentation (fever, lymphadenopathy, hepatosplenomegaly, diarrhea, rash)
- Polymorphic infiltrate that includes small EBV-positive T-cells or NK-cells involving multiple sites including lymph nodes, bone marrow, liver, spleen, skin
- Clinical course ranges from indolent disease to overt lymphoma, hemophagocytic syndrome, multiorgan failure

Hydroa Vacciniforme-Like Lymphoproliferative Disorder

- Skin papules and vesicles that may progress to ulceration and scarring
- Perivascular/periadnexal dermal infiltrate of small- to medium-sized cytotoxic T-cells (usually CD8+) or NK-cells
- Classic form: self-limited seasonal eruption in sun-exposed areas
- Severe form: lesions in sun-exposed and sun-protected areas with systemic symptoms

Severe Mosquito Bite Allergy

- Severe reaction to mosquito bites with erythema, intraepidermal bullae, ulceration, necrosis, and scarring
- Dense polymorphous inflammatory infiltrate with EBV-positive NK-cells
- Systemic symptoms include fever, malaise, lymphadenopathy, and liver dysfunction
- Can progress to hemophagocytic syndrome or overt NK-cell leukemia/lymphoma

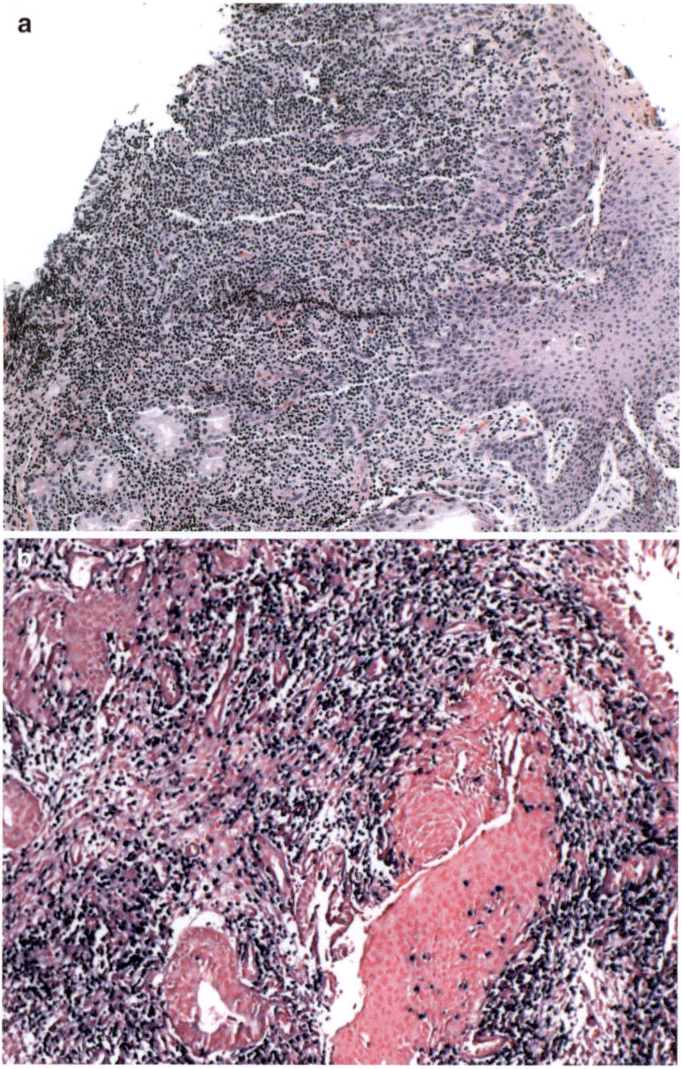

EBV+ T-cell lymphoproliferative disease of childhood (**a**) H&E of skin lesion; (**b**) numerous small EBER-ISH positive lymphocytes (blue signal)

Adult T-Cell Leukemia/Lymphoma (ATLL)

Snapshot

- Blood, lymph node, and/or skin involvement by markedly pleomorphic T-cells in a patient with remote HTLV-1 infection

Clinical Features

- Causally related to HTLV-1 infection, occurring in areas with endemic HTLV-1
- Systemic disease with variable presentation (see clinical variants below)
- Can have secondary immunodeficiency and infection

Morphologic Features

- Highly pleomorphic cells of variable size with coarse chromatin and distinct nucleoli
- Circulating "flower cells" have multilobed nuclei
- Lymph nodes effaced by dense infiltrate; may include EBV+ Reed-Sternberg-like B-cells
- Skin shows epidermal and superficial dermal infiltrate; Pautrier-like microabscesses

Immunophenotype

- POSITIVE: CD3, CD2, CD4, CD5, CD25, CD52, CCR4, FOXP3, CD30 (large cells).
- NEGATIVE: CD7, CD8, ALK
- Uncommonly may be CD4+/CD8+ or CD4−/CD8+

Genetics

- Clonal integration of HTLV-1, with expression of viral oncoproteins TAX and HBZ

Clinical Variants

Acute

- (Most common): many circulating cells, extensive lymphadenopathy, rash, lytic bone lesions, hepatosplenomegaly

Lymphomatous

- Extensive lymphadenopathy, rash

Chronic

- Modest number of circulating cells, rash

Smoldering

- Few circulating cells, rash, pulmonary lesions

Differential Diagnosis

- *Anaplastic large cell lymphoma*: Often CD3 negative. HTLV-1 negative. ALK expression in ALK+ ALCL
- *Cutaneous T-cell lymphoma, Sezary syndrome*: CD25 negative. HTLV-1 negative. Sezary cell nucleiare cerebriform, not multilobated

Caveats and Pearls

- Flower cells are best observed on peripheral blood smear

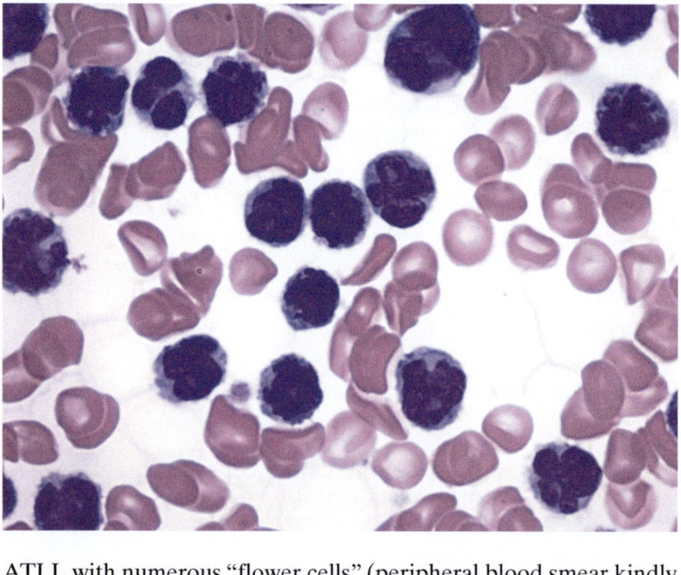

ATLL with numerous "flower cells" (peripheral blood smear kindly provided by Dr. Zenggang Pan, Yale Pathology)

Extranodal NK-/T-Cell Lymphoma, Nasal Type

Snapshot
- Dense infiltrate of atypical lymphocytes in upper aerodigestive tract, with necrosis and angiocentricity/angiodestruction

Clinical Features
- More common in Asian and indigenous Central/South American populations
- Involves upper aerodigestive tract, especially nasal cavity
- Local spread and dissemination to skin, GI tract, testes, and other tissues
- Hemophagocytic syndrome may occur

Morphologic Features
- Dense diffuse angiocentric lymphoid infiltrate often with necrosis and mucosal ulceration

Immunophenotype
- POSITIVE: cytoplasmic CD3ε, CD2, CD43, CD45RO, CD56 (+/−), CD94, cytotoxic antigens (TIA, granzyme B, perforin), EBV
- NEGATIVE: surface CD3, CD16 (−/+), CD57
- Uncommonly may express T-cell antigens: CD4, CD5, CD7, CD8

Genetics
- Alterations in *JAK/STAT* pathway, *TP53*, *KIT*, *RAS* family, *CDK* family, *MYC*, *FAS*, others
- 1p−, 6q−, 11q−, 13q−, 17p−, 1q+, 2q+, others

Variant

Extranasal NK-/T-Cell Lymphoma
- Skin, GI tract, testes, soft tissue with no involvement of upper aerodigestive tract

Differential Diagnosis

- *Aggressive NK-cell leukemia* (involves peripheral blood and bone marrow in addition to organs/tissues)
- *Lymphomatoid granulomatosis* (predominantly lung disease, polymorphous infiltrate with large EBV+ B-cells)

Caveats and Pearls

- CD16 and CD56 are expressed by NK-cells, whereas CD57 is expressed by T-LGL

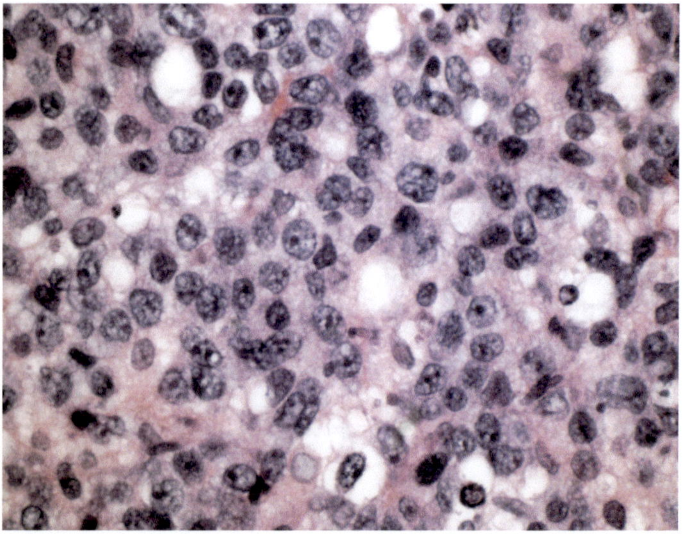

Extranodal NK/T lymphoma, nasal type. Monomorphic large cell infiltrate

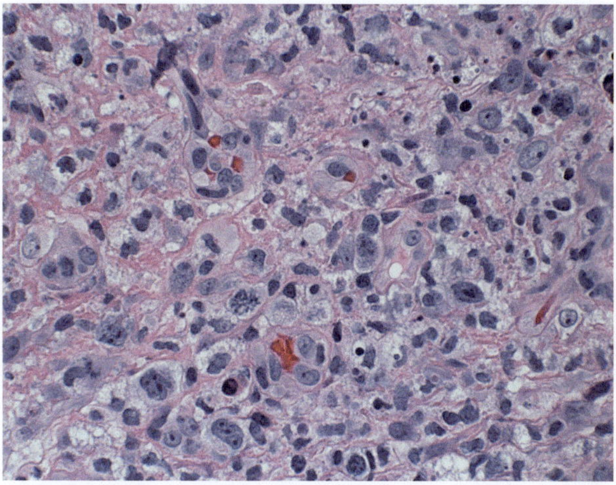

Extranodal NK/T lymphoma, nasal type. Polymorphic large cell infiltrate

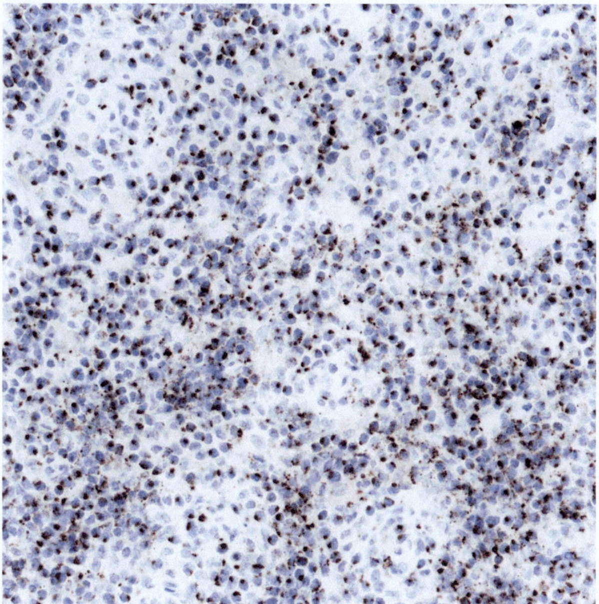

Extranodal NK/T lymphoma, nasal type. Granzyme B-positive infiltrate

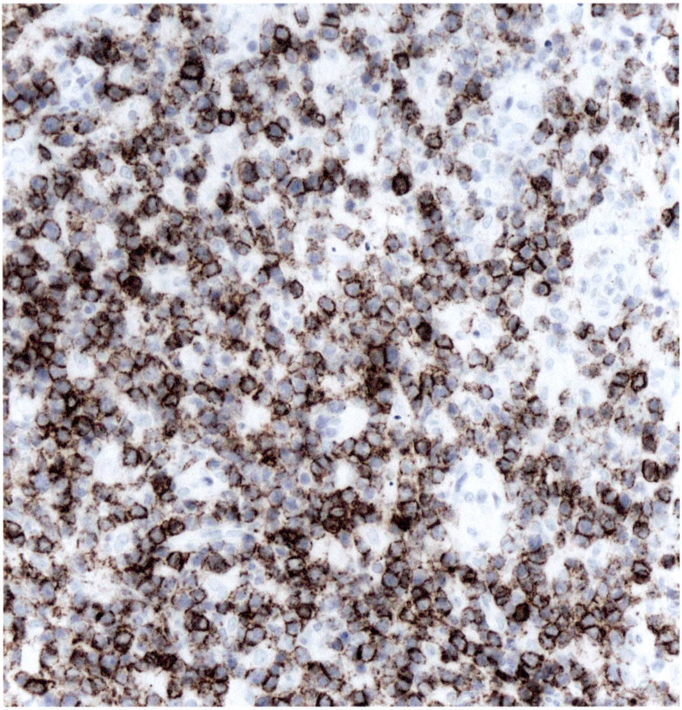

Extranodal NK/T lymphoma, nasal type. CD56-positive infiltrate

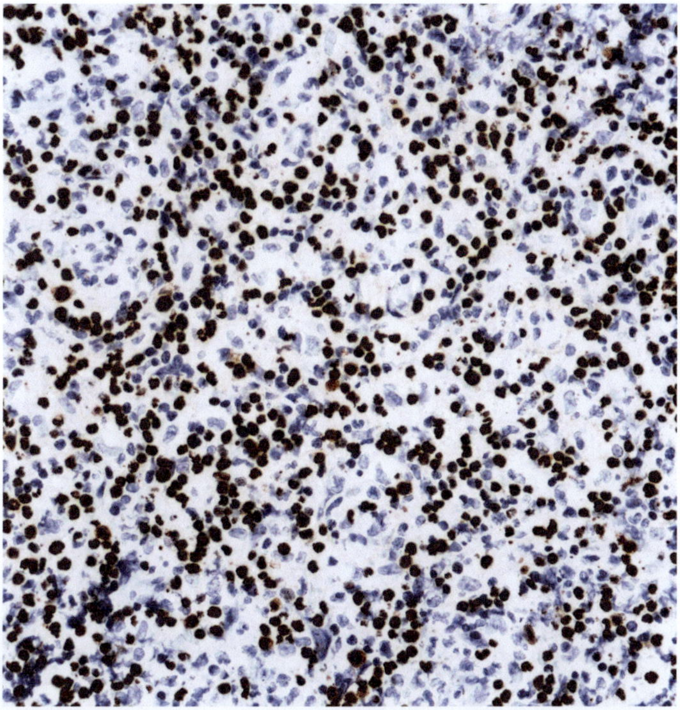

Extranodal NK/T lymphoma, nasal type. EBV (EBER ISH)-positive infiltrate

Intestinal T-Cell Lymphoma

Enteropathy-Associated T-Cell Lymphoma (EATL)

Snapshot

- Pleomorphic intraepithelial lymphocytes that form small intestinal mass lesions with necrosis, ulceration, and a polymorphous inflammatory background

Clinical Features

- Rare complication of gluten-sensitive enteropathy (GSE) (*aka* celiac disease)
- Involves small intestine, occasionally stomach or large intestine, with lymph node spread
- Abdominal pain, weight loss, diarrhea, hemorrhage, obstruction, and B symptoms

Morphologic Features

- Medium to large, pleomorphic intraepithelial lymphocytes with round or angulated nuclei, distinct nucleoli, and moderate to abundant pale cytoplasm
- Forms one or more ulcerating plaques, nodules/masses, and strictures
- Admixed histiocytes and eosinophils, necrosis, and angiocentricity/angioinvasion
- Uninvolved mucosa often shows features of GSE

Immunophenotype

- POSITIVE: CD3, CD2, CD7, CD30 (+/−, large cells), CD103, TIA1, granzyme B, perforin
- NEGATIVE: CD4, CD5, CD8 (−/+), CD56
- Increased Ki67 proliferation index (>50%)

Genetics

- Gains of 1q, 5q, 6q, and 9q. Loss of 16q
- Association with HLA-DQA1*0501 and HLA-DQB1*0201 (similar to GSE)

Differential Diagnosis

- *Monomorphic epitheliotropic intestinal T-cell lymphoma*: Small, monomorphic cells, positive for CD56. No association with gluten-sensitive enteropathy (GSE)
- *Indolent T-cell lymphoproliferative disease of the gastrointestinal tract*: Monotonous small, round T-cells expanding the lamina propria with no epithelial destruction or necrosis. Immunophenotype: CD8+, CD4 −/+, CD5+, CD7 +/−, low Ki67 proliferation index

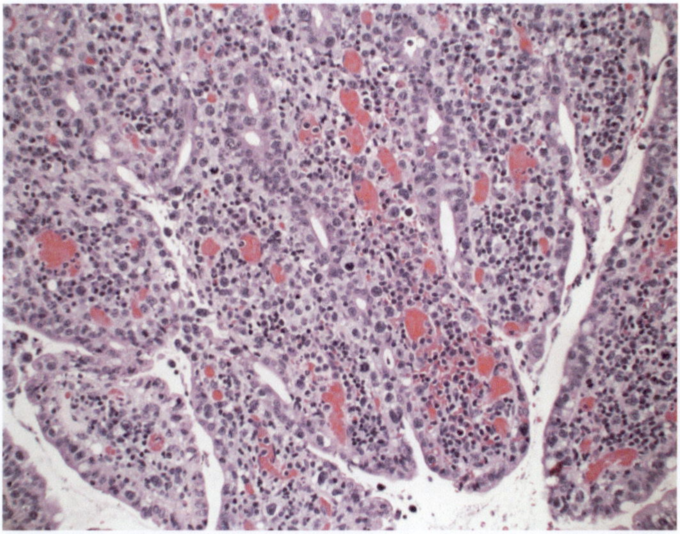

Enteropathy-associated T-cell lymphoma (EATCL) with T-cell infiltrate within the lamina propria

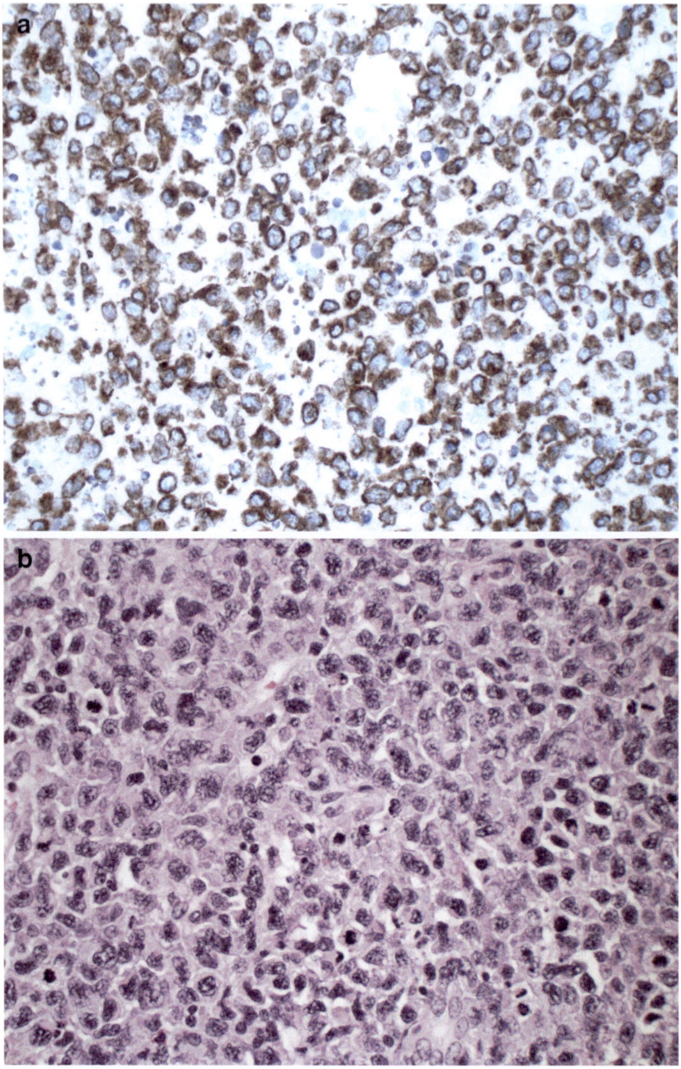

Enteropathy-associated T-cell lymphoma (EATCL): (**a**) CD3-positive infiltrate; (**b**) neoplastic T-cells with medium-large cells with irregular nuclear contour

Monomorphic Epitheliotropic Intestinal T-Cell Lymphoma (MEITL)

Snapshot
- Small- to medium-sized, round intraepithelial lymphocytes that form mass lesions in the small intestine

Clinical Features
- Not associated with gluten-sensitive enteropathy (celiac disease)
- Involves small intestine, occasionally stomach or large intestine, with lymph node spread
- Abdominal pain, weight loss, diarrhea, hemorrhage, obstruction, and B symptoms

Morphologic Features
- Small- to medium-sized, monomorphic intraepithelial lymphocytes with round nuclei and a rim of pale cytoplasm
- Forms one or more ulcerating mass lesions; may have focal necrosis
- Prominent epitheliotropism and crypt destruction

Immunophenotype
- POSITIVE: CD3, CD8, CD56, TIA1, granzyme B, perforin, MATK
- NEGATIVE: CD4 (rarely +), CD5, CD20 (−/+), CD30
- Increased Ki67 proliferation index (can be >50%)

Genetics
- Gain of 8q (MYC) and 9q
- Mutations of *STAT5B* and *SETD2*

Differential Diagnosis

- *Enteropathy-associated T-cell lymphoma*: Pleomorphic cells, negative for CD56. Mixed inflammatory background. Associated with GSE
- *Indolent T-cell lymphoproliferative disease of the gastrointestinal tract*: Monotonous small, round T-cells expanding the lamina propria without epithelial destruction or necrosis. CD8+, CD4 −/+, CD5+, CD7 +/−, low Ki67 proliferation index

Hepatosplenic T-Cell Lymphoma (HSTL)

Snapshot

- Sinusoidal infiltration of the spleen, liver, and bone marrow by monomorphic medium-sized lymphocytes with a rim of pale cytoplasm

Clinical Features

- Typically affects young adults, sometimes in the setting of chronic immunosuppression
- Marked splenomegaly and often hepatomegaly, but no lymphadenopathy
- Pancytopenia and B symptoms

Morphologic Features

- Monomorphic medium-sized lymphocytes with round to ovoid nuclei, partially condensed chromatin, and a rim of pale cytoplasm
- Spleen: Diffuse infiltration of the red pulp cords and sinuses; diminished white pulp
- Liver: Infiltration in a mostly sinusoidal distribution
- Bone marrow: Infiltration and distension of the sinuses; aspirate shows occasional atypical lymphocytes with cytoplasmic projections

Immunophenotype

- POSITIVE: CD3, CD2, CD7 (+/−), CD56 (+/−), TIA1, granzyme M, TCRγδ
- NEGATIVE: CD4, CD5, CD8 (−/+), CD25, CD30, CD57, granzyme B, perforin, TCRαβ
- Uncommonly some cases are TCRαβ+ and TCRγδ−

Genetics

- Isochrome 7q
- *STAT5B* mutations

Differential Diagnosis

- *Aggressive NK-cell leukemia* (EBV [EBER]-positive; bone marrow infiltration is interstitial or diffuse)
- *Primary cutaneous γδ T-cell lymphoma, other T-cell lymphomas expressing* TCRγδ (different clinicopathologic features, particularly the absence of sinusoidal infiltration exclusive to the spleen, liver, and bone marrow)
- *Hairy cell leukemia, HCL-variant, splenic diffuse red pulp small B-cell lymphoma* (morphologic similarities, but easily distinguished by B-cell immunophenotype)

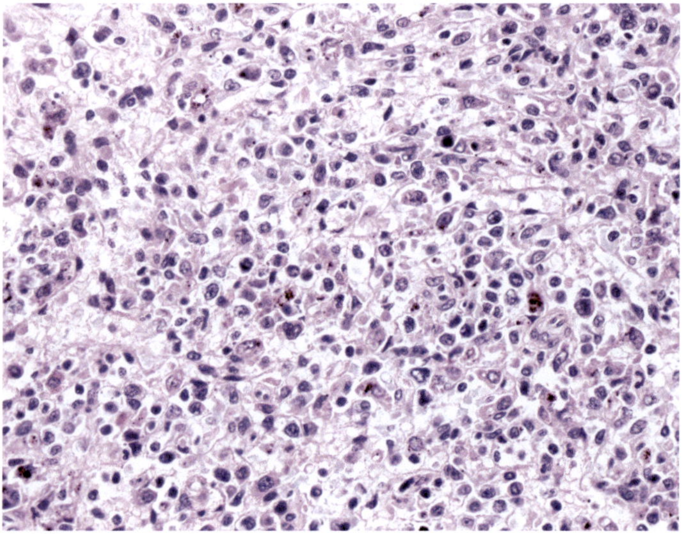

Hepatosplenic T-cell lymphoma (HSTL) in spleen

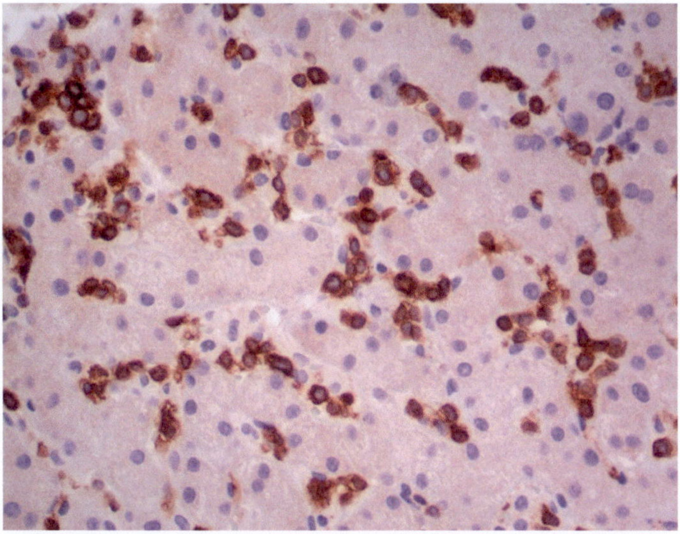

Hepatosplenic T-cell lymphoma (HSTL) with sinusoidal infiltrate in liver (CD3 IHC)

Subcutaneous Panniculitis-Like T-Cell Lymphoma (SPTCL)

Snapshot

- Pleomorphic lymphocytes infiltrating subcutaneous fat lobules with rimming of adipocytes, necrosis, and admixed histiocytes

Clinical Features

- Subcutaneous nodules and plaques on the trunk and extremities
- Some cases associated with autoimmune conditions or immunosuppression
- Cytopenias and increased liver function tests
- Uncommonly seen with fever, weight loss, malaise, or hemophagocytic syndrome

Morphologic Features

- Fat lobules contain nodular or diffuse infiltrate of small, medium, or large pleomorphic cells with hyperchromatic nuclei, irregular nuclear contours, and a rim of pale cytoplasm
- Neoplastic cells form rims around individual adipocytes
- Sparing of septa, dermis, and epidermis
- Admixed vacuolated histiocytes, necrosis, and karyorrhectic debris

Immunophenotype

- POSITIVE: CD3, CD8, TIA1, granzyme B, perforin, βF1
- NEGATIVE: CD4, CD30, CD56, TCRγ

Differential Diagnosis

- *Lupus erythematosus panniculitis (*admixed plasma cells and B-cell aggregates; no aggregates of CD8+ T-cells)
- *Primary cutaneous γδ T-cell lymphoma* (involves dermis, epidermis, and subcutaneous tissue; TCRγ and CD56-positive)

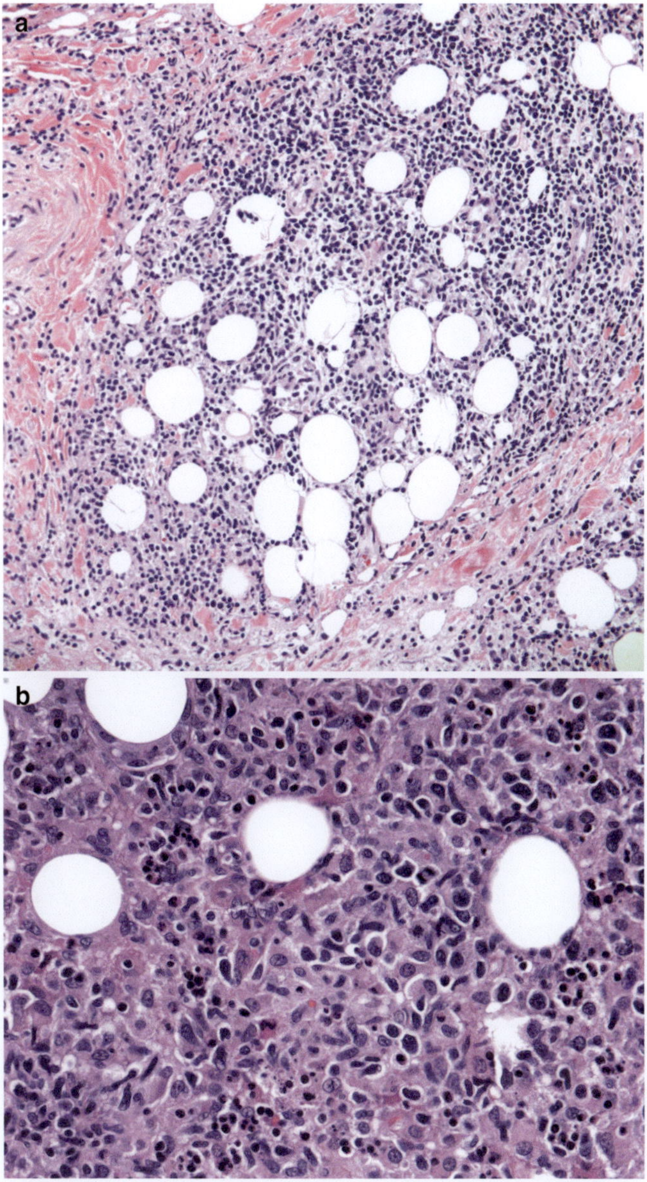

Subcutaneous panniculitis-like T-cell lymphoma (SPTCL): (**a**) subcutaneous lymphoid infiltrate; (**b**) pleomorphic population of T-cells; (**c**) rimming of adipocytes

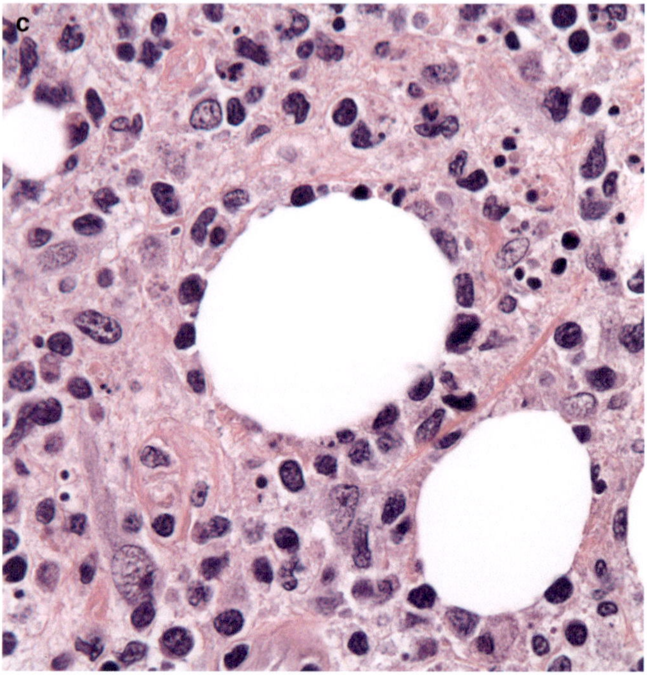

(continued)

Mycosis Fungoides

Snapshot

- Skin infiltrates of small- to medium-sized CD4 + T-lymphocytes with cerebriform nuclei that progress from patches to plaques and tumors

Clinical Features

- Indolent lymphoma that begins as scaly patches, evolves into thickened plaques, and finally develops tumor nodules with frequent ulceration
- Longstanding disease may spread systemically

Morphologic Features

- Early lesions consist of small- to medium-sized cells with cerebriform nuclei
- More evolved lesions contain increasingly larger and more atypical cells
- Patches: Lichenoid dermal infiltrate with spread into the basal layer of the epidermis
- Plaques: Extension into the reticular dermis; Pautrier microabscesses in the epidermis
- Tumors: Nodules/sheets of neoplastic cells in the reticular dermis; less epidermotropism

Immunophenotype

- POSITIVE: CD3, CD4, CD2, CD5, βF1
- NEGATIVE: CD8, CD7 (−/+)
- Uncommonly, may be CD8+, CD4−, TCRγ+
- Large neoplastic cells may express CD30

Variants

Folliculotropic MF

- Involves hair follicles, with sparing of interfollicular epidermis
- Follicular mucinous degeneration is common
- Usually found on head, neck, and upper trunk

Pagetoid Reticulosis

- Pronounced epidermotropism and a verrucous appearance
- Occurs on extremities

Granulomatous Slack Skin

- Abundant infiltration by histiocytes and giant T-cells with destruction of elastic fibers, leading to pendulous folds of skin
- Typically in the axilla and groin

Differential Diagnosis

- *Various inflammatory, spongiotic, and other dermatitides; drug eruption* (the differential diagnosis for patch stage MF includes many benign skin conditions that can have similar morphology; clinical features and morphologic details are important for diagnosis)
- *Peripheral T-cell lymphoma, NOS; primary cutaneous CD4+ small/medium T-cell lymphoproliferative disorder; primary cutaneous anaplastic large cell lymphoma* (MF may be indistinguishable from other T-cell lymphomas based on a single biopsy; clinical history is important for diagnosis, particularly other skin lesions)

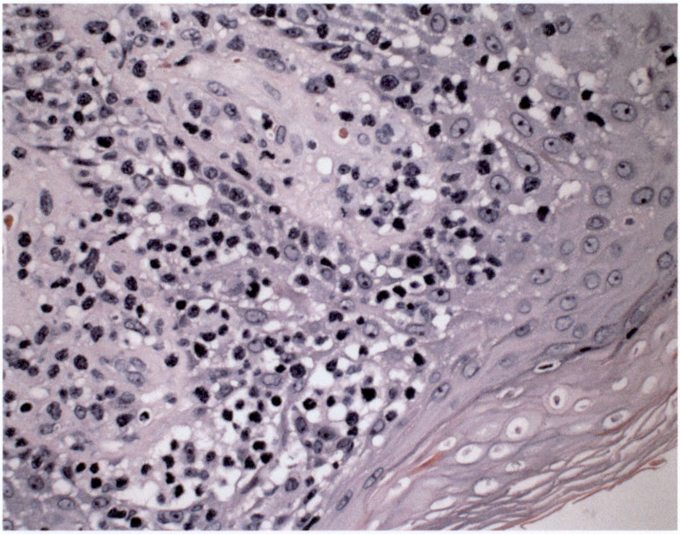

Mycosis fungoides. Atypical T-cells infiltrate within lamina propria with epidermotropism

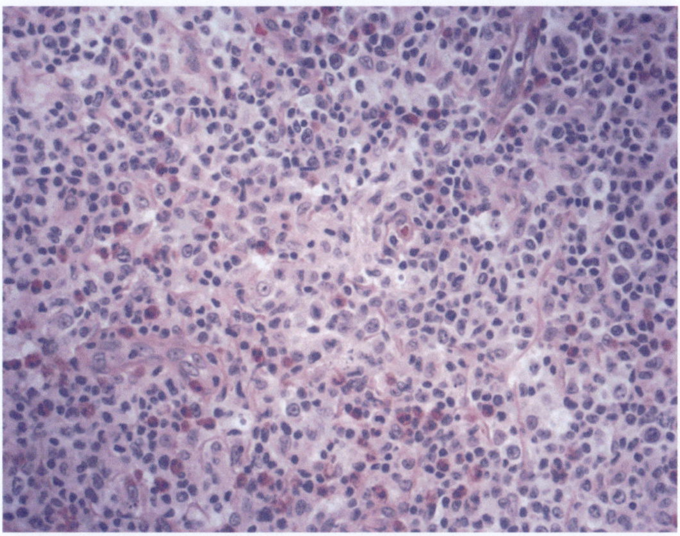

Mycosis fungoides. Paracortical lymphoid infiltrate and eosinophilia (lymph node)

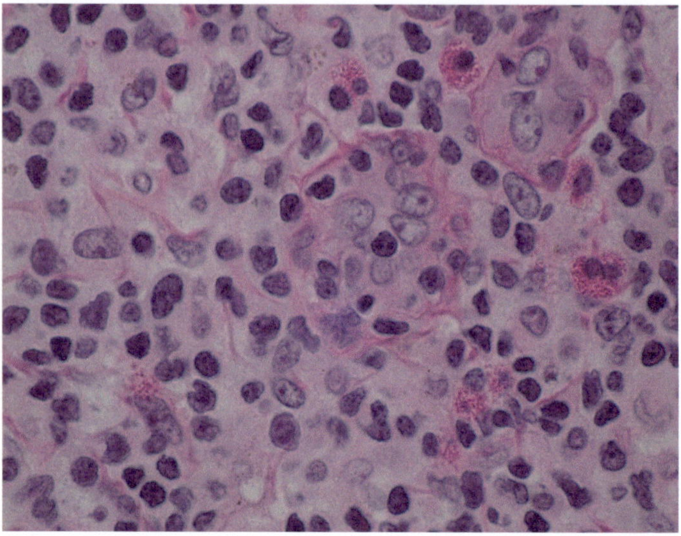

Mycosis fungoides. Infiltrate of T-cells with cerebriform nuclear irregularities and eosinophils

Sezary Syndrome

Snapshot

- Monotonous lymphocytes with cerebriform nuclei in the blood, skin, and lymph nodes in the setting of erythroderma and lymphadenopathy

Clinical Features

- Generalized lymphadenopathy
- Erythroderma: diffusely red and scaly skin
- Hyperkeratosis of the palms and soles

Morphologic Features

- Monotonous small to medium (sometimes large) cells with convoluted cerebriform nuclei
- Skin demonstrates a lichenoid infiltrate, +/– epidermotropism
- Lymph node architecture is effaced by a diffuse infiltrate of lymphocytes

Immunophenotype

- POSITIVE: CD3, CD4, CD2, CD5, PD1
- NEGATIVE: CD8, CD7, CD26

Genetics

- Clonal T-cell population detected in peripheral blood

Differential Diagnosis

- *Erythrodermic psoriasis* (parakeratosis with neutrophils; dilated vessels and edema in the dermis)
- *Mycosis fungoides* (does not have the triad of erythroderma, diffuse lymphadenopathy, and circulating Sezary cells)

Caveats and Pearls

Flow cytometric analysis should meet one of the following criteria:

1. Sezary cell count >1000/μL
2. CD4:CD8 ratio greater than 10
3. Abnormal CD4+ T-cell population that shows loss of CD7 or CD26

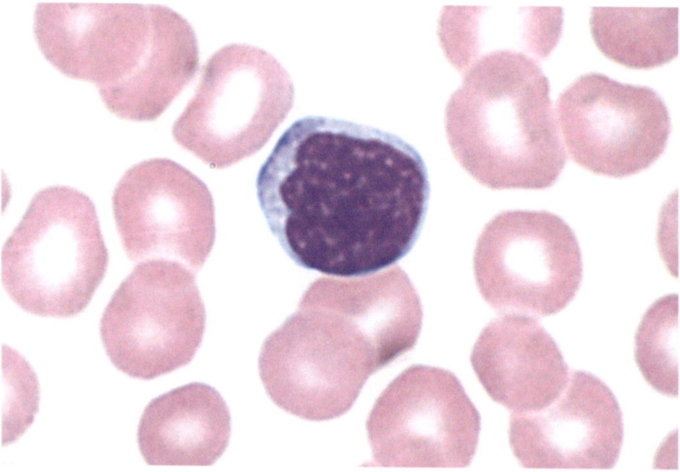

Sezary T-cell with convoluted nucleus (blood smear)

Primary Cutaneous CD30-Positive T-Cell Lymphoproliferative Disorders

Snapshot

- Dermal infiltrate of atypical CD30+ T-cells classified, using morphologic and clinical features, as lymphomatoid papulosis or primary cutaneous anaplastic large cell lymphoma
- Cases that cannot be distinguished may be referred to as borderline lesions

Lymphomatoid Papulosis (LyP)

Chronic benign skin disease with papules or nodules on the trunk and extremities that resolve after 1–3 months and may leave scarring

Six common histologic subtypes:

- *Type A*: Large atypical cells, which may include Reed-Sternberg (RS)-like cells and immunoblasts. Admixed reactive lymphocytes, neutrophils, and/or eosinophils
- *Type B*: Small- to medium-sized cells with irregular nuclear contours (sometimes cerebriform). Frequent epidermotropism
- *Type C*: Sheets of large cells without significant inflammation
- *Type D*: Small- to medium-sized cells with prominent epidermotropism
- *Type E*: Small- to medium-sized pleomorphic cells. Angioinvasion and necrosis
- *LyP with 6p25.3 rearrangement*: Small- to medium-sized epidermal infiltrate with nodules of large blast-like cells in the dermis

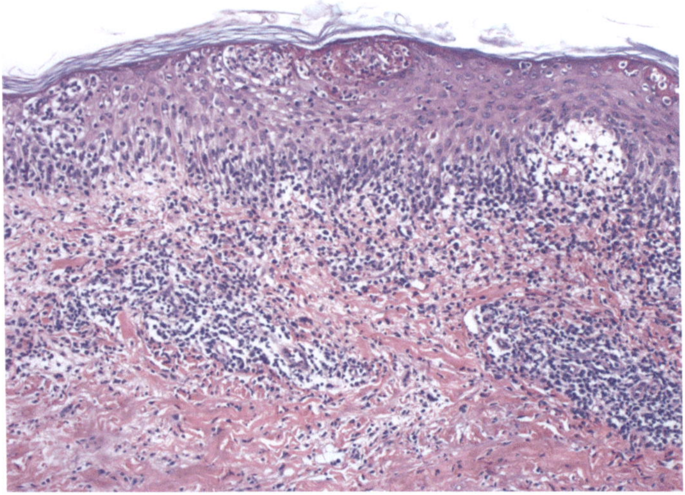

Lymphomatoid papulosis (LyP). Periadnexal infiltrate with epidermotropism (LyP type D)

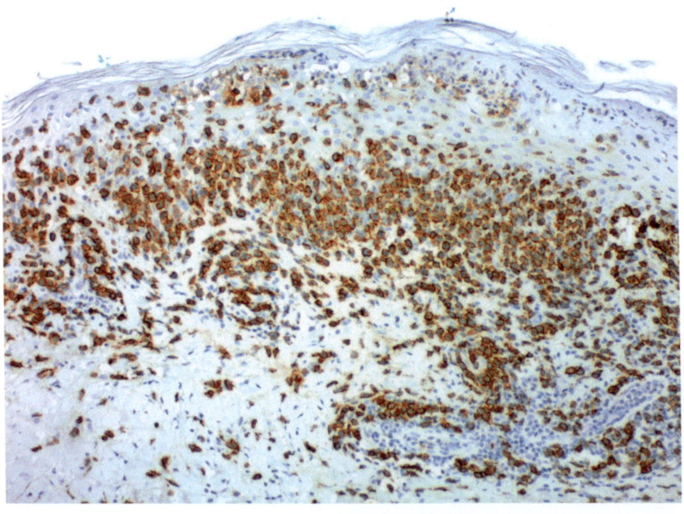

Lymphomatoid papulosis (LyP). CD30-positive infiltrate (LyP type D)

Primary Cutaneous Anaplastic Large Cell Lymphoma (PC-ALCL)

- Solitary or few skin nodules or tumors, involving the face, trunk, or extremities
- Dense dermal infiltrate of large anaplastic cells with ovoid or irregular nuclear contours, prominent eosinophilic nucleoli, and abundant cytoplasm
- May demonstrate epidermotropism and/or ulceration
- Occasionally spreads to local lymph nodes

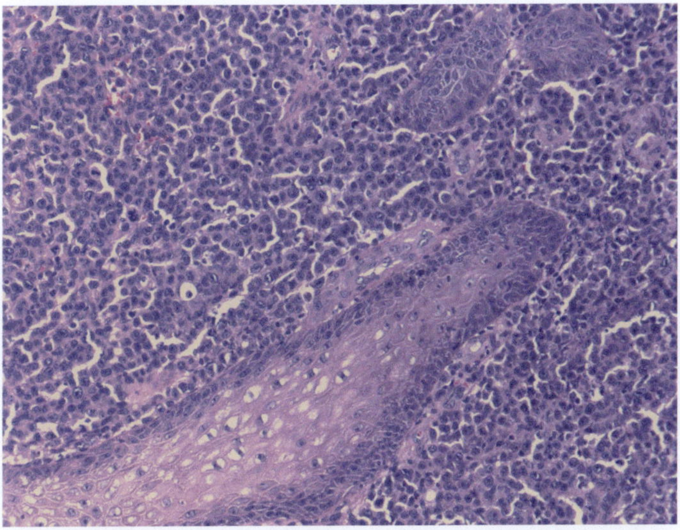

Primary cutaneous anaplastic T-cell lymphoma (PC-ALCL). Dense monotonous T-cell infiltrate in dermis

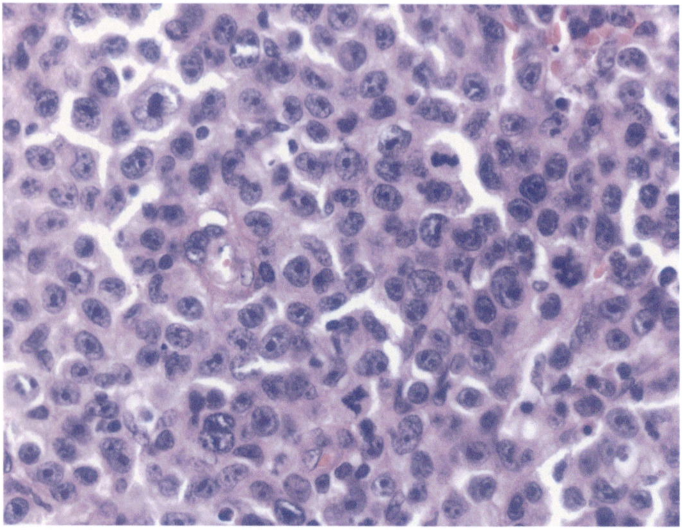

Primary cutaneous anaplastic T-cell lymphoma (PC-ALCL) with monomorphic infiltrate of medium-large cells with immunoblastic/plasmablastic features

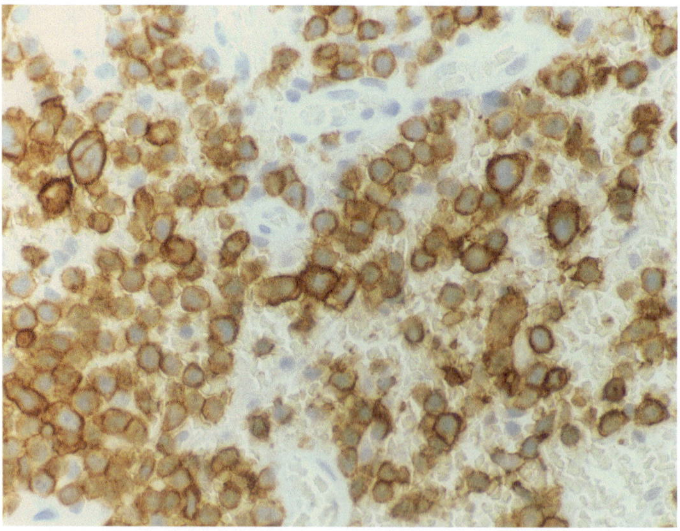

Primary cutaneous anaplastic T-cell lymphoma (PC-ALCL) with strong CD30 expression

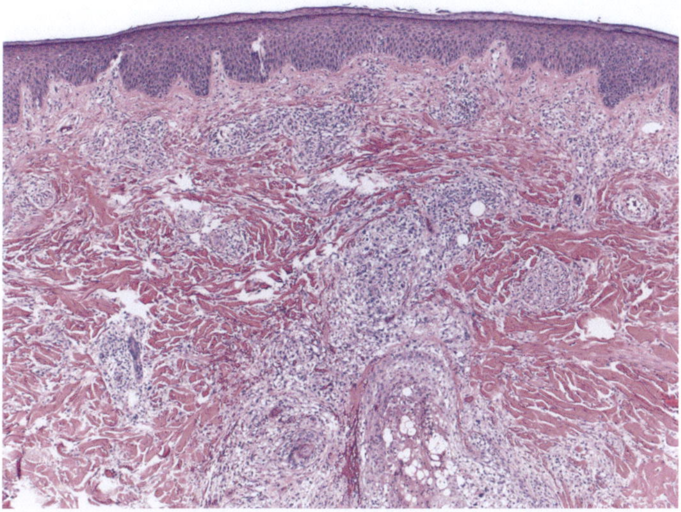

Primary cutaneous anaplastic T-cell lymphoma (PC-ALCL) with periadnexal infiltrate

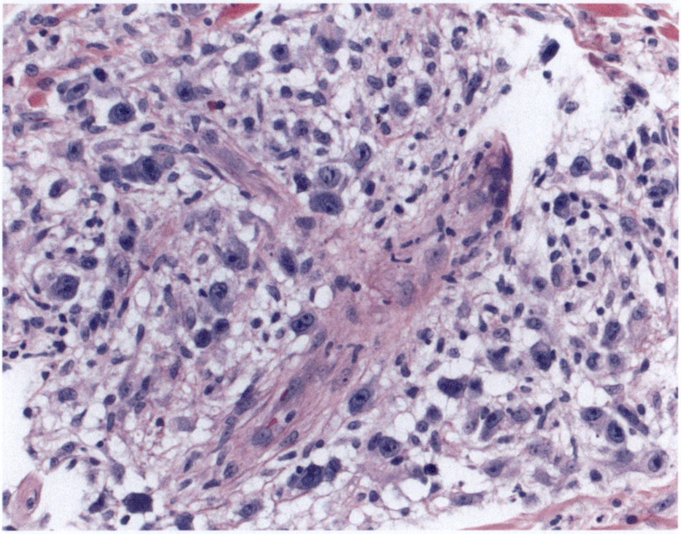

Primary cutaneous anaplastic T-cell lymphoma (PC-ALCL). Highly pleomorphic anaplastic large cells

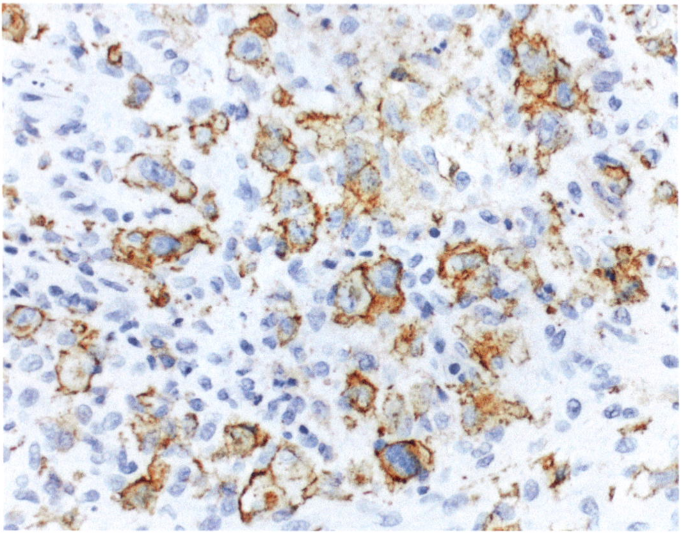

Primary cutaneous anaplastic T-cell lymphoma (PC-ALCL). Scattered CD30-positive anaplastic large cells

Immunophenotype (LyP and PC-ALCL)

- POSITIVE: CD30, CD4, CD25, CD45, TIA1, granzyme B, perforin
- Variable: CD3, CD2, CD5, CD7
- NEGATIVE: CD8, ALK, EMA, EBV (EBER), CD15, PAX5
- Note: CD4−/CD8+ phenotype occurs in LyP types D, E, and 6p25.3 rearrangement

Differential Diagnosis

- *Systemic anaplastic large cell lymphoma (ALK+ or ALK−)* (cells may be positive for ALK and/or EMA; no epidermotropism; involves distant lymph nodes and other extranodal tissues)
- *Mycosis fungoides* (usually retains CD3, CD2, and CD5; progression from scaly patches to plaques to tumors; no RS-like cells)
- *Classic Hodgkin lymphoma* (RS cells are PAX5 dim+ and CD45−; sometimes EBV (EBER)-positive)

Primary Cutaneous T-Cell Lymphomas, Rare Subtypes

Primary Cutaneous γδ (gamma-delta) T-Cell Lymphoma

- Frequent systemic manifestations, including B symptoms and hemophagocytic syndrome
- Localized (often extremities) or generalized, plaques or nodules
- Can involve any/all layers of skin; may involve mucosal tissue
- Medium to large cells; may show adipocyte rimming, necrosis, angioinvasion, and angiodestruction
- POSITIVE: CD3, CD2, CD7 (+/−), CD56, TIA1, granzyme B, perforin, TCRγ
- NEGATIVE: CD4, CD8 (−/+), CD5

Primary Cutaneous CD+ Aggressive Epidermotropic Cytotoxic T-Cell Lymphoma

- Plaques or nodules with prominent epidermotropism, ulceration, necrosis, and destruction of adnexal structures
- Wide range of cell size, with pleomorphic or blast-like nuclei
- POSITIVE: CD3, CD8, CD7, TIA1, granzyme B, perforin, βF1
- NEGATIVE: CD2(−/+), CD5 (−/+), CD30

Primary Cutaneous Acral CD8+ T-Cell Lymphoma

- Slow-growing, usually solitary nodule of acral sites
- Dense dermal infiltrate of monotonous medium-sized cells with irregular nuclei; may spread to subcutaneous tissue; no epidermal involvement
- POSITIVE: CD3, CD8, CD2+/−, CD5+/−, CD7+/−, CD68, TIA1, βF1
- NEGATIVE: CD4, CD56, granzyme B, perforin, CD30

Primary Cutaneous CD4+ Small/Medium T-Cell Lymphoproliferative Disorder

- Solitary plaque or nodule on the face, neck, or trunk
- Dense infiltrate of small- or medium-sized pleomorphic lymphocytes within the dermis and superficial subcutaneous tissue, sometimes with focal epidermotropism
- POSITIVE: CD3, CD4, CD2, CD5, CD7, βF1 (in some cases, TFH markers PD1, BCL6, and CXCL13)
- NEGATIVE: CD8, CD10, CD30

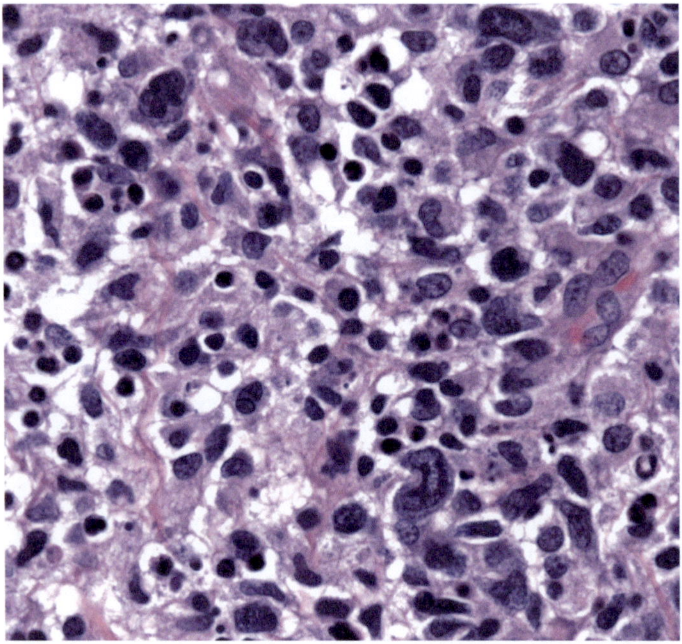

Primary cutaneous γδ (gamma-delta) T-cell lymphoma with cellular pleomorphism

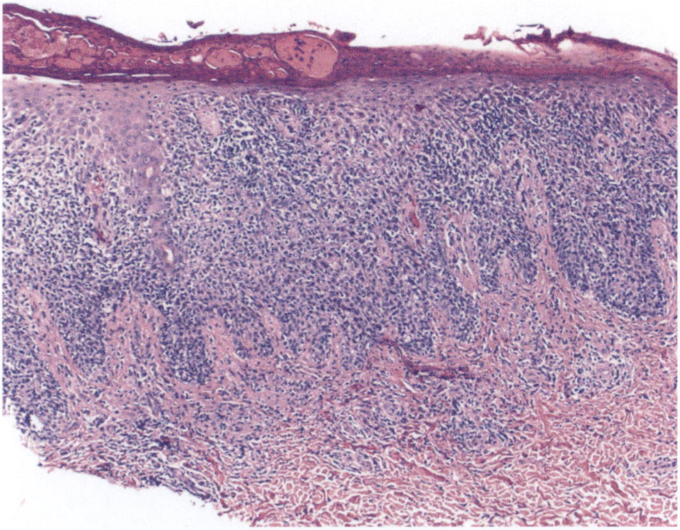

Primary cutaneous CD8 aggressive cytotoxic T-cell lymphoma. Dense lymphoid infiltrate in lamina propria

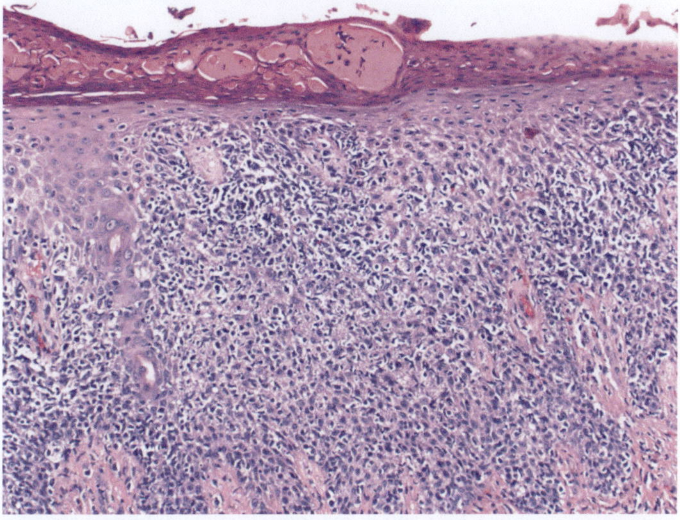

Primary cutaneous CD8 aggressive cytotoxic T-cell lymphoma. Atypical lamina propria infiltrate with epidermotropism

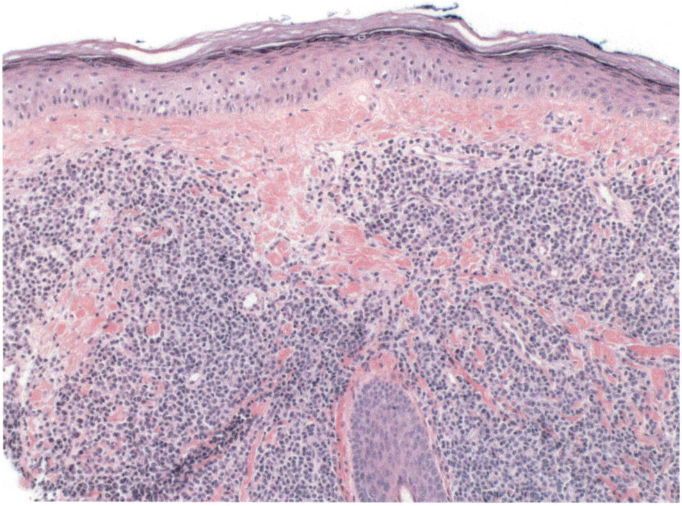

Primary cutaneous acral CD8+ T-cell lymphoma

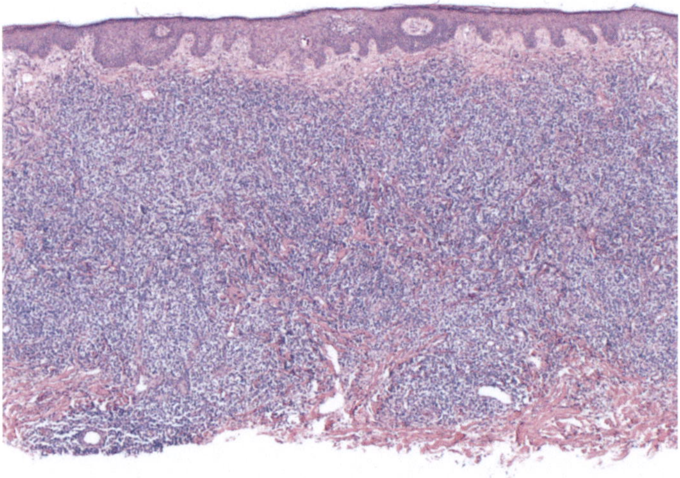

Primary cutaneous CD4+ small-/medium-T-cell lymphoproliferative disorder

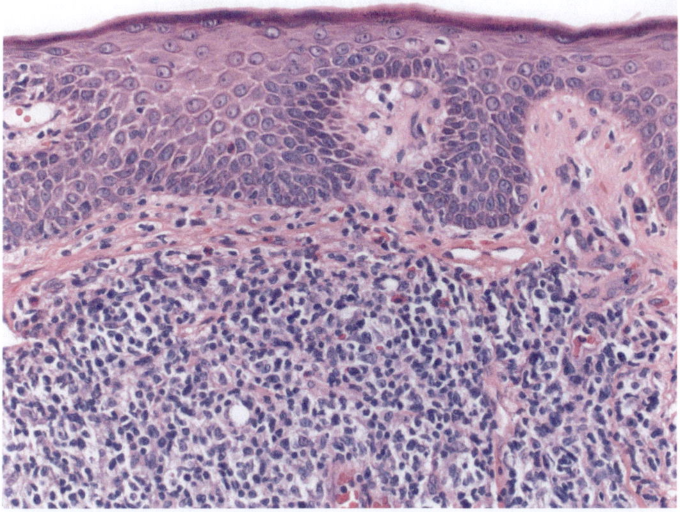

Primary cutaneous acral CD8+ T-cell lymphoma. Dense small lymphocytic infiltrate in dermis

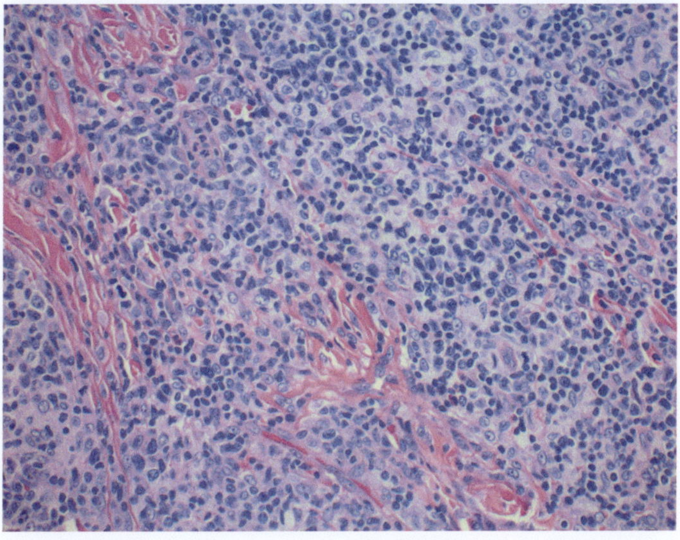

Primary cutaneous acral CD8+ T-cell lymphoma. Diffuse small lymphocytic infiltrate in dermis

Peripheral T-Cell Lymphoma, NOS (PTCL, NOS)

Snapshot

- Nodal and/or extranodal infiltrate of pleomorphic T-cells with a mixed inflammatory background that does not meet the criteria for other T-cell lymphomas

Clinical Features

- Lymphadenopathy and B symptoms
- May also involve bone marrow, liver, spleen, skin, GI tract, lung, or CNS
- Extranodal presentation can occur in skin or GI tract

Morphologic Features

- Variable due to heterogeneous nature of PTCL, NOS
- Diffuse, nodular, or other patterns of infiltration by often pleomorphic cells of variable size with irregular nuclear contours and distinct nucleoli
- Frequently has mitotic figures; may include Reed-Sternberg-like cells or clear cells
- Background of polymorphic inflammatory cells that can include small reactive lymphocytes, histiocytes, plasma cells, and eosinophils

Immunophenotype

- POSITIVE: CD3, CD2, CD4, beta F1, CD30 (+/−, subset)
- Usually negative: CD5, CD7, CD8
- Uncommonly may be CD4+/CD8+, CD4−/CD8+, or CD4−/CD8−

Genetics

- Complex karyotype

Variants

Lymphoepithelioid lymphoma (Lennert lymphoma)

- Lymph nodes with a diffuse or interfollicular infiltrate of predominantly small lymphocytes admixed with abundant reactive epithelioid histiocytes

T-Zone Lymphoma

- Interfollicular T-cell proliferation surrounding preserved B-cell follicles

Differential Diagnosis

- *Reactive T-cell hyperplasia*: No cytologic atypia. No architectural alteration or extranodal extension
- *Follicular T-cell lymphoma (aka nodal peripheral T-cell lymphoma with TFH phenotype)*: Expresses 2+ TFH markers: CD10, PD1/CD279, CXCL13, BCL6, ICOS, SAP, CXCR5
- *Other specified T-cell lymphomas*: Exclude other T-cell lymphomas by morphologic and immunophenotypic criteria

Caveats and Pearls

- PTCL, NOS is a diagnosis of exclusion

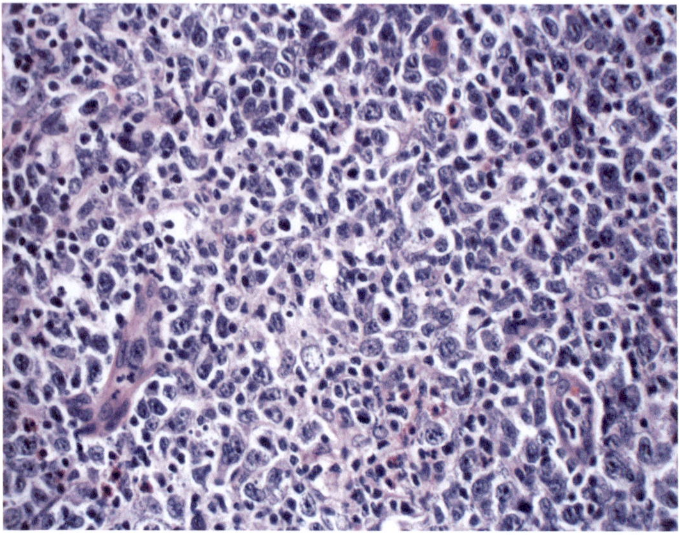

Peripheral T-cell lymphoma (PTCL), NOS, with diffuse infiltrate of medium-large pleomorphic immunoblast-like cells and admixed small lymphocytes

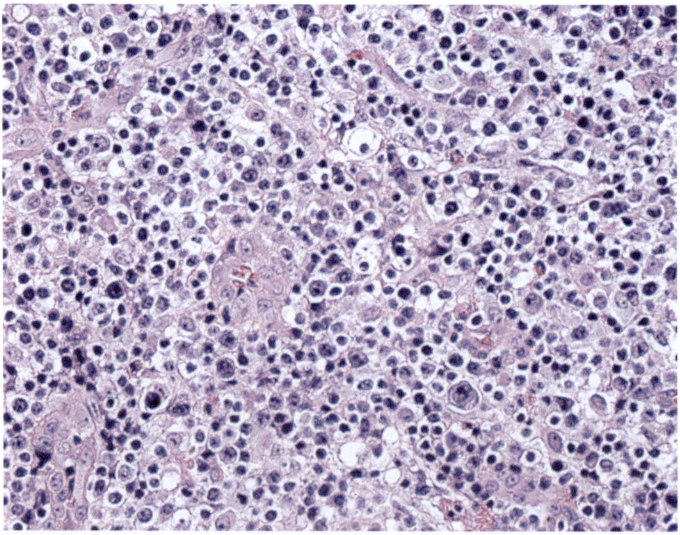

Peripheral T-cell lymphoma (PTCL), NOS, with clear cell morphology

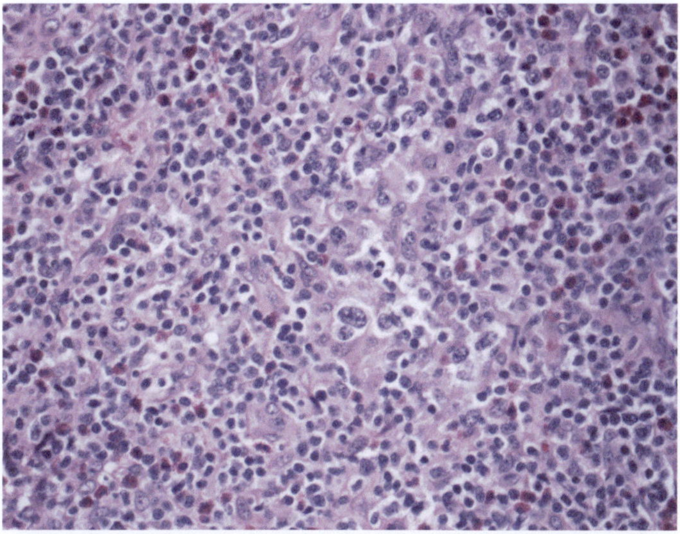

Peripheral T-cell lymphoma (PTCL), NOS, with a mixed infiltrate of small T-cells, plasma cells, eosinophils, and increased vascularity

Angioimmunoblastic T-Cell Lymphoma (AITL)

Snapshot

- Proliferation of small- to medium-sized T-cells with clear cytoplasm in a polymorphic inflammatory background with large EBV+ B-cells and prominent arborizing vessels

Clinical Features

- Systemic disease involving lymph nodes, liver, spleen, skin, and bone marrow
- May have arthritis, effusions, polyclonal hypergammaglobulinemia, immunodeficiency

Morphology

- Partial effacement of lymph nodes (sinuses spared)
- Polymorphic inflammatory infiltrate with atypical small- to medium-sized lymphocytes with round to irregular nuclei, clear cytoplasm
- Scattered large EBV-positive B-cells
- Proliferation of arborizing high endothelial venules
- Extranodal extension

Immunophenotype

- Neoplastic CD4-positive T-cells with intact pan-T-cell markers and at least two TFH markers: CD10, PD1, CXCL3, BCL6, ICOS, SAP, and CCR5
- Expanded and distorted follicular dendritic cell networks highlighted by CD21 and/or CD23

Genetics

- Trisomy 3, trisomy 5, +X
- *TET2, IDH2, DNMT3A, RHOA*, and CD28 mutations; *ITK-SYK* and *CTLA4*-CD28 fusions

- Clonal immunoglobulin gene rearrangement may be detected if numerous EBV+ B-cells are present

Related Entity/Variant

Follicular T-Cell Lymphoma (Nodal Peripheral T-Cell Lymphoma with TFH Phenotype)

- Nodular proliferation of intermediate-sized T-cells with a moderate amount of pale cytoplasm that express TFH markers. Lacks the polymorphous background and angio-proliferation of AITL

Differential Diagnosis

- *Atypical T-zone hyperplasia* (intact lymph node architecture; lymphocytes lack clear cytoplasm; no arborizing vessels)
- *Peripheral T-cell lymphoma, NOS* (weak/absent CD5 and/or CD7; no expansion of follicular dendritic cell networks)
- *Classic Hodgkin lymphoma* (typical HRS cell immunophenotype: CD30+, CD15+/−, PAX5 dim+, CD20−/+, CD45−

Caveats and Pearls

- May develop a concomitant B-cell lymphoma

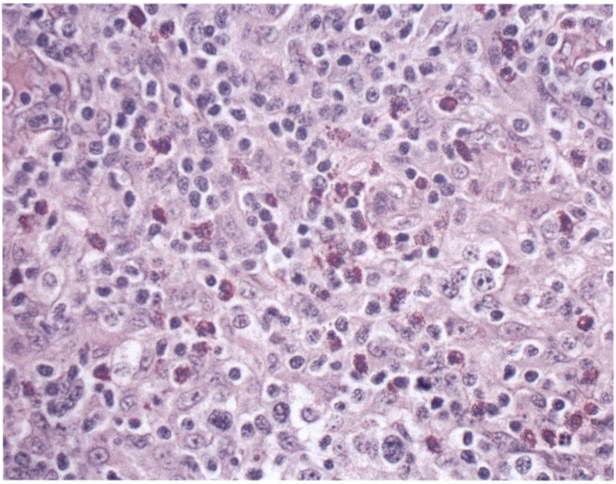

Angioimmunoblastic T-cell lymphoma (AITL) with scattered large cells, increased vascularity, and eosinophilia

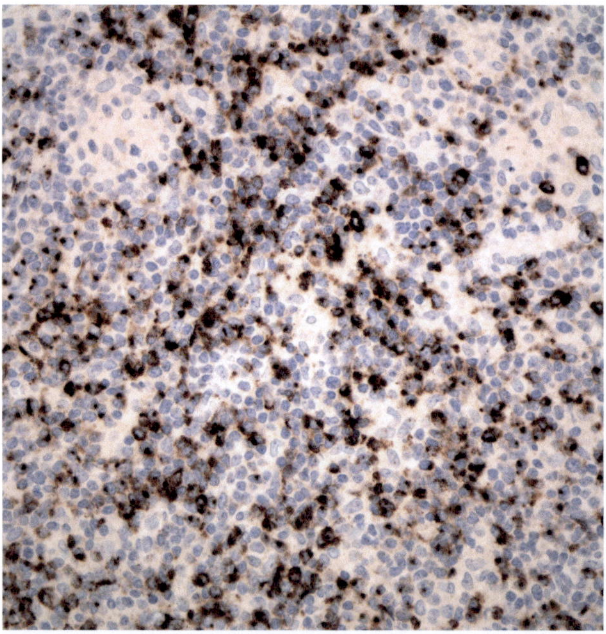

Angioimmunoblastic T-cell lymphoma (AITL). Numerous CXCL13-positive T-cells

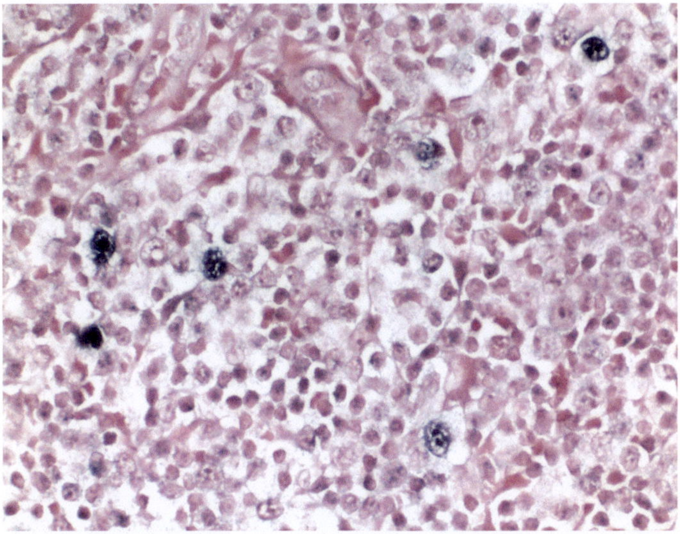

Angioimmunoblastic T-cell lymphoma (AITL). Scattered large EBV-positive B cells (EBER ISH)

Anaplastic Large Cell Lymphoma, ALK Positive (ALCL, ALK+)

Snapshot

- Infiltrate of pleomorphic cells of variable size, with prominent nucleoli, abundant cytoplasm, and co-expression of CD30 and ALK

Clinical Features

- Occurs predominantly in children and young adults with B symptoms
- Involves lymph nodes and extranodal tissues (skin, bone, lungs, liver, soft tissue)

Morphology

Several distinctive histologic patterns:

- *Common Pattern.* Large pleomorphic cells (including multinucleated) with prominent nucleoli and abundant cytoplasm
- *Lymphohistiocytic Pattern.* Tumor cells admixed with numerous histiocytes
- *Small-Cell Pattern.* Small- to medium-sized cells; can have "fried-egg" appearance
- *Hodgkin-Like Pattern.* RS-like cells with fibrotic bands
- Other patterns include sarcomatoid, signet ring-like, and composite (more than one type)
- All patterns show hallmark cells, large cells with eccentric horseshoe- or kidney-shaped nuclei

Immunophenotype

- POSITIVE: ALK, CD30, CD25, EMA (+/–)
- VARIABLY POSITIVE: CD2, CD4, TIA1, granzyme B, perforin (less commonly CD3, CD5, CD7, CD8)
- NEGATIVE: CD45 (–/+), EBV (EBER), CD15 (rarely +), PAX5

Genetics

- Rearrangements of ALK, most commonly t(2;5); usually clonal TCR-positive

Differential Diagnosis

- *Other ALCLs (ALK-negative; primary cutaneous; breast-implant-associated)* (ALK-*negative*; different epidemiology or locations)
- *ALK-positive large B-cell lymphoma* (CD30-negative; positive for CD138, kappa or lambda, and often IgA)
- *Reactive lymphadenopathy/lymphadenitis with prominent histiocytes* (CD30 and ALK fail to demonstrate neoplastic cells)
- *Peripheral T-cell lymphoma, NOS* (small- or medium-sized neoplastic cells may weakly express CD30/ALK, but no large cells that strongly express CD30/ALK or exhibit hallmark cell morphology)
- *Classic Hodgkin lymphoma* (RS cells are ALK-*negative* and PAX5 dim+)

Caveats and Pearls

- Some cases have null-cell phenotype, lacking expression of all T-cell markers

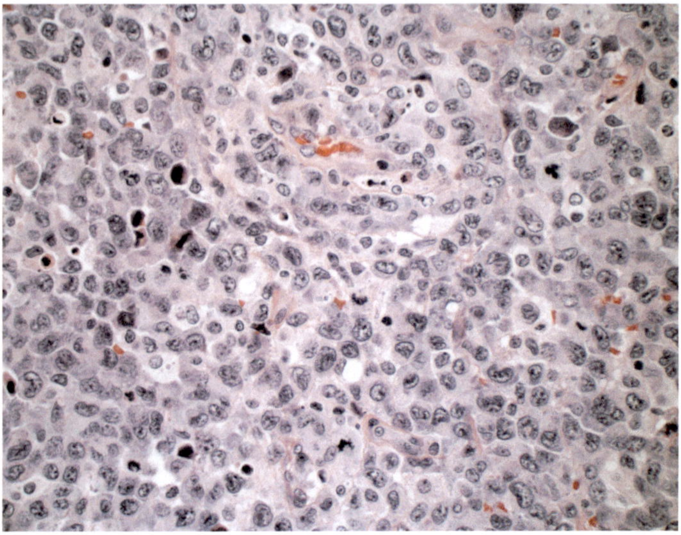

Anaplastic large cell lymphoma, ALK-positive (ALCL, ALK+). Sheets of large cells with abundant cytoplasm, including few Hallmark cells

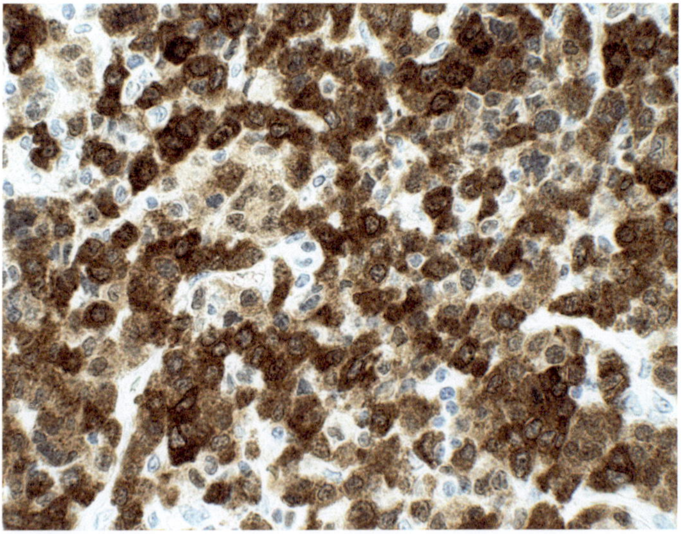

Anaplastic large cell lymphoma, ALK-positive (ALCL, ALK+). Strong ALK1 positivity

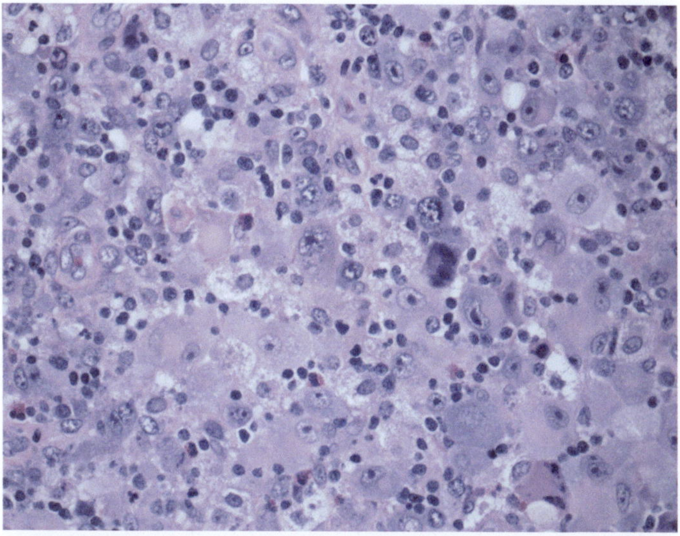

Anaplastic large cell lymphoma, ALK-positive (ALCL, ALK+). Large cells with prominent nucleoli and abundant amphophilic cytoplasm and admixed multinucleated giant cells

Anaplastic Large Cell Lymphoma, ALK Negative (ALCL, ALK−)

Snapshot

- Large pleomorphic CD30+ T-cells in sheet-like or intrasinusoidal distribution

Clinical Features

- Occurs predominantly in middle-aged adults with frequent B symptoms
- Involves lymph nodes and, less often, extranodal tissues (skin, bone, soft tissue)

Morphology

- Cohesive aggregates or sheets of large pleomorphic cells with distinct-prominent nucleoli and abundant cytoplasm
- Multinucleated cells, and hallmark cells with eccentric horseshoe- or kidney-shaped nuclei often seen
- Intrasinusoidal pattern seen in lymph nodes
- Sclerosis and increased eosinophils may be seen

Immunophenotype

- POSITIVE: CD30, EMA (+/−)
- Most express one or more T-cell markers: CD3, CD2, CD4, CD43, TIA1, granzyme B, perforin > CD5, CD7, CD8
- NEGATIVE: ALK, EBV (EBER), CD15, PAX5 (rarely +)

Genetics

- *JAK/STAT3* mutations; *DUSP22* and *TP63* rearrangements; usually clonal TCR-positive

Differential Diagnosis

- *ALCL, ALK+* (smaller, less polymorphic ALK+ tumor cells)
- *Primary cutaneous ALCL; breast-implant-associated ALCL* (site-specific neoplasms)
- *Peripheral T-cell lymphoma, NOS* (small- to medium-sized T-cells, lack of intrasinusoidal growth pattern)

- *Classic Hodgkin lymphoma* (*PAX5*-dim+ RS cells, nodular sclerosis, eosinophilia)

Caveats and Pearls

- Some cases with null-cell phenotype, lacking expression of all T-cell markers

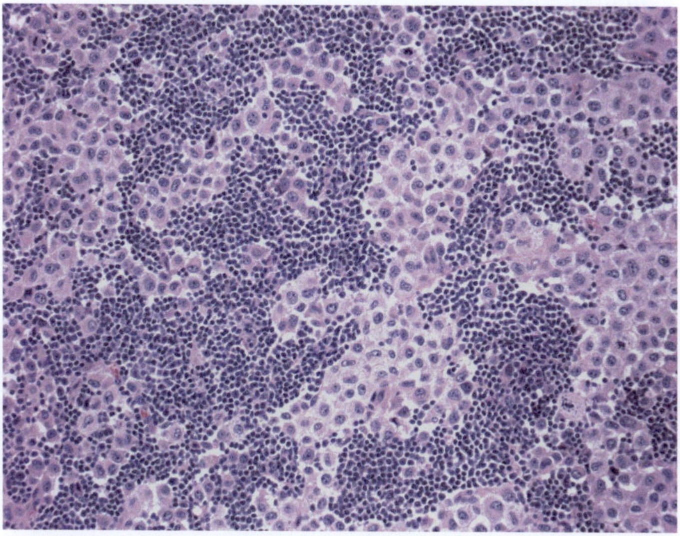

Anaplastic large cell lymphoma, ALK-negative (ALCL, ALK-). Prominent sinusoidal infiltrate of large cells with abundant cytoplasm (lymph node)

Breast Implant-Associated Anaplastic Large Cell Lymphoma (iALCL)

Snapshot

- Peri-implant effusion and/or capsule with large, pleomorphic CD30+ lymphocytes

Clinical Features

- Occurs rarely, on average a decade after breast implantation
- Involves peri-implant effusion and fibrous capsule surrounding the implant
- Uncommonly spreads to adjacent tissues or axillary lymph nodes

Morphology

- Large, pleomorphic cells with distinct nucleoli and abundant cytoplasm
- Usually includes hallmark cells with horseshoe- or kidney-shaped nuclei
- Tumor may have admixed eosinophils, sometimes with RS-like cells

Immunophenotype

- POSITIVE: CD30, EMA (+/−)
- Most express one or more T-cell markers:

  CD3, CD2, CD4, CD43, TIA1, granzyme B, perforin > CD5, CD7, CD8

- NEGATIVE: CD45 (−/+), ALK, EBV (EBER), CD15 (rarely +), PAX5

Differential Diagnosis

- *ALCL, ALK-; peripheral T-cell lymphoma, NOS* (systemic involvement or non-breast primary)
- *Classic Hodgkin lymphoma* (systemic involvement or non-breast primary; PAX5 dim+ RS cells)

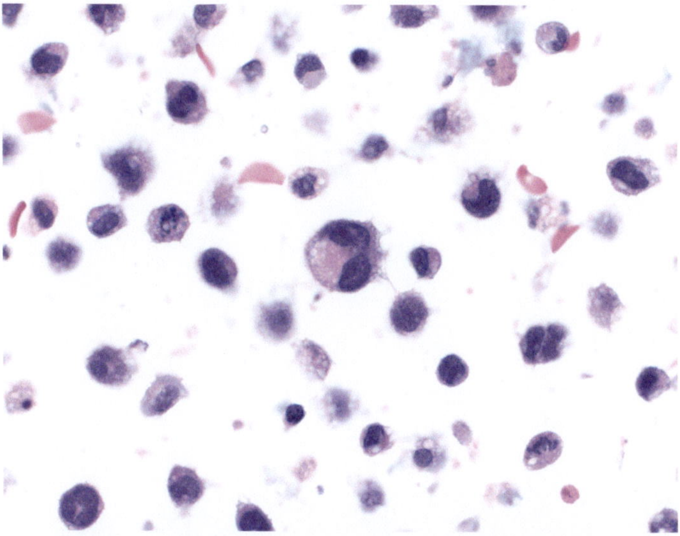

Breast implant-associated anaplastic large cell lymphoma (iALCL). Seroma with pleomorphic large cells, including multinucleated forms

Chapter 12
Hodgkin Lymphomas

Nodular Lymphocyte Predominant Hodgkin Lymphoma

Snapshot

- Lymph node effacement by a vaguely nodular small lymphocytic infiltrate with scattered large mononuclear B-cells with multilobate nuclei (lymphocyte predominant [LP] cells)

Clinical Features

- Most common in adult males who present with asymptomatic peripheral lymphadenopathy (cervical, axillary, inguinal)

Morphology

- Nodal effacement by large nodular lymphoid aggregates composed primarily of small B-cells with scattered large B-cells with irregular multilobate nuclei (often resembling popcorn kernels); histiocytes may be numerous; rare diffuse pattern with background of small T-cells
- Variant morphologic patterns include cases with irregular serpiginous nodules, numerous extranodular LP cells, nodular or diffuse T-cell-rich background, and diffuse B-cell-rich background

© Springer Nature Switzerland AG 2019

S. D. Hudnall et al., *Pocket Guide to Diagnostic Hematopathology*, https://doi.org/10.1007/978-3-030-10630-0_12

- May progress to diffuse large B-cell lymphoma or undergo T-cell/histiocyte-rich large B-cell lymphoma-like transformation

Immunophenotype
- POSITIVE (LP CELLS): CD20, CD45, PAX5, OCT2, J chain, CD75, EMA (+/−)
- NEGATIVE (LP CELLS): CD3, CD15, MUM1, fascin, EBER, ALK, CD75, CD30 (−/wk+)
- CD57+/PD1+ T-cell rosettes surround LP cells
- Dual CD4/CD8-positive T-cells often detected by flow cytometry

Genetics
- Clonal IgH rearrangement sometimes detected by IgH PCR

Differential Diagnosis
- *T-cell/histiocyte-rich large B-cell lymphoma* (diffuse infiltrate with scattered large abnormal centroblastic B-cells in a background of numerous CD8+ cytotoxic T-cells, absent small B-cells, and few CD57+ T-cells)
- Rare *diffuse variant of NLPHL* particularly difficult to distinguish from T-cell/histiocyte-rich large B-cell lymphoma

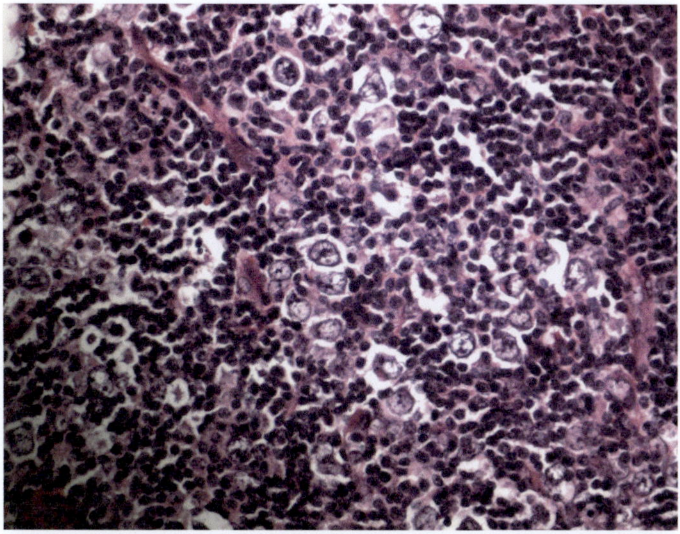

Nodular lymphocyte predominant (LP) Hodgkin lymphoma. Large LP (popcorn) cells scattered among small lymphocytes

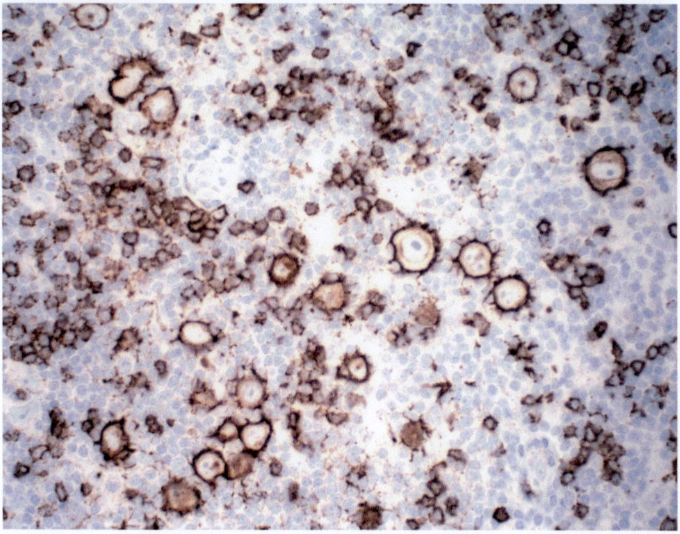

Nodular lymphocyte predominant (LP) Hodgkin lymphoma. CD20-positive large LP cells and small B-cells

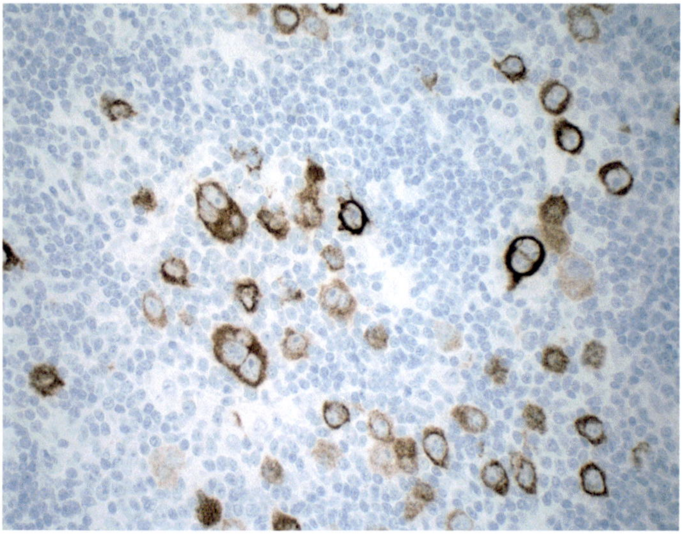

Nodular lymphocyte predominant (LP) Hodgkin lymphoma. EMA-positive large LP cells

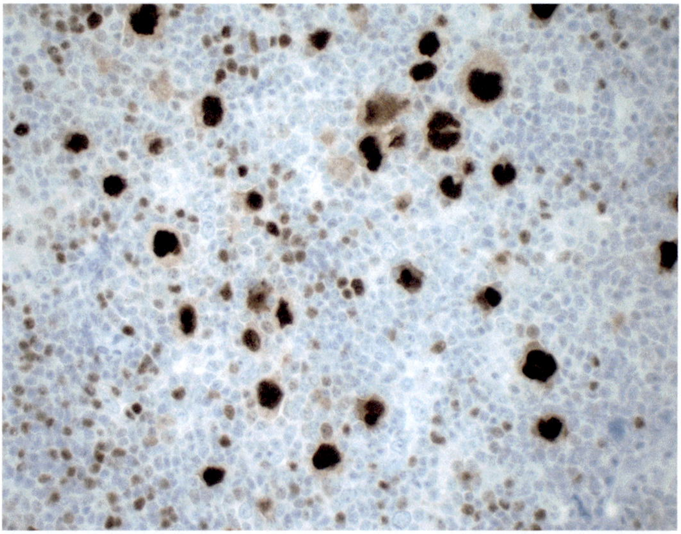

Nodular lymphocyte predominant (LP) Hodgkin lymphoma, with OCT2 positive large LP cells

Classic Hodgkin Lymphoma, Nodular Sclerosis Variant

Snapshot

- Nodular lymphocytic infiltrate with broad bands of collagenous fibrosis and scattered large mononuclear lacunar cells

Clinical Features

- Most common in adolescents and young adults with mediastinal mass or cervical lymphadenopathy; sometimes accompanied by fever, night sweats, and weight loss

Morphology

- Nodal effacement by a nodular infiltrate of inflammatory cells (small T-cells, histiocytes, eosinophils), admixed with large mononuclear cells often within lacuna, mummified cells, and relatively few large multinucleated cells with prominent inclusion-like nucleoli (classic Reed-Sternberg [RS] cells); in some cases, necrosis may be prominent and large cells may form sheets or aggregates (*syncytial variant*)
- *Fibrohistiocytic variant* with predominance of fibroblasts and histiocytes within nodules
- Marrow involvement seen as irregular lymphoid aggregates composed of small T-cells, histiocytes, scattered eosinophils, and, usually rare, large Hodgkin cells

Immunophenotype

- POSITIVE: CD30, CD15 (+/−), PAX5 (wk), MUM1, fascin, EBER (−/+)
- NEGATIVE: CD3, CD20 (−/+), CD45, ALK, EMA, CD75, J chain

Genetics

- Clonal IgH rearrangement may be detected

Differential Diagnosis

- *Anaplastic large cell lymphoma* (CD3+, ALK+, TIA1+, CD2+)
- *Diffuse large B-cell lymphoma* (CD20+, CD79a+, *OCT2*+, PAX5 ++, CD45+)
- *Nodular lymphocyte predominant Hodgkin lymphoma* (CD20+, PAX5++, OCT2+, EMA+)

Caveats and Pearls

- In staging marrow biopsies with suspicious but non-diagnostic lymphoid aggregates, levels may be useful in detecting rare classic Hodgkin cells

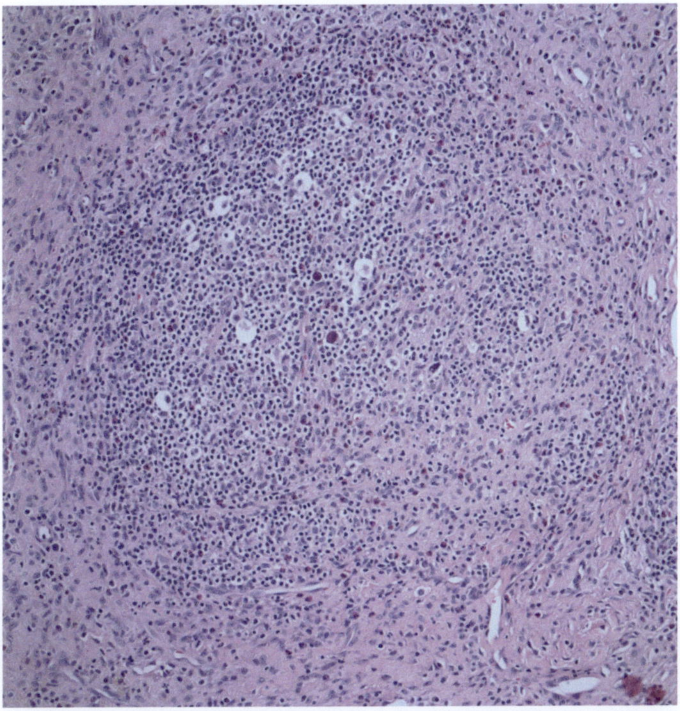

Classic Hodgkin lymphoma, nodular sclerosis variant. Lymphoid nodule surrounded by fibrosis (note lacunar cells and few mummified cells)

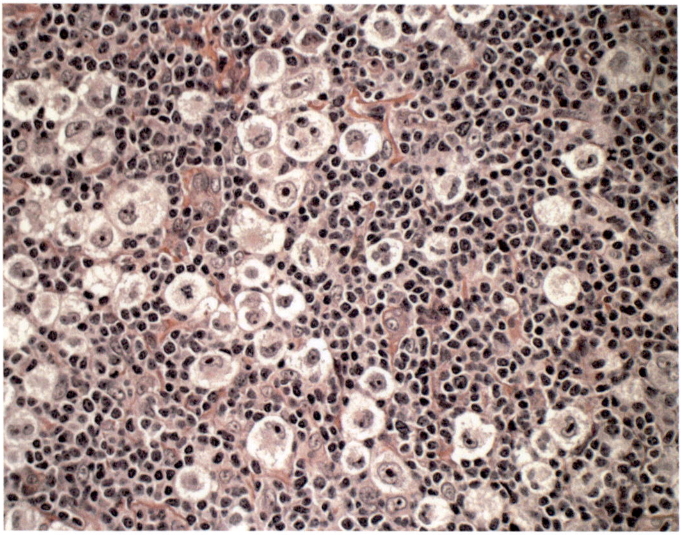

Classic Hodgkin lymphoma, nodular sclerosis variant. Numerous lacunar cells

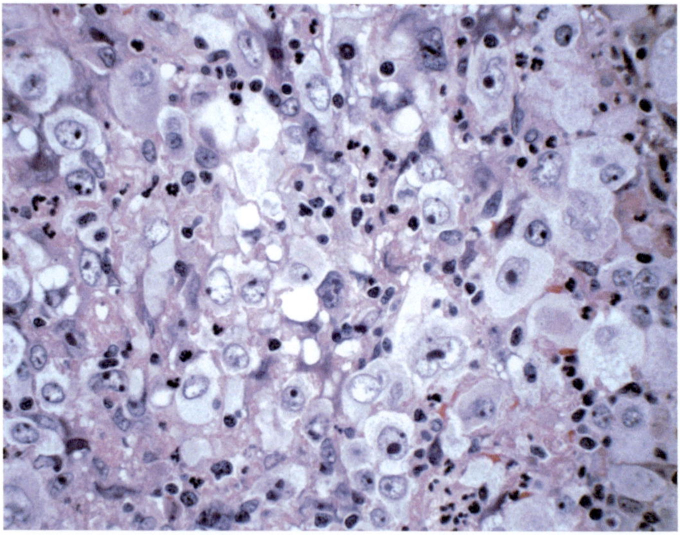

Classic Hodgkin lymphoma, nodular sclerosis variant. Sheets of lacunar cells (syncytial variant)

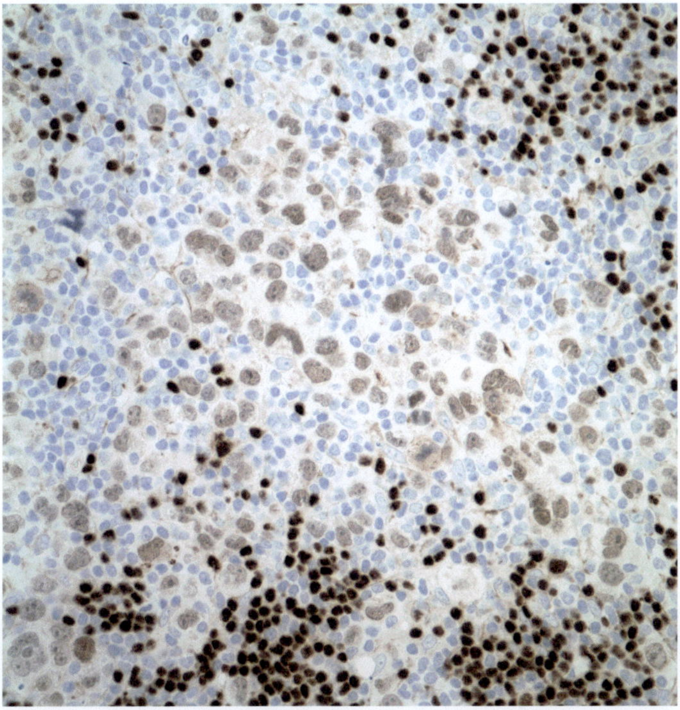

Classic Hodgkin lymphoma, nodular sclerosis variant. Weak *PAX5*-positive Reed-Sternberg cells

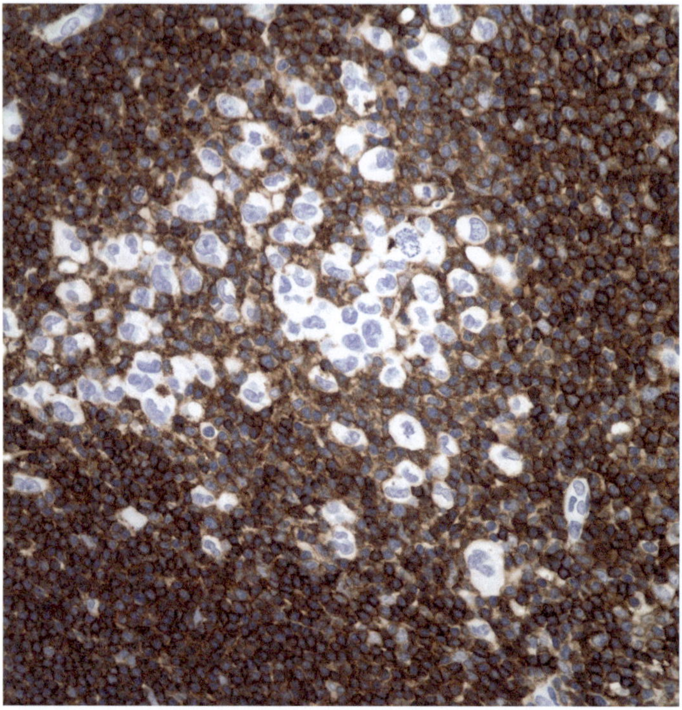

Classic Hodgkin lymphoma, nodular sclerosis variant. CD45-negative Reed-Sternberg cells

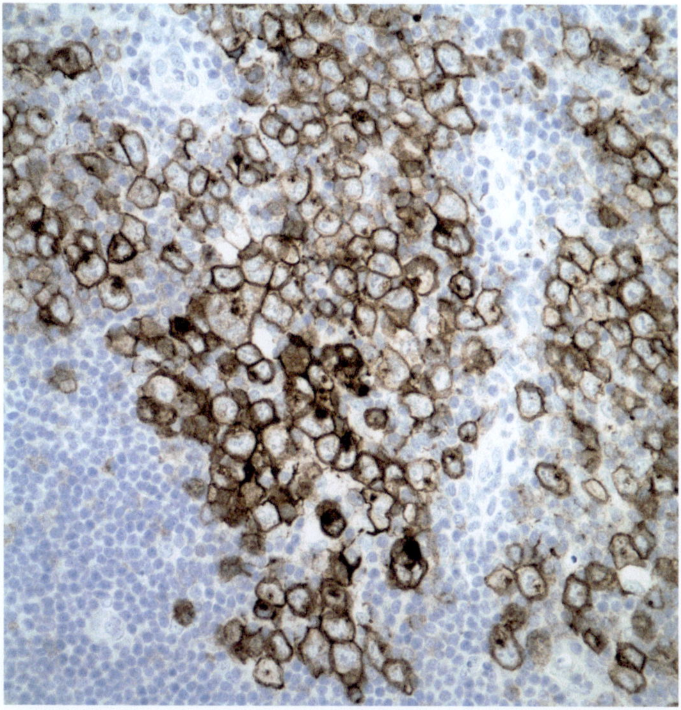

Classic Hodgkin lymphoma, nodular sclerosis variant. CD30-positive Reed-Sternberg cells

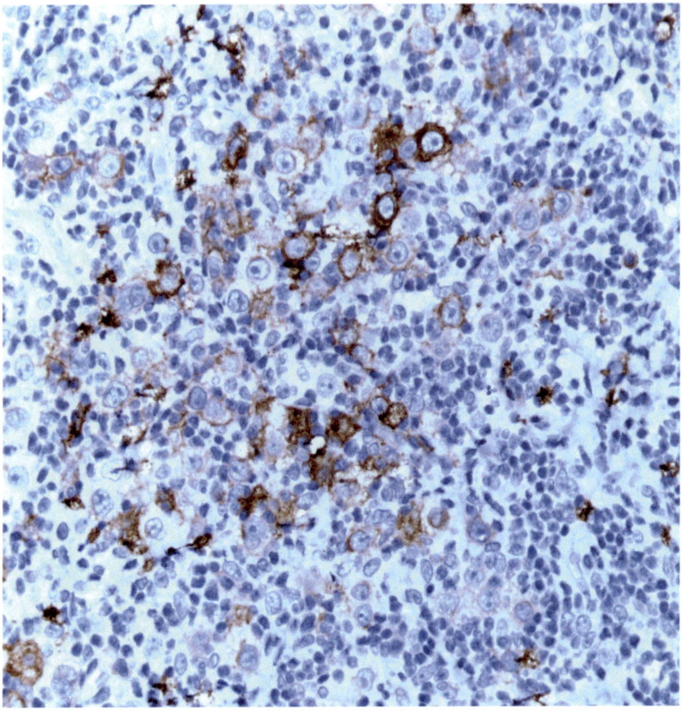

Classic Hodgkin lymphoma, nodular sclerosis variant. CD15-positive Reed-Sternberg cells

Classic Hodgkin Lymphoma, Lymphocyte-Rich Variant

Snapshot

- Large classic RS cells scattered within expanded B-cell-rich mantle zones

Clinical Features

- Most common in middle-aged adult males with asymptomatic peripheral lymphadenopathy

Morphology

- Scattered classic RS cells within irregular nodular expansions of B-cell-rich mantle zones, often with associated small regressed germinal centers; few-absent neutrophils and eosinophils
- Rare diffuse pattern with T-cell predominance and scattered histiocytes

RS Cell Immunophenotype

- POSITIVE: CD30, CD15 (+/−), PAX5 (weak), MUM1, fascin, EBV (+/−)
- NEGATIVE: CD3, CD20 (−/+), CD45, EMA, ALK, OCT2, CD75, J chain

Differential Diagnosis

- *Nodular lymphocyte predominant Hodgkin lymphoma* (LP popcorn cells; CD20+, PAX5+ [strong], OCT2+, EMA+/− EBV- phenotype)
- *T-cell/histiocyte-rich large B-cell lymphoma* (large CD20+ PAX5+ [strong], OCT2+ EBV- B-cells)

Caveats and Pearls

- Distinction from NLPHL dependent upon demonstration of classic RS cell phenotype
- Presence of fibrotic bands favors nodular sclerosis variant
- Numerous eosinophils or neutrophils favor mixed-cellularity variant

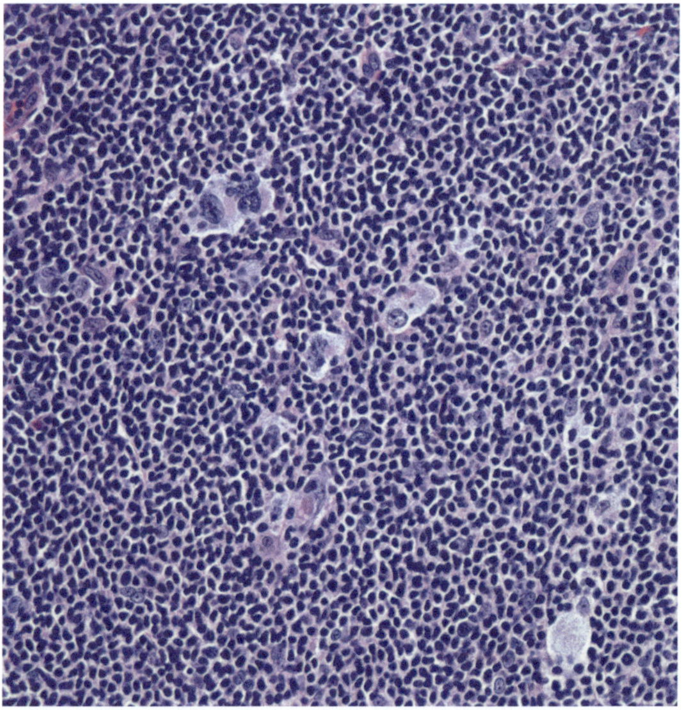

Classic Hodgkin lymphoma, lymphocyte-rich variant. Few scattered large Reed-Sternberg cells in lymphocyte-rich background

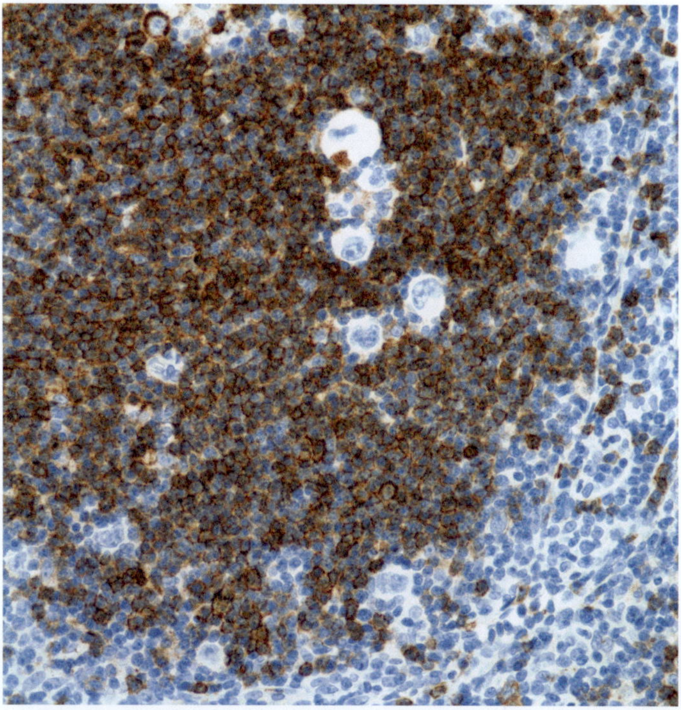

Classic Hodgkin lymphoma, lymphocyte-rich variant. Large CD20-negative Reed-Sternberg cells amid numerous small CD20+ B-cells

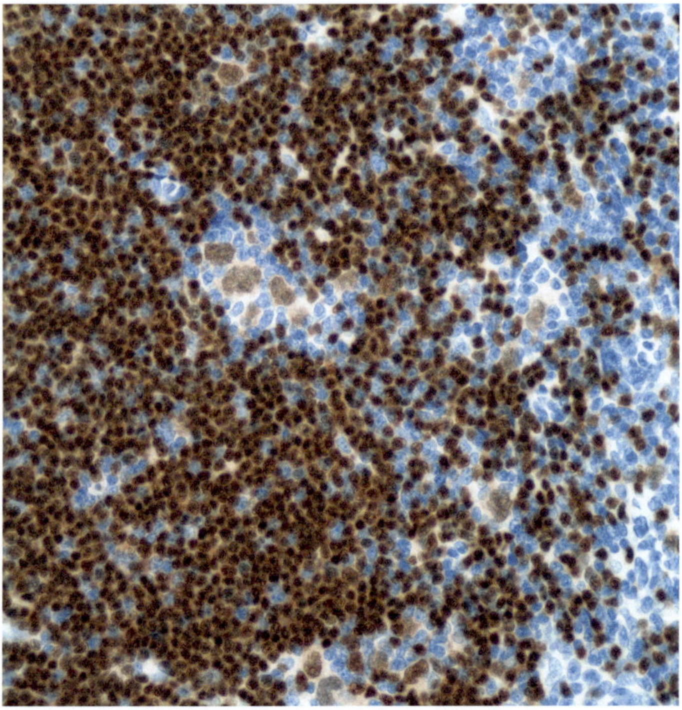

Classic Hodgkin lymphoma, lymphocyte-rich variant. Weak PAX5-positive Reed-Sternberg cells surrounded by numerous small strong PAX5-positive B-cells

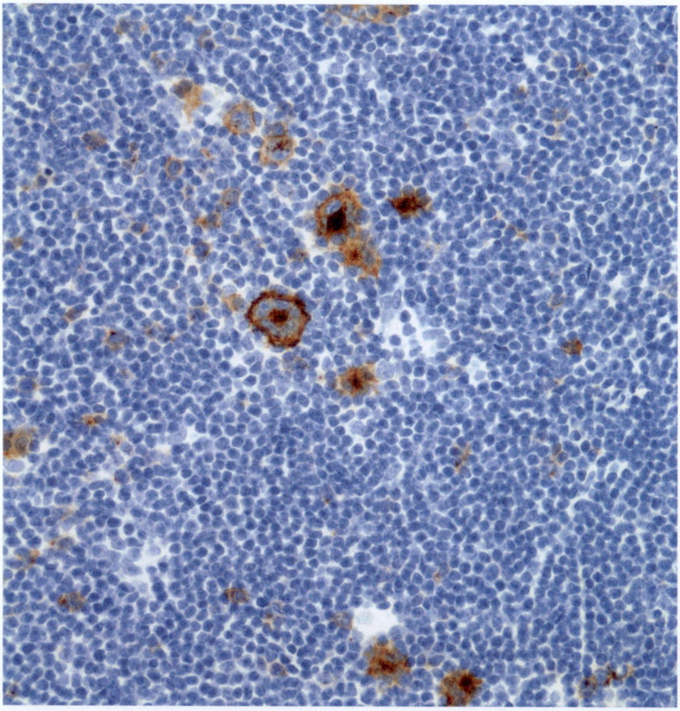

Classic Hodgkin lymphoma, lymphocyte-rich variant. Scattered CD30-positive Reed-Sternberg cells

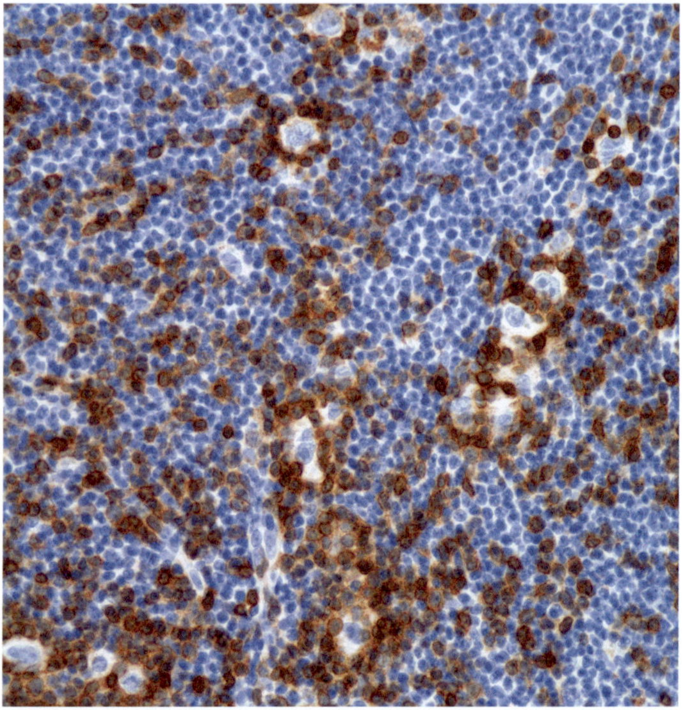

Classic Hodgkin lymphoma, lymphocyte-rich variant. CD3-positive T-cell rosettes surrounding Reed-Sternberg cells

Classic Hodgkin Lymphoma, Mixed-Cellularity Variant

Snapshot

- Diffuse polymorphic infiltrate of small lymphocytes, histiocytes, eosinophils, granulocytes, classic RS cells (including mononuclear variants)

Clinical Features

- Most common in middle-aged adults who present with lymphadenopathy often accompanied by fever, night sweats, and weight loss

Morphology

- Effacement by a diffuse infiltrate of inflammatory cells (small T-cells, histiocytes, eosinophils, granulocytes), admixed with large cells with prominent inclusion-like nucleoli (classic Hodgkin RS cells)
- While classic RS cells are binucleated, multinucleated, and mononuclear, degenerated (mummified) forms may also be present
- Some cases may be accompanied by prominent granulomatous inflammation
- Marrow involvement seen as irregular lymphoid aggregates composed of small T-cells, histiocytes, scattered eosinophils, and (usually rare) large Hodgkin cells

Immunophenotype (RS Cells)

- POSITIVE: CD30, CD15 (+/−), PAX5 (weak), MUM1, fascin, EBER (+/−)
- NEGATIVE: CD3, CD20 (−/+), CD45, CD75, ALK, EMA, OCT2, J chain

Genetics

- Clonal IGH rearrangement may be detected

Differential Diagnosis

- Anaplastic large cell lymphoma (CD3+, ALK+, TIA1+, CD2+)
- Diffuse large B-cell lymphoma (CD20+, CD79a+, OCT2+, PAX5 ++, CD45+)
- Nodular lymphocyte predominant Hodgkin lymphoma (CD20+, PAX5++, OCT2+, EMA+)

Caveats and Pearls

- In contrast to nodular sclerosis variant, mediastinal involvement is uncommon
- Cases with broad bands of collagenous fibrosis are best classified as nodular sclerosis variant
- In cases with interfollicular pattern or prominent granulomatous inflammation, classic RS cells may be difficult to identify on H&E (need IHC)

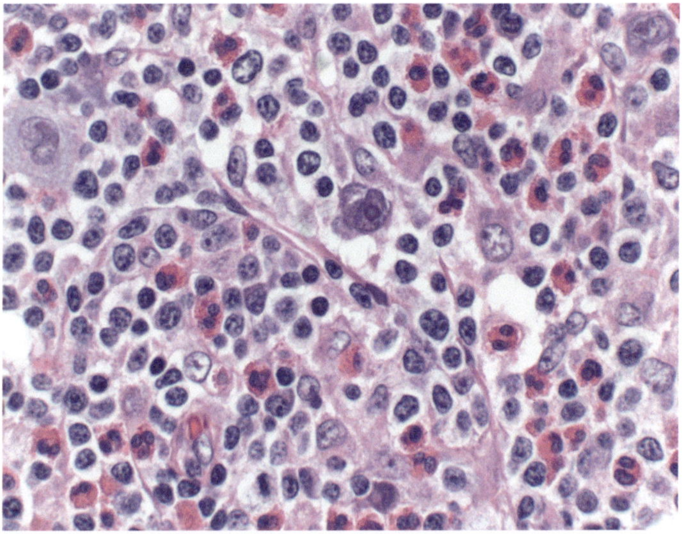

Classic Hodgkin lymphoma, mixed-cellularity variant. Mixed inflammatory infiltrate

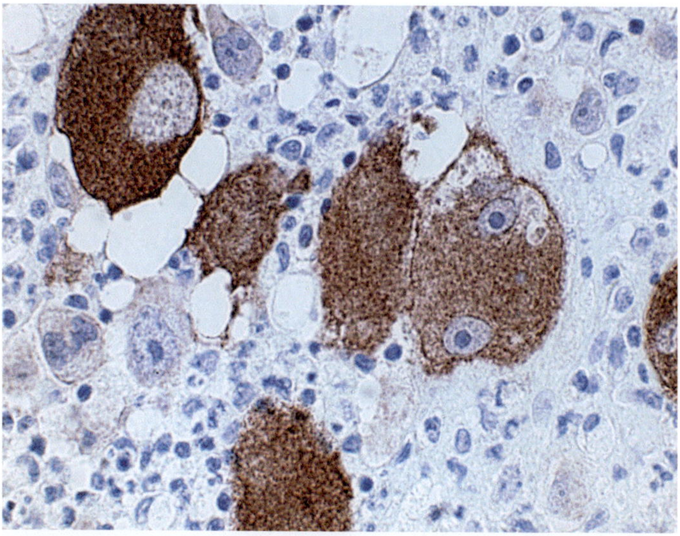

Classic Hodgkin lymphoma, mixed-cellularity variant. Fascin-positive Reed-Sternberg cells

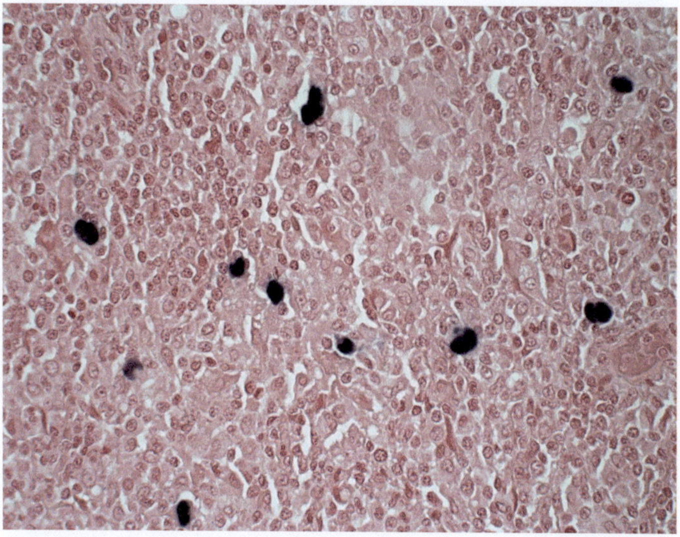

Classic Hodgkin lymphoma, mixed-cellularity variant. EBER ISH-positive Reed-Sternberg cells

Classic Hodgkin Lymphoma, Lymphocyte-Depleted Variant

Snapshot

- Lymph node effacement by a diffuse infiltrate of large pleomorphic RS cells often within a fibrotic lymphocyte-depleted background

Clinical Features

- More common in developing countries and in association with HIV infection
- Abdominal and retroperitoneal lymphadenopathy with marrow involvement
- Often accompanied by fever, night sweats, and weight loss

Morphology

- Nodal effacement by a diffuse infiltrate of large often pleomorphic cells with multilobate nuclei within a fibrotic lymphocyte-poor background

Patterns

- *Reticular.* Predominance of pleomorphic RS cells
- *Diffuse Fibrosis.* Prominent fibroblastic infiltrate with scattered pleomorphic RS cells

Immunophenotype

- POSITIVE (large cells): CD30, CD15 (+/−), PAX5 (weak), MUM1, fascin, EBER (+/−)
- NEGATIVE (large cells): CD3, CD20 (−/+), OCT2, CD45, ALK, EMA, CD75, J chain

Genetics

- Clonal IGH rearrangement may be detected

Differential Diagnosis

- *Anaplastic large cell lymphoma* (CD3+, ALK+, TIA1+, CD2+)
- *Diffuse large B-cell lymphoma* (CD20+, CD79a+, OCT2+, PAX5 [strong], CD45+)
- *Nodular lymphocyte predominant Hodgkin lymphoma* (CD20+, PAX5 [strong], OCT2+, BOB1+, EMA+)
- *Nodular sclerosis Hodgkin lymphoma* (sclerosing fibrosis with nodular aggregates of tumor, lacunar RS cells)

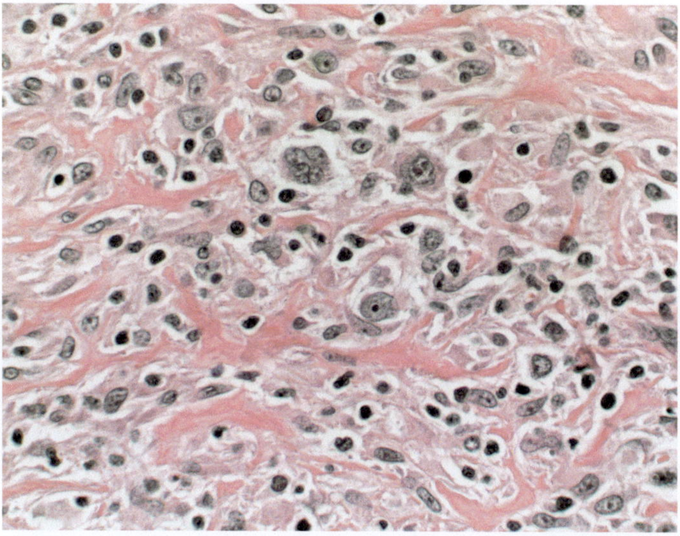

Classic Hodgkin lymphoma, lymphocyte-depleted diffuse fibrosis variant

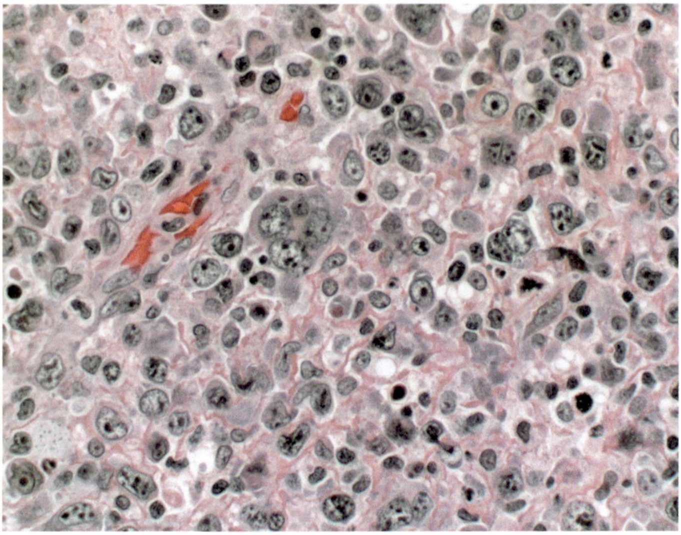

Classic Hodgkin lymphoma, lymphocyte-depleted reticular variant

Chapter 13
Histiocytic and Dendritic Cell Neoplasms

Histiocytic Sarcoma

Snapshot

- A diffuse infiltrate of large, often pleomorphic, histiocytic cells with a variable admixture of inflammatory cells

Clinical Features

- Adults with localized mass most often in intestine, skin, or soft tissue
- Fever and weight loss are common. Rarely systemic
- Rare cases seen with mediastinal germ cell tumor

Morphology

- Diffuse infiltrate of large cells with oval nuclei, indistinct nucleoli, and abundant eosinophilic cytoplasm. Multinucleated cells are common

Immunophenotype

- POSITIVE: CD68, CD163, lysozyme, +/− CD45
- NEGATIVE: CD3, CD20, MPO, CD1a, CD21, HMB45, cytokeratin

© Springer Nature Switzerland AG 2019

S. D. Hudnall et al., *Pocket Guide to Diagnostic Hematopathology*, https://doi.org/10.1007/978-3-030-10630-0_13

Genetics

- Isochromosome 12p in cases with mediastinal germ cell tumor

Differential Diagnosis

- *Diffuse large B-cell lymphoma* (CD20-positive)
- *Melanoma* (HMB-45, melan-A-positive)
- *Carcinoma* (cytokeratin, EMA-positive)

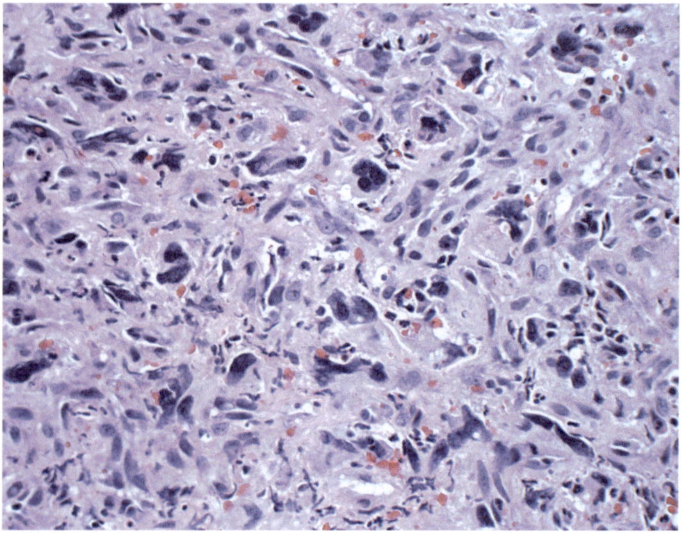

Histiocytic sarcoma—low power

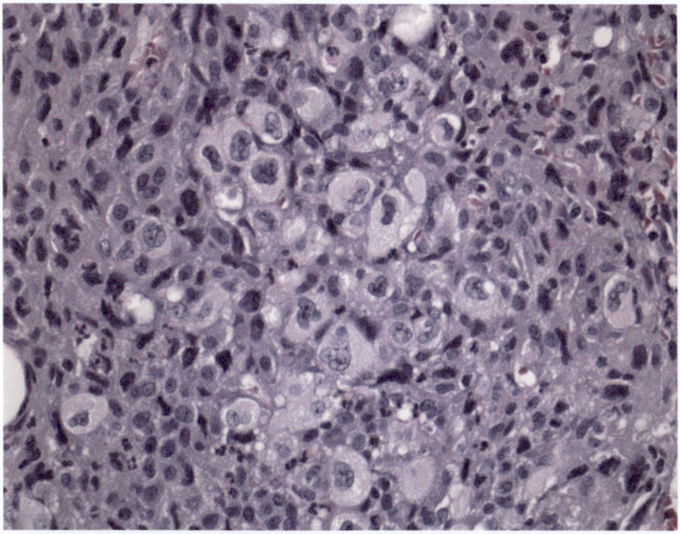

Histiocytic sarcoma—high power

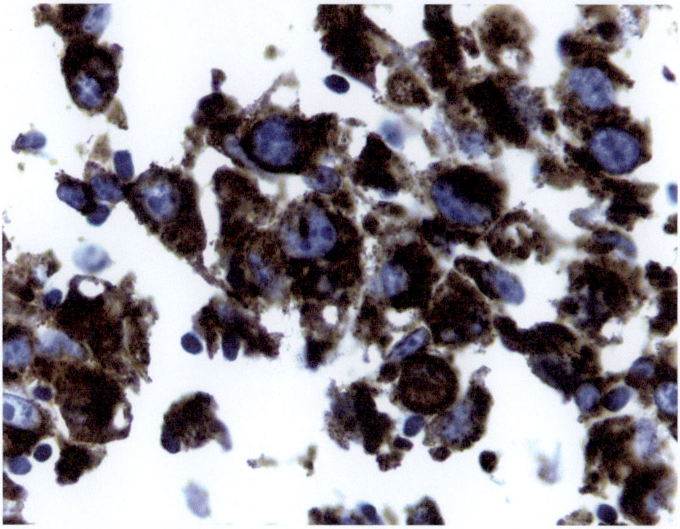

Histiocytic sarcoma. CD68-positive large cells

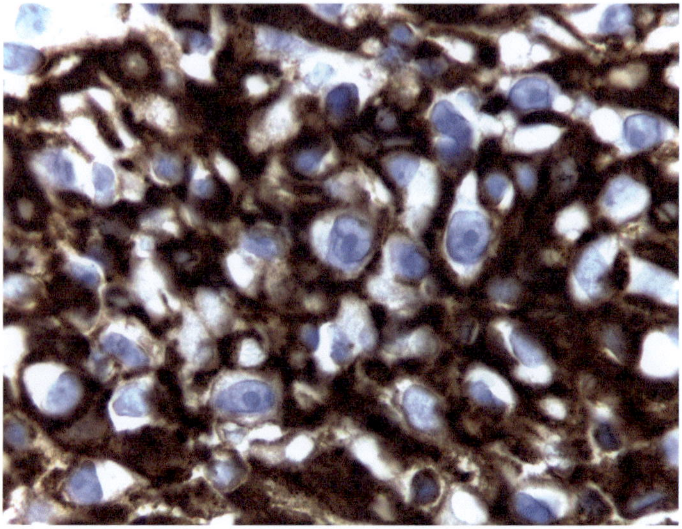

Histiocytic sarcoma. CD163-positive large cells

Tumors Derived from Langerhans Cells

- *Langerhans Cell Histiocytosis (LCH)*
- *Langerhans Cell Sarcoma (LCS)*

Snapshot

- Infiltrate of medium to large histiocytic cells with highly characteristic longitudinal nuclear grooves, sometimes accompanied by eosinophils

Clinical Features

Langerhans Cell Histiocytosis

- Children (white males most common) with lytic bone lesions and soft tissue tumors. Infants with systemic disease (fever, hepatosplenomegaly, skin and bone lesions, and cytopenia). Adult smokers with primary nonclonal pulmonary disease

Langerhans Cell Sarcoma

- Adults with skin, bone, or multisystem involvement

Morphology

Langerhans Cell Histiocytosis

- Nonpleomorphic infiltrate of medium to large ovoid cells with elongated grooved nuclei, indistinct nucleoli, and abundant cytoplasm. Variable admixture of eosinophils (with microabscess), histiocytes, lymphocytes, and granulocytes

Langerhans Cell Sarcoma

- Pleomorphic infiltrate of medium-large cells with prominent nucleoli, +/− grooved nuclei, rare eosinophils, high mitotic rate

Immunophenotype

- POSITIVE: S100, CD1a, langerin, CD68
- NEGATIVE: CD3, CD20, MPO, lysozyme, CD21, CD23, CD30

Differential Diagnosis

- *Histiocytic sarcoma* (positive for lysozyme)
- *Myeloid sarcoma* (positive for lysozyme, MPO)
- *Non-Hodgkin lymphoma* (positive for CD3, CD20, or CD30)
- *Non-Langerhans dendritic cell tumors* (negative for langerin)

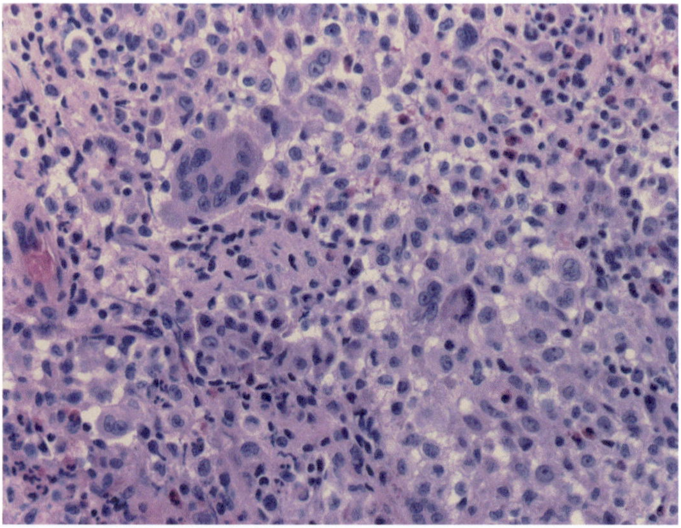

Langerhans cell histiocytosis. Scattered multinucleated giant cells

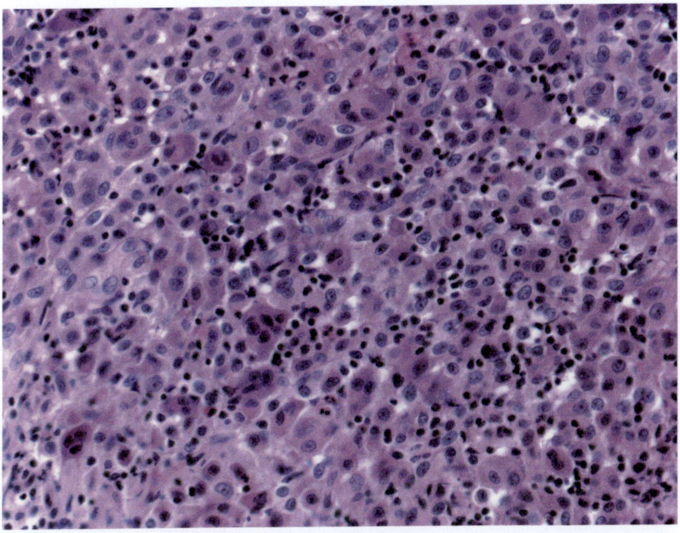

Langerhans cell histiocytosis. Admixed small lymphocytes

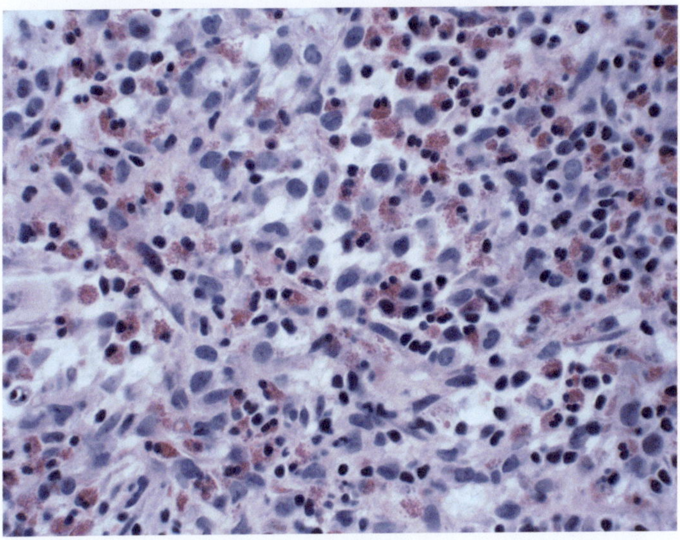

Langerhans cell histiocytosis. Eosinophilia

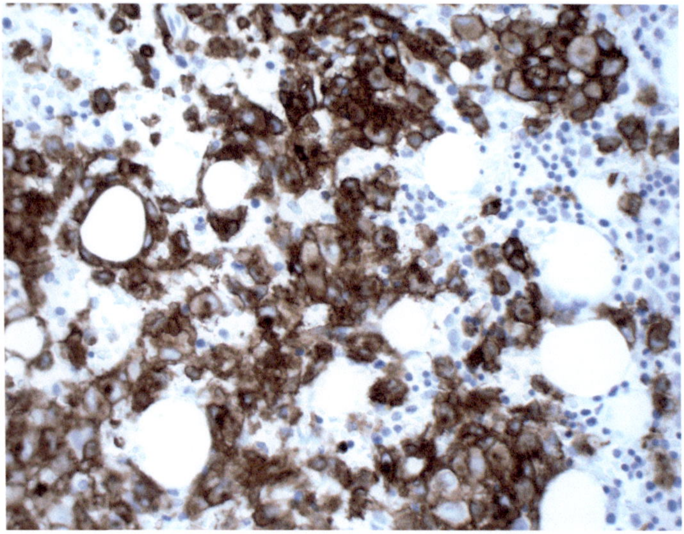

Langerhans cell histiocytosis. CD1a-positive Langerhans cells

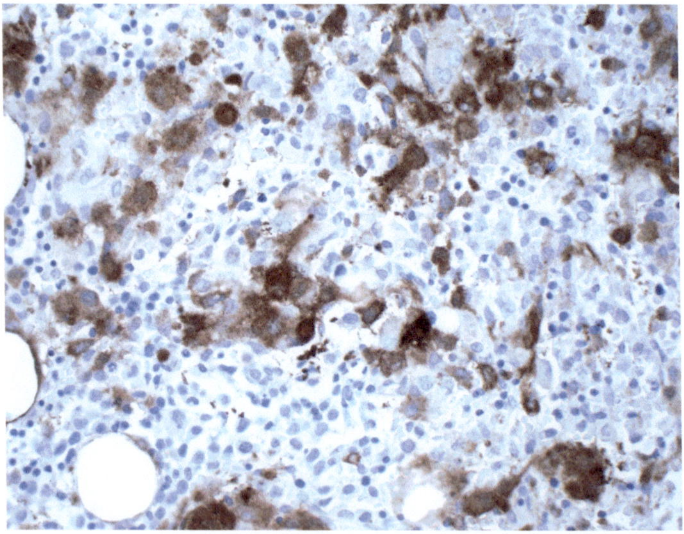

Langerhans cell histiocytosis. S100-positive Langerhans cells

Rare Dendritic Cell Tumors

Fibroblastic Reticular Cell Tumor (S100−)

- Mass in lymph node, spleen, or soft tissue
- Plump spindle cells in whorls
- VARIABLY POSITIVE: SMA, desmin, cytokeratin, CD68
- NEGATIVE: S-100, langerin, CD21

Indeterminate Dendritic Cell Tumor (S100+ CD1a+)

- Skin lesions (papules, nodules, plaques) most common presentation
- Langerhans-like cellular morphology with nuclear grooves
- No Birbeck granules; eosinophils typically not prominent
- POSITIVE: S-100, CD1a
- NEGATIVE: CD21, langerin

Interdigitating Dendritic Cell Sarcoma (S100+ CD1a−)

- Asymptomatic lymph node mass; skin and soft tissue involvement may be seen
- Fascicles of plump spindle/ovoid cells or sheets of round cells with admixed T-cells
- POSITIVE: S-100, fascin, CD68 (+/−), lysozyme (+/−)
- NEGATIVE: CD1a, langerin, CD21, CD23, CD35

Differential Diagnosis

- *Follicular dendritic cell sarcoma* (CD21, CD23, and/or CD35-positive)
- *Langerhans cell histiocytosis* (admixed eosinophils, langerin-positive)

Follicular Dendritic Cell Sarcoma

Snapshot

- Sheets or fascicles of large plump spindle/ovoid cells with scattered small lymphocytes, often with binucleated or multinucleated cells

Clinical Features

- Adults with asymptomatic lymphadenopathy (cervical nodes most common), often with extranodal involvement
- Associated with hyaline-vascular Castleman disease

Immunophenotype

- POSITIVE: CD21, CD23, CD35, clusterin
- VARIABLY POSITIVE: for S100, CD68
- NEGATIVE: lysozyme, MPO, CD1a

Differential Diagnosis

- *Langerhans cell histiocytosis* (numerous eosinophils, CD1a-positive)

Variant

Inflammatory Pseudotumor-Like Follicular/Fibroblastic Dendritic Cell Sarcoma

- Females with spleen and/or liver involvement (rarely GI tract)
- EBV-positive tumor cells
- Necrosis, numerous eosinophils, granulomas may be present
- Variably positive for CD21, CD35, SMA

Caveats and Pearls

- Clonal immunoglobulin gene rearrangements may be detected

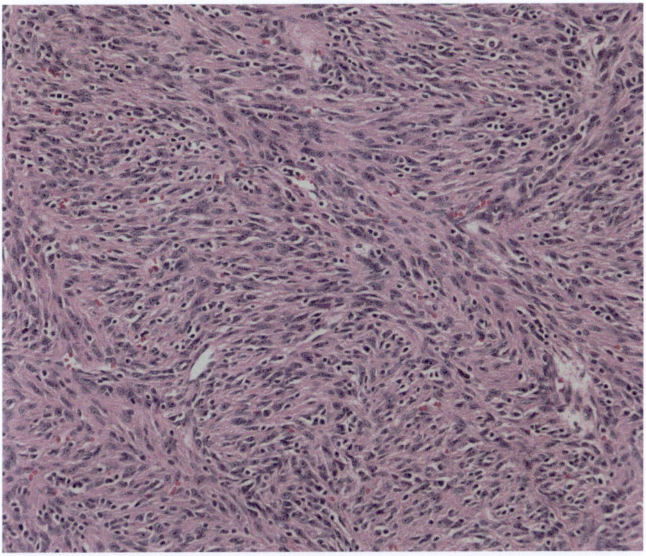

Follicular dendritic cell sarcoma. Fascicles of plump spindle-shaped cells

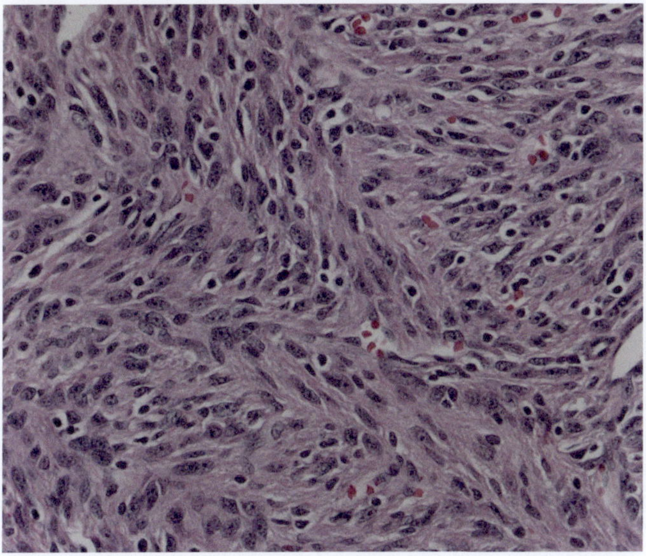

Follicular dendritic cell sarcoma—high power

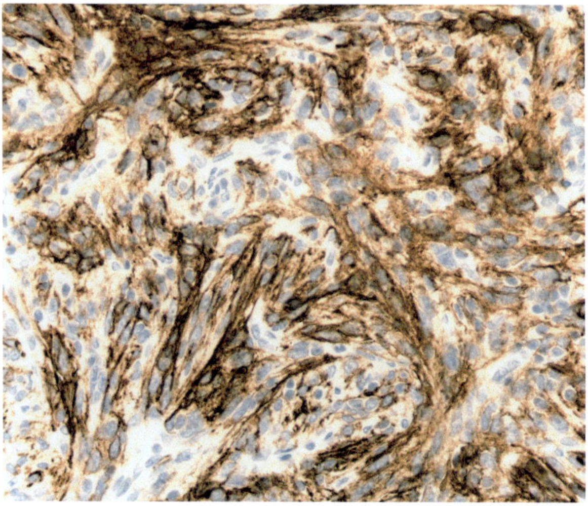

Follicular dendritic cell sarcoma. CD21-positive follicular dendritic cells

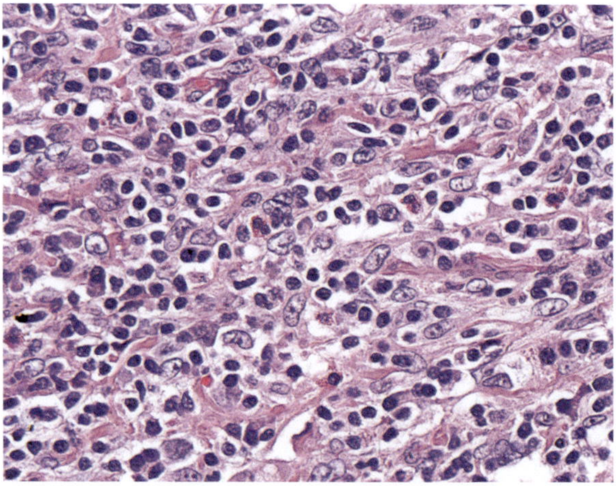

Inflammatory pseudotumor (IPT)-like follicular dendritic cell sarcoma (spleen). Note the plump spindle-shaped tumor cells with a background population of small lymphocytes, plasma cells, and eosinophils. (Courtesy of Daniel A Arber, MD, Department of Pathology, University of Chicago, Chicago, Illinois, USA)

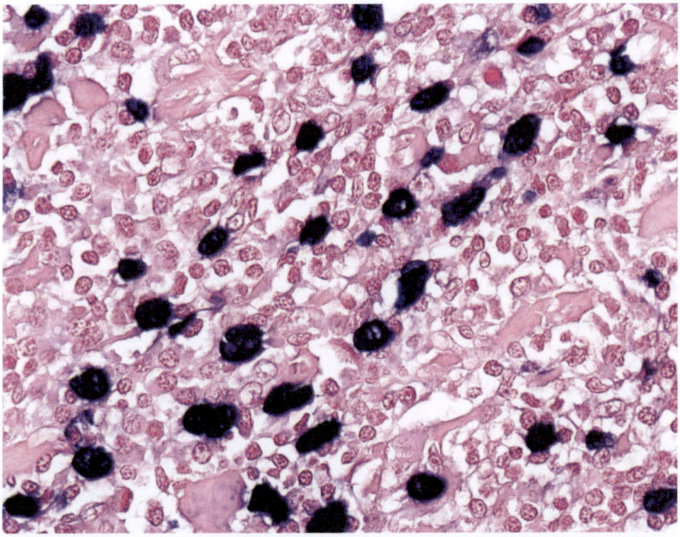

Inflammatory pseudotumor-like follicular dendritic cell sarcoma with EBV-positive tumor cells (EBER ISH). (Courtesy of Daniel A Arber, MD, Department of Pathology, University of Chicago, Chicago, Illinois, USA)

Disseminated Juvenile Xanthogranuloma

Snapshot

- Dense infiltrate of oval histiocytes, large foamy histiocytes, and Touton giant cells

Clinical Features

- Most often seen in children <10 years of age
- Associated with neurofibromatosis type 1
- Multiple sites of involvement, including skin and soft tissue
- Anemia, thrombocytopenia, hepatosplenomegaly

Morphology

- Dense infiltrate of small oval histiocytes, large foamy (xanthomatous) histiocytes, Touton giant cells, and inflammatory cells; older lesions may be fibrotic

Immunophenotype

- POSITIVE: CD14, CD68 (PGM1), CD163, factor XIIIa, fascin
- NEGATIVE: CD1a, langerin, and S100 (most cases)

Differential Diagnosis

- *Langerhans cell histiocytosis* (positive for S100, CD1a, and langerin)
- *Erdheim-Chester disease* (adults with bone involvement, *BRAF* mutation)
- *Juvenile xanthogranuloma* (solitary dermal lesion, indolent disease)

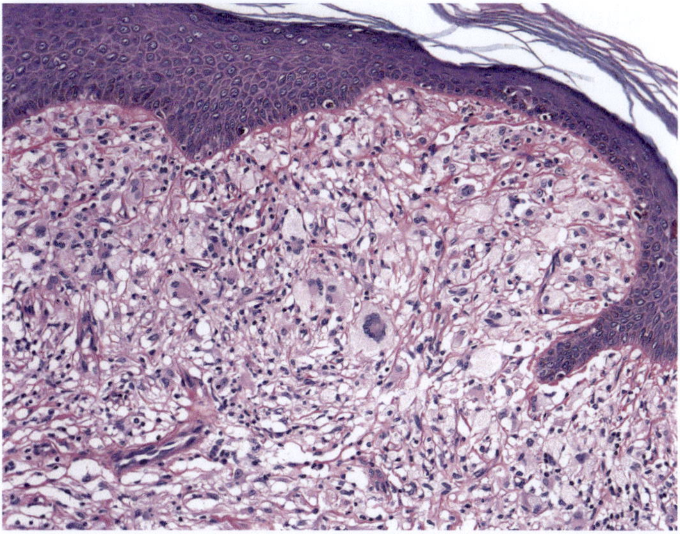

Subcutaneous infiltrate of foamy histiocytes and Touton-type giant cells

Erdheim-Chester Disease

Snapshot

- Infiltrate of foamy histiocytes with Touton-type giant cells, nearly always involving long bones

Clinical Features

- Adult male predominance
- Bilateral osteosclerosis of long bones
- Skin (xanthelasma), periaortic, perinephric, and CNS involvement

Pathologic Features

- Collections of foamy histiocytes with admixed inflammatory cells, Touton giant cells, and fibrosis

Immunophenotype

- POSITIVE: CD14, CD68, CD163, factor XIIIa, fascin, and *BRAF* (if mutation present)
- USUALLY NEGATIVE: CD1a, langerin, and S-100

Genetics

- *BRAF* V600E mutation (most cases)
- *NRAS* and *PIK3CA* mutations (uncommon)

Differential Diagnosis

- *Disseminated juvenile xanthogranuloma* (children with no bone disease or *BRAF* mutation)

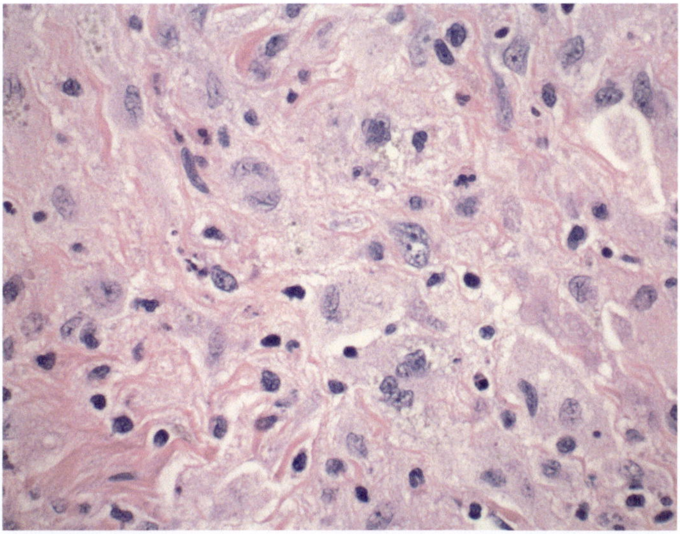

Erdheim-Chester disease with enlarged histiocytes and few multinucleated cells

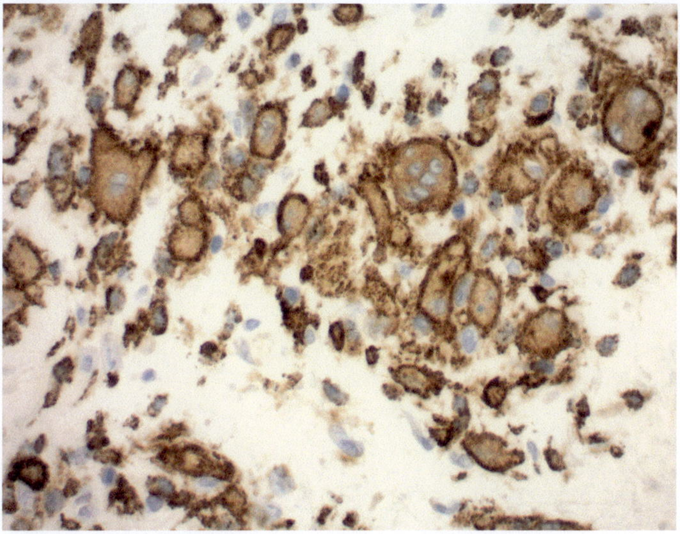

CD163-positive histiocytes in Erdheim-Chester disease

Chapter 14
Non-neoplastic Marrow Findings

Parvovirus Infection

Snapshot
- Nuclear inclusions within enlarged proerythroblasts in bone marrow due to parvovirus B19 infection

Clinical Features
- Can affect healthy individuals
- May also affect immunodeficient patients (often in HIV-positive individuals)
- Causes normochromic, normocytic anemia

Diagnosis
- Causes erythroblast hypoplasia/red cell aplasia with scattered infected erythroblasts
- Giant erythroblasts with prominent intranuclear inclusions
- Can be confirmed with parvovirus B19 IHC or in situ hybridization
- Serum PCR may be positive for parvovirus B19

Differential Diagnosis
- *Congenital dyserythropoietic anemias* (multinucleated erythroid precursors, absence of giant erythroblasts with nuclear inclusions)

© Springer Nature Switzerland AG 2019

S. D. Hudnall et al., *Pocket Guide to Diagnostic Hematopathology*, https://doi.org/10.1007/978-3-030-10630-0_14

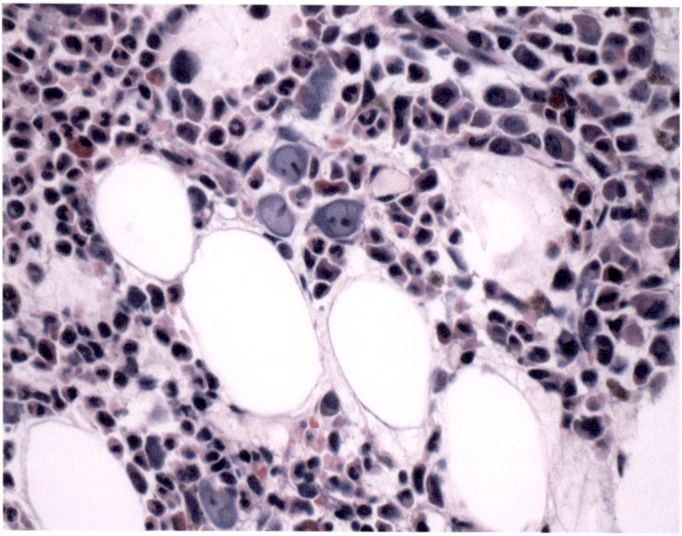

Parvovirus infection. Marrow showing scattered enlarged erythroblasts with glassy nuclei due to parvovirus infection

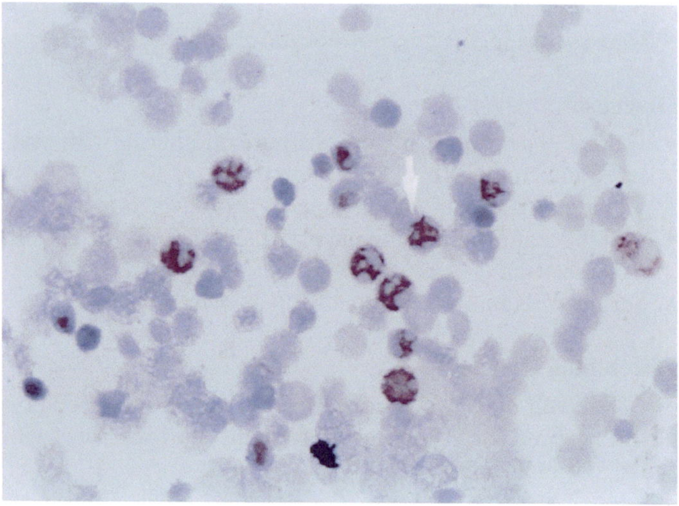

Parvovirus infection. Immunohistochemical stain for parvovirus B19

Cryptococcus Infection

Snapshot

- Pancytopenia with bone marrow involvement by *Cryptococcus neoformans*

Clinical Features

- Generally found in patients with underlying immunodeficiency, most commonly HIV
- Can cause meningitis
- Pulmonary, skin, and bone lesions

Diagnosis

- Round yeast forms of variable size with thick capsule (in most cases)
- Infection of blood/marrow neutrophils and monocytes
- Rare granulomas in marrow
- Can be seen in the aspirate using a Wright stain
- *Cryptococcal* organisms are positive in tissue using both PAS and silver stains
- Serum antibody testing may be positive

Differential Diagnosis

- *Histoplasma infection* (marrow granulomas; smaller non-encapsulated forms of uniform size; urine antigen is positive for histoplasma)

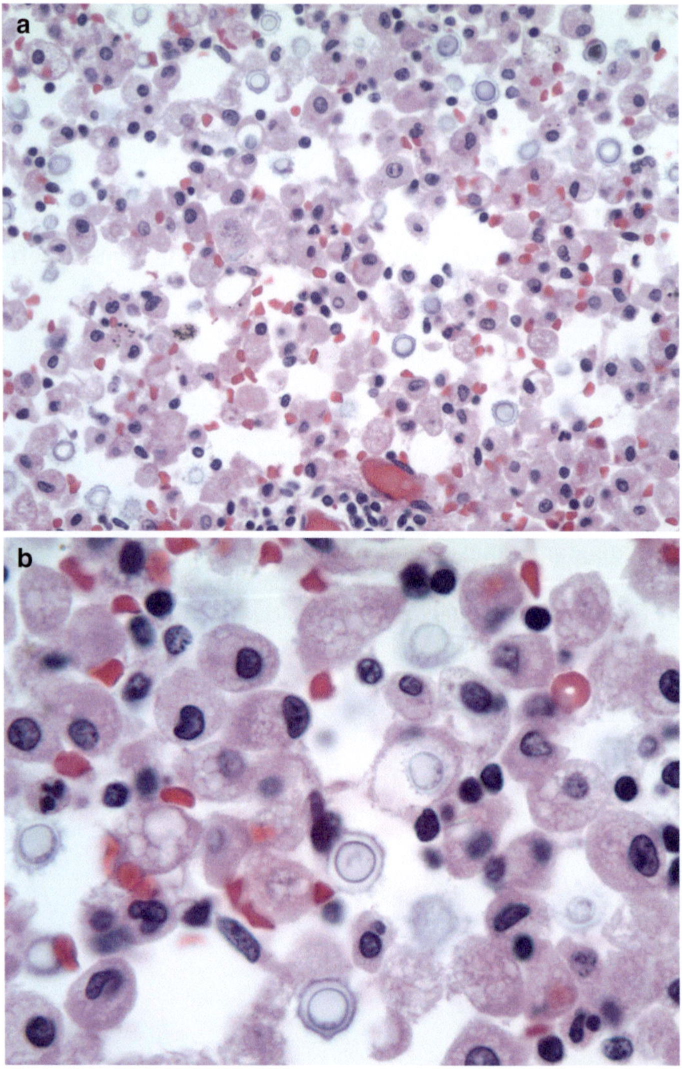

Cryptococcus infection. (**a**, **b**) Cryptococcus organisms with a thick capsule

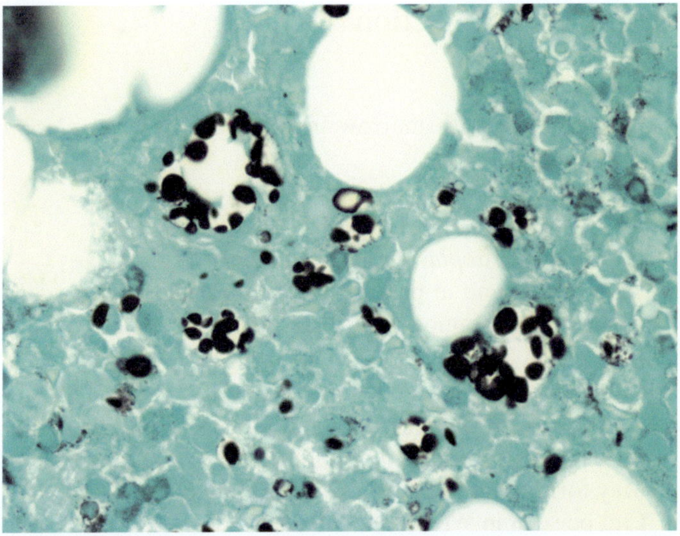

Cryptococcus infection. Grocott's methenamine silver (GMS) stain highlighting numerous cryptococcal organisms

Histoplasma Infection

Snapshot

- Pancytopenia with marrow involvement by *Histoplasma capsulatum*

Clinical Features

- Caused by *Histoplasmosis capsulatum*
- Generally found in patients with underlying immunodeficiency, most commonly HIV

Diagnosis

- Small (2–4 μm) helmet-shaped intracellular budding yeast forms in neutrophils and monocytes
- May form granulomas in marrow
- Can be seen in Wright-stained aspirate smears
- Histoplasma organisms are positive for PAS and silver stains
- Urine and serum histoplasma antigen testing can be performed, as well as culture

Differential Diagnosis

- *Cryptococcus infection* (round uniform yeast forms with wide capsule)

Caveats and Pearls

- May be associated with hemophagocytic syndrome

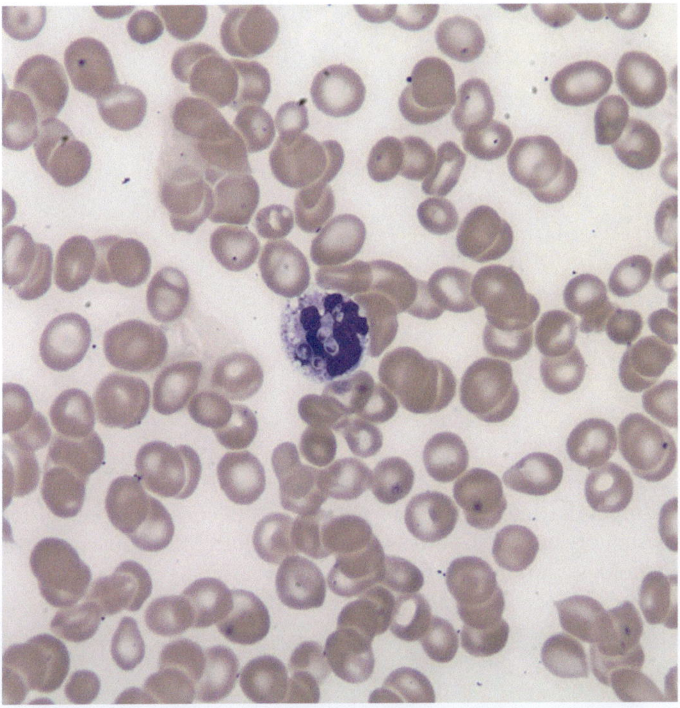

Histoplasma infection. Circulating monocyte containing numerous histoplasma yeast forms

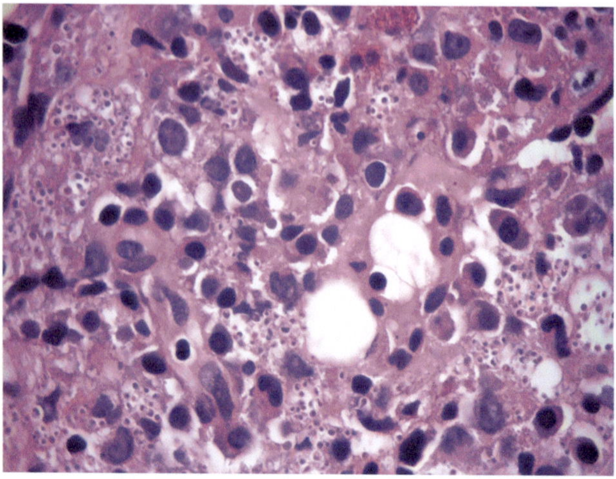

Histoplasma infection. Bone marrow containing abundant histoplasma organisms. (Courtesy of Megan Selbst, MD, Department of Pathology, Florida Hospital, Tampa, Florida, USA)

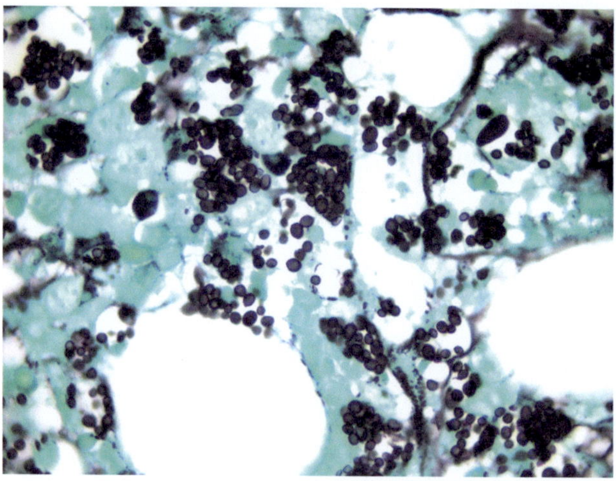

Histoplasma infection. Grocott's methenamine silver (GMS) highlighting histoplasma within marrow. (Courtesy of Megan Selbst, MD Department of Pathology, Florida Hospital, Tampa, Florida, USA)

Leishmania Infection

Snapshot

- Bone marrow infection by *Leishmania* species

Clinical Features

- Cutaneous form with skin ulcers; mucocutaneous form may be severe
- Visceral form with fever, hepatosplenomegaly, pancytopenia, marrow involvement
- Can be found endemically or as an opportunistic infection in immunocompromised individuals (most commonly with HIV or bone marrow transplantation)

Diagnosis

- *Leishmania* amastigotes can be seen in marrow histiocytes as small round parasites with a large nucleus, small rod-like kinetoplast, and thin cell membrane
- May have granulomas in marrow
- Reactive plasmacytosis

Differential Diagnosis

- *Trypanosoma cruzi* (amastigotes are morphologically indistinguishable from *Leishmania spp.*, found in heart, brain, GI tract, placenta; typically, not in marrow, lymph node, or spleen)
- *Cryptococcus neoformans/gattii* (usually larger than *Leishmania* with a thick capsule; no kinetoplast, serum antigen testing usually positive)
- *Histoplasma capsulatum* (yeast forms are similar in size but have no kinetoplast)

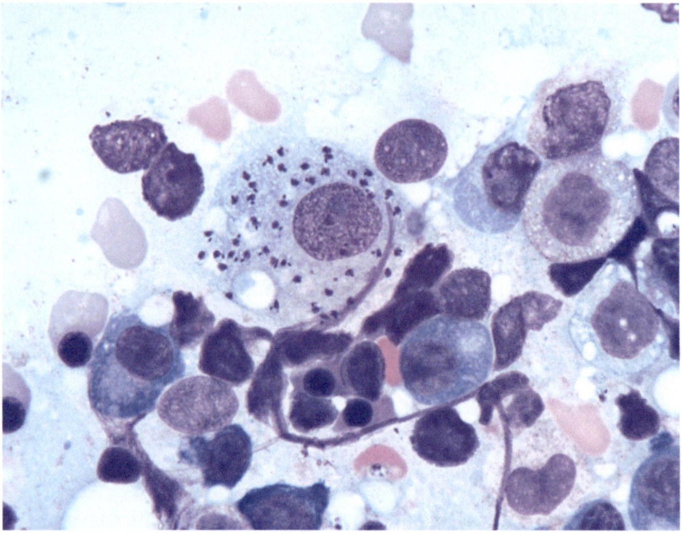

Leishmania infection. Marrow histiocyte containing numerous leishmania parasites

Gaucher Disease

Snapshot

- Lysosomal storage disease characterized by bone marrow infiltration of Gaucher histiocytes containing glycosphingolipids

Clinical Features

- Can be an incidental (asymptomatic)
- Autosomal recessive disorder
  - *Type 1*—Involvement of bone marrow, skeletal muscle, liver, and spleen
  - *Type 2*—Fatal within first few years of life due to significant neurologic disease
  - *Type 3*—Later onset of neurologic symptoms

Morphology

- Macrophages with abundant crinkled "tissue-paper" cytoplasm
- Gaucher histiocytes are PAS+ and TRAP+, sometime positive with iron stain

Genetics

- Various mutations in the *GBA1* gene

Differential Diagnosis

- *Other storage diseases* (Neiman-Pick with macrophages containing small lipid vacuoles)
- *Hemophagocytic syndrome* (primary and secondary HLH need to be excluded based on clinical symptoms; should not have the classic macrophages of storage disorders)
- *Sinus histiocytosis with massive lymphadenopathy* (histiocytes are S-100+, CD68+, and CD1a-, and generally involve lymph nodes)

Caveats and Pearls

- May be associated with hemophagocytic syndrome

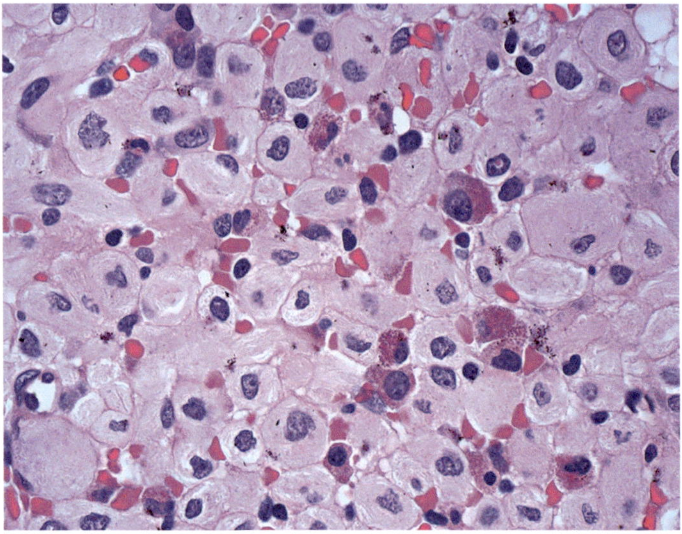

Gaucher disease. Marrow with sheets of enlarged histiocytes with abundant eosinophilic cytoplasm

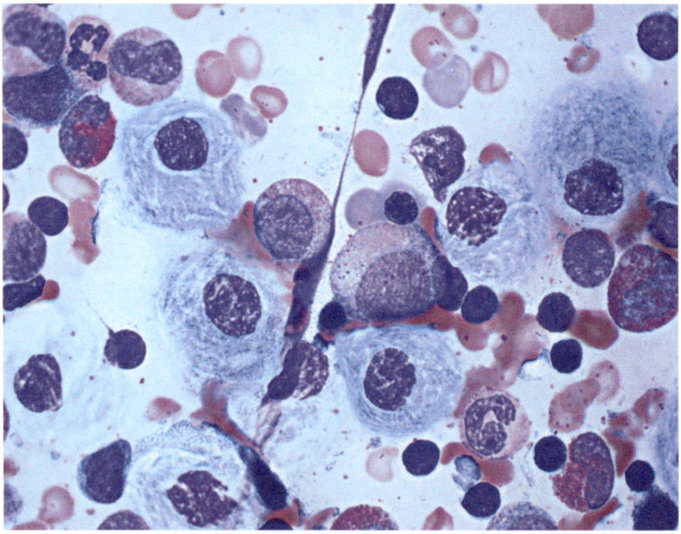

Gaucher disease. Marrow aspirate showing "tissue-paper" cells

Aplastic Anemia

Snapshot

- Pancytopenia with a markedly hypocellular marrow

Clinical Features

- Anemia with reticulocytopenia, neutropenia, and thrombocytopenia
- Commonly idiopathic
- May be secondary to viral infection (hepatitis virus), drug effect, or toxin exposure
- May evolve from paroxysmal nocturnal hemoglobinuria (PNH)

Diagnosis

- Markedly hypocellular marrow (<25% of normal age-adjusted marrow cellularity)
- Relatively numerous lymphocytes, plasma cells, and macrophages; reactive lymphoid aggregates; evidence of stromal damage

Differential Diagnosis

- *Hairy cell leukemia* (numerous CD20+ B-cells)
- *Hypocellular MDS/AML* (variable myelodysplasia, variably increased CD34+ blasts, Auer rods, abnormal cytogenetics)
- *Hypocellular acute lymphoblastic leukemia (ALL)* (increased CD34+ TdT+ blasts)
- *Inherited bone marrow failure syndrome* (including Fanconi anemia, Shwachman-Diamond syndrome, and dyskeratosis congenita)

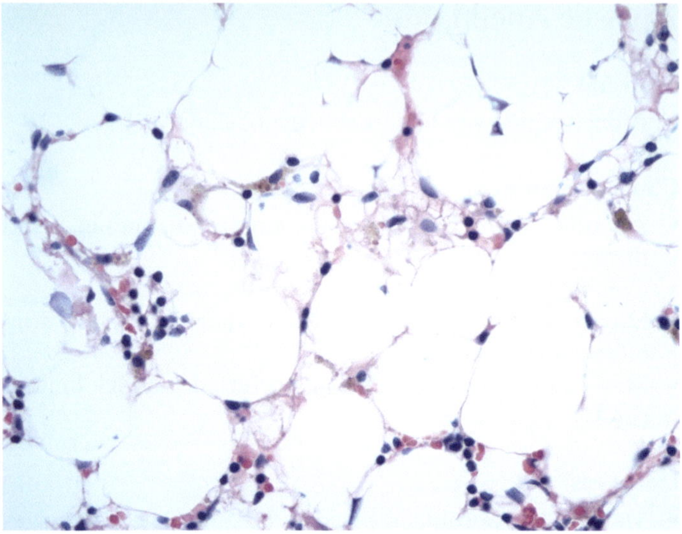

Aplastic anemia. Hypocellular marrow with hemosiderin

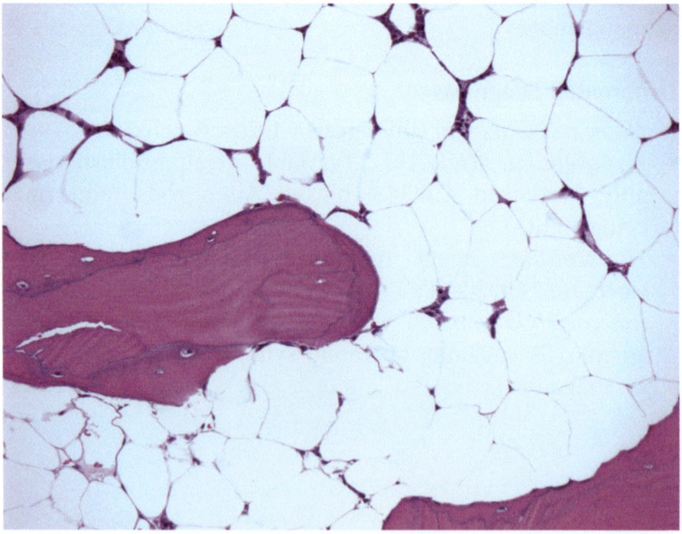

Aplastic anemia. Markedly hypocellular marrow with rare hematopoietic elements

Hemophagocytic Lymphohistiocytosis

Snapshot

- Cytopenias with infiltrate of benign hemophagocytic histiocytes

Clinical Features

- Bone marrow failure and cytopenias
- Primary forms are associated with genetic mutations
- Secondary forms are due to infections (frequently EBV or HIV), autoimmune disease, malignancy, and immunosuppression

Diagnostic Criteria

Must meet five of eight criteria:

1. Fever
2. Splenomegaly
3. Cytopenia of at least 2 of 3 marrow lineages (neutrophils $<1.0 \times 10^9$/L, hemoglobin <90 g/L, platelets $<100 \times 10^9$/L)
4. Hypertriglyceridemia or hypofibrinogenemia
5. Morphologic hemophagocytosis in marrow, lymph nodes, or spleen
6. Decreased NK-cell activity
7. Elevated serum ferritin (≥500 μg/L)
8. Elevated serum soluble CD25 (≥2400 U/mL)

Morphology

- Benign-appearing histiocytes with phagocytosis of erythrocytes and/or neutrophils

Genetics

- Mutations of *STXBP2*, *UNC13D*, *PRF1*, *LYST*, *STX11*, *RAB27A*, *SH2D1A*, *XIAP*, *AP3B1*, among others, in primary HLH

Differential Diagnosis

- *Sinus histiocytosis with massive lymphadenopathy* (histiocytes are S-100+, CD68+, and CD1a-, and generally involve lymph nodes)
- *Bone marrow failure syndromes* (Fanconi anemia, Shwachman-Diamond syndrome, dyskeratosis congenita, etc.)

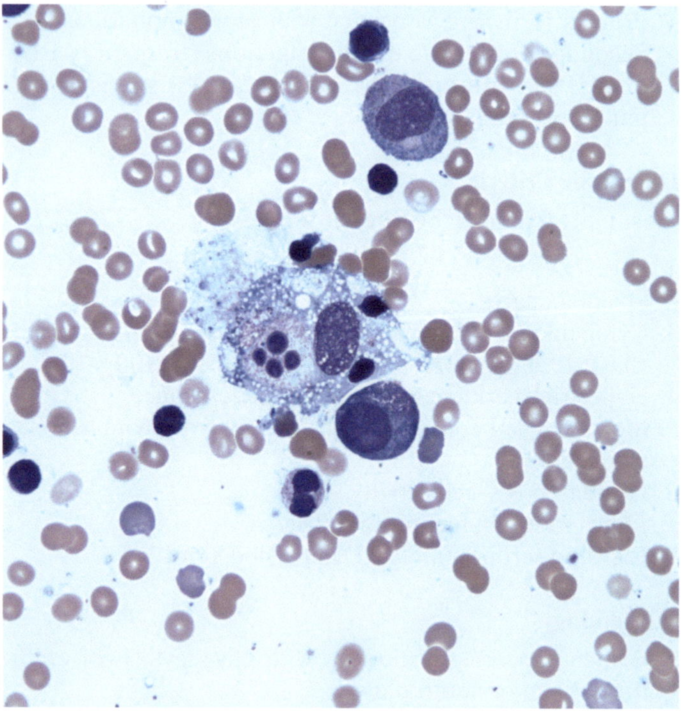

Hemophagocytic lymphohistiocytosis. Histiocyte that has engulfed a neutrophil

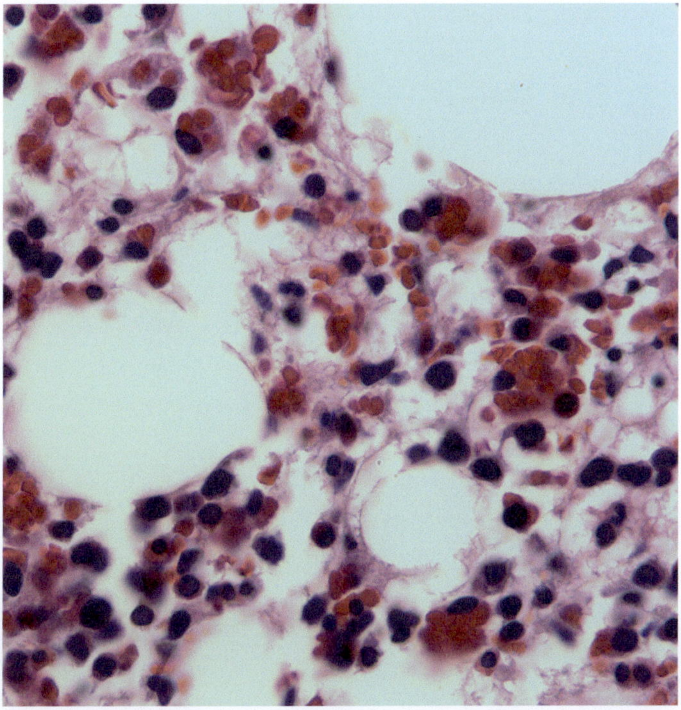

Hemophagocytic lymphohistiocytosis. Marrow showing histiocytes containing abundant erythrocytes

Chapter 15
Non-neoplastic Lymph Node and Spleen Lesions

Reactive Lymphoid Hyperplasia

Snapshot

- Reversible enlargement of lymphoid tissue due to antigenic stimulation

Clinical Features

- Can be caused by a variety of local or systemic processes

Morphology

- May exhibit a variety of patterns such as follicular hyperplasia, sinusoidal hyperplasia, paracortical hyperplasia, and mixed

Differential Diagnosis

- *Follicular lymphoma* (would have *BCL-2*-positive follicles and/or t(14;18) and lack of tingible-body macrophages)

© Springer Nature Switzerland AG 2019

S. D. Hudnall et al., *Pocket Guide to Diagnostic Hematopathology*, https://doi.org/10.1007/978-3-030-10630-0_15

Progressive Transformation of Germinal Centers

Snapshot

- A pattern of reactive lymph node hyperplasia causing expanded germinal centers being infiltrated by B-cells

Clinical Features

- Generally presents as localized lymphadenopathy, most commonly cervical
- Can be associated with lymphocyte predominant Hodgkin lymphoma

Morphology

- Lymph node only focally involved
- Enlargement and disruption of follicles by mantle zone B- and interfollicular T-cells entering the germinal center
- Affected germinal centers lose polarization and may lose tingible-body macrophages

Differential Diagnosis

- *Reactive lymphoid hyperplasia* (can have overlapping features, but germinal centers remain intact)

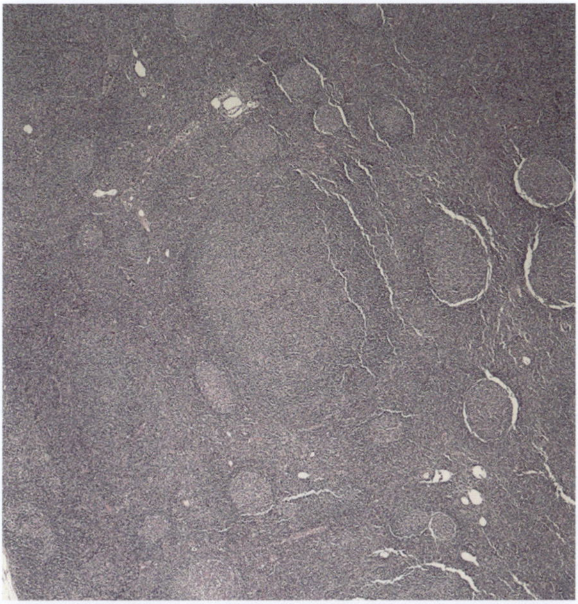

Progressive transformation of germinal centers. Single enlarged follicle in center of image, with scattered normal secondary follicles

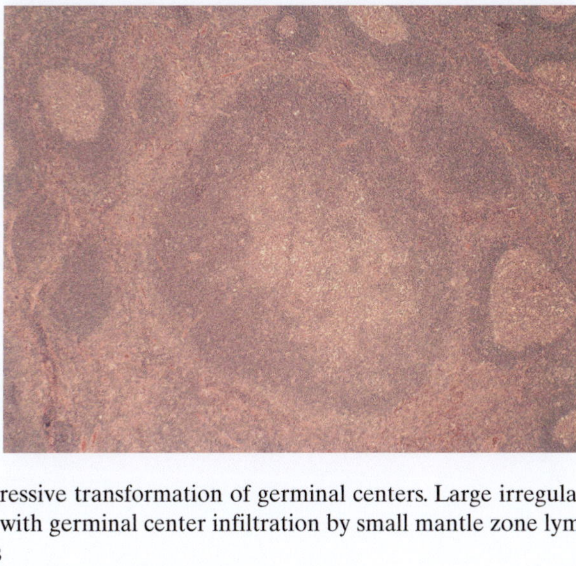

Progressive transformation of germinal centers. Large irregular follicle with germinal center infiltration by small mantle zone lymphocytes

Sarcoidosis Lymphadenopathy

Snapshot

- Granulomatous disease involving lymph nodes and extra-nodal sites

Clinical Features

- Often involves numerous organ systems, including lymph nodes (commonly hilar)
- Can present with fever and weight loss
- Often spontaneously regresses
- Laboratory studies show elevated ACE, ESR, hypergammablobulinemia, hypercalcemia, and elevated liver function tests

Morphology

- Lymph nodes are effaced by small epithelioid granulomas with multinucleated giant cells
- Absent necrosis
- Giant cells can contain asteroid bodies or Schaumann bodies

Differential Diagnosis

- *Mycobacterial lymphadenitis* (granulomas are often caseating; AFB stain positive)

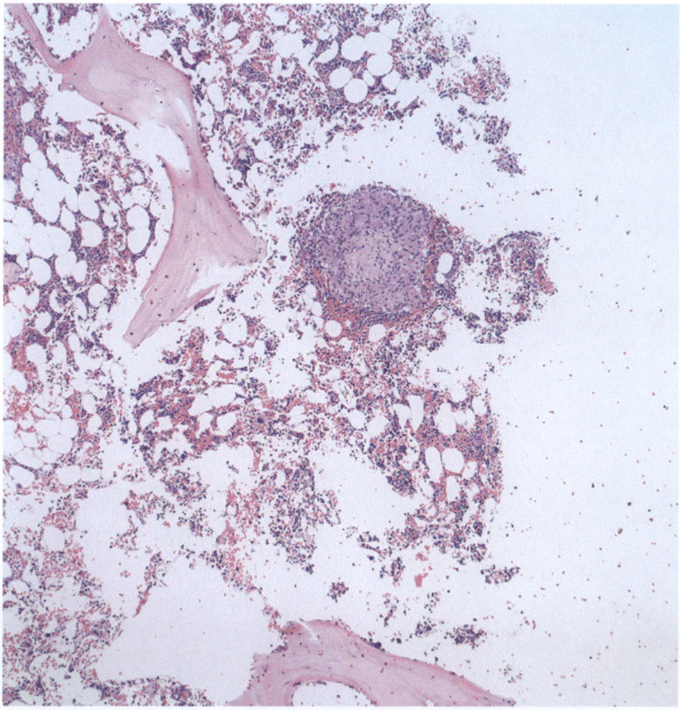

Sarcoidosis lymphadenopathy. Marrow containing a large non-caseating granuloma with epithelioid histiocytes

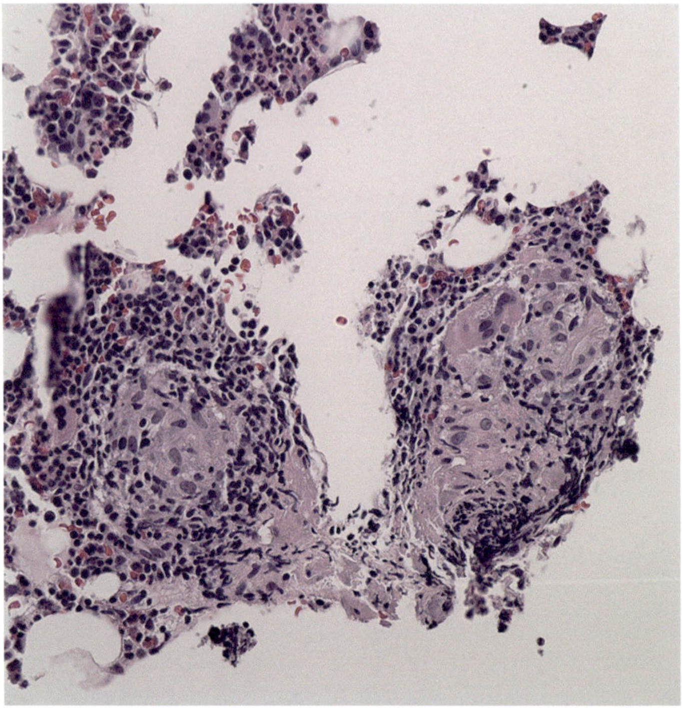

Sarcoidosis lymphadenopathy. Granulomas with scattered multinucleated giant cells

Sinus Histiocytosis with Massive Lymphadenopathy (Rosai-Dorfman Disease)

Snapshot

Lymphadenopathy due to a proliferation of histiocytes, which engulf lymphocytes and other hematopoietic cells; also called Rosai-Dorfman disease

Clinical Features

- Involves lymph nodes and can affect any extranodal site
- Generally asymptomatic
- Undergoes spontaneous regression (may take years)

Morphology

- Enlarged lymph nodes, which may be matted
- Capsular fibrosis
- Marked sinsusoidal dilation containing large histiocytes, many of which exhibit emperipolesis of lymphocytes, plasma cells, and erythrocytes
- Histiocytes are positive for S-100, CD68, and CD163, while negative for CD1a

Differential Diagnosis

- *Reactive sinus histiocytosis* (should not have emperipolesis; histiocytes are generally S-100-negative)
- *Langerhans cell histiocytosis* (generally has associated eosinophilia, and histiocytes are positive for CD1a as well as S-100)

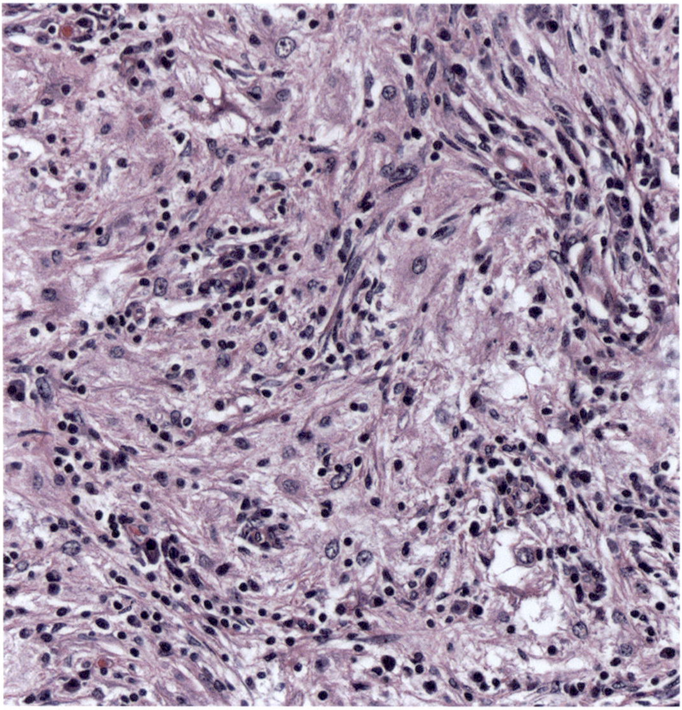

Sinus histiocytosis with massive lymphadenopathy. Numerous histiocytes with scattered lymphocytes and plasma cells

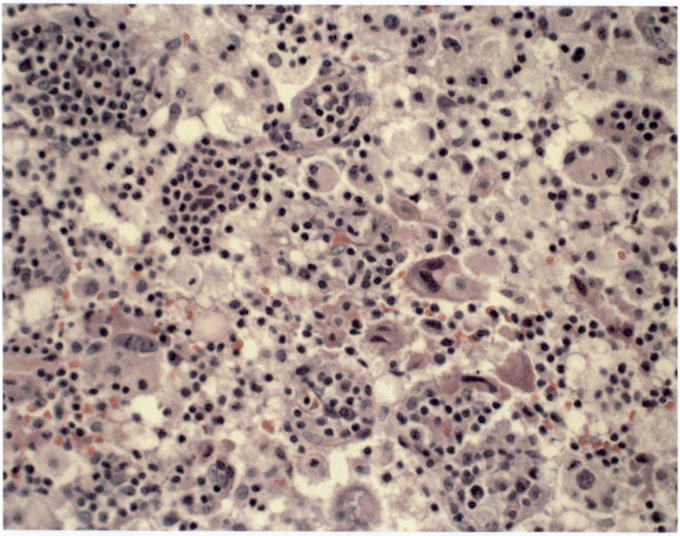

Sinus histiocytosis with massive lymphadenopathy. Enlarged histiocytes containing many intact intracytoplasmic lymphocytes (emperipolesis)

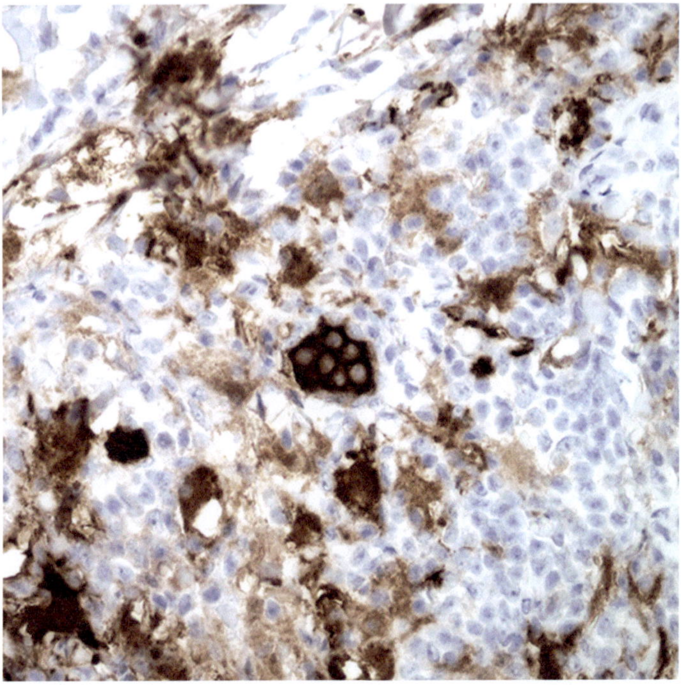

Sinus histiocytosis with massive lymphadenopathy. S-100 stain highlighting a histiocyte containing numerous mononuclear cells

Kikuchi Lymphadenopathy

Snapshot

- Histiocytic necrotizing lymphadenopathy, commonly in Asian populations

Clinical Features

- Painless regional lymphadenopathy
- Can present with fever, malaise, and skin rash
- May have liver or spleen involvement
- Spontaneous resolution

Morphology

- Intact follicular architecture with reactive germinal centers
- Patches of irregular fibrinoid necrosis lacking neutrophils and eosinophils
- Necrotic areas are surrounded by CD68+ histiocytes
- Clsuters of CD123+ plasmacytoid dendritic cells are common

Differential Diagnosis

- *Cat-scratch lymphadenitis* (may have areas of necrosis, but Warthin-Starry may highlight bacilli)
- *Lupus lymphadenitis* (may have areas of necrosis, but neutrophils will also be present)

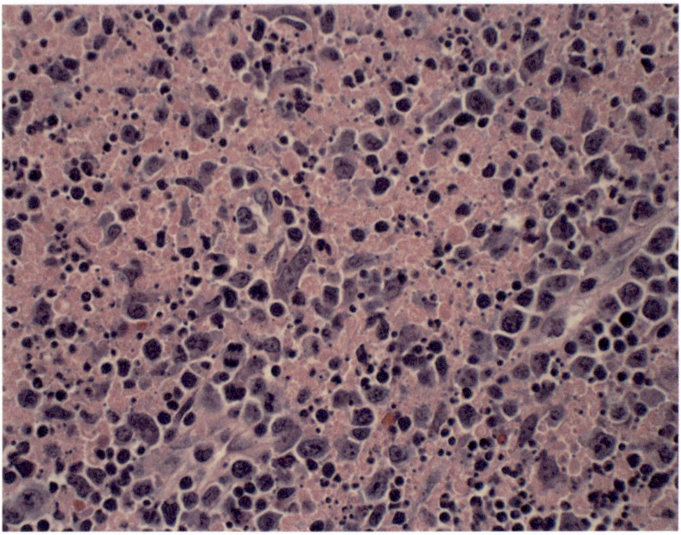

Kikuchi lymphadenopathy. Prominent necrosis and apoptotic debris with lack of neutrophils

Kimura Lymphadenopathy

Snapshot

- An inflammatory lymphadenopathy associated with prominent eosinophilia and most commonly occurring in Asian populations

Clinical Features

- Involves lymph nodes and subcutaneous tissue, frequently of the head and neck regions
- Usually associated with peripheral blood eosinophilia and elevated IgE levels

Morphology

- Lymph nodes are enlarged with hyperplastic follicles
- Eosinophilic microabcesses are prominent, and eosinophils infiltrate the follicles, sometimes causing disruption and folliculolysis
- Eosinophilic crystals may be present in histiocytes or stroma (Charcot-Leyden crystals)
- Warthin-Finkeldey cells and vascular proliferation are frequent

Differential Diagnosis

- *Classic Hodgkin lymphoma* (may have significant eosinophilia; Reed-Sternberg cells are absent in Kimura disease)
- *Castleman disease* (can have hyalinized and vascularized follicles; however, should not have prominent eosinophilia)

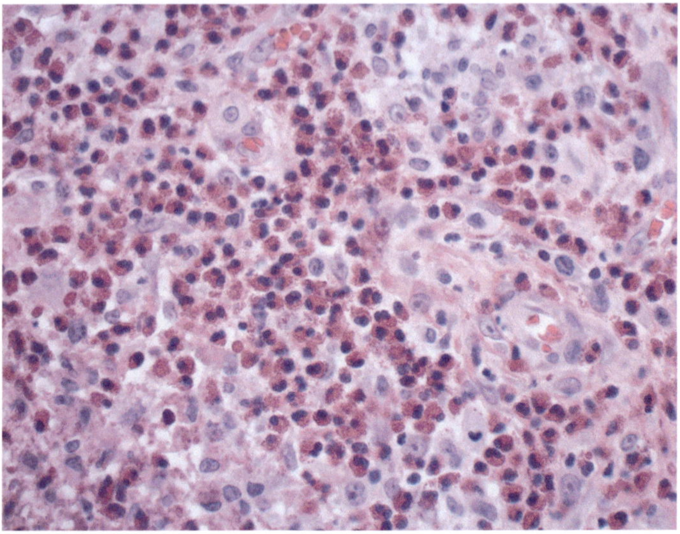

Kimura lymphadenopathy. Abundant eosinophils infiltrate the lymphoid tissue, creating eosinophilic abscesses

Castleman Disease

Snapshot

- Lymph node enlargement due to Castleman disease of either the hyaline vascular variant or the plasma cell variant

Clinical Features

Hyaline Vascular Variant

- Accounts for the majority of localized disease, often in the mediastinum
- Symptoms are generally due to mass effect
- May cause an elevated LDH

Plasma Cell Variant

- Rarely causes localized disease
- Multicentric disease often associated with HIV
- Can lead to fever, weight loss, night sweats, hepatosplenomegaly
- Patients may be anemic and/or thrombocytopenic
- Serum IL-6 elevated

Morphology

Hyaline Vascular Variant

- Lymphoid follicles are increased in number and can contain one or two germinal centers ("twinning")
- Germinal centers are atrophic and contain hyaline deposits and perpendicularly penetrating blood vessels ("lollipop lesions")
- Follicular dendritic cells can be enlarged and numerous
- Mantle zones contain concentric rings of lymphocytes, making them appear like onionskin
- Interfollicular regions may contain clusters of monocytes, and sinuses are generally absent

Plasma Cell Type

- May be associated with HHV-8 in some cases (HHV-8 immunostain positive)
- Interfollicular areas are expanded by numerous plasma cells
- Vascular proliferation is present
- Sinuses are patent

Differential Diagnosis

- *Reactive lymphoid hyperplasia* (can have subtle features overlapping with hyaline vascular Castleman disease; however, not all features are present)
- *HIV lymphadenitis* (Patterns B and C can have atrophic germinal centers, but will also have prominent lymphocyte depletion)

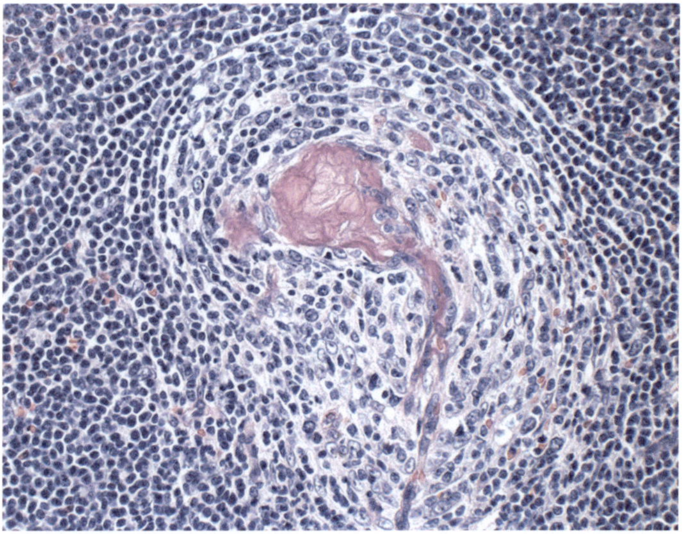

Castleman disease. Atrophic germinal center with a perpendicularly oriented capillary (lollipop) in hyaline vascular variant

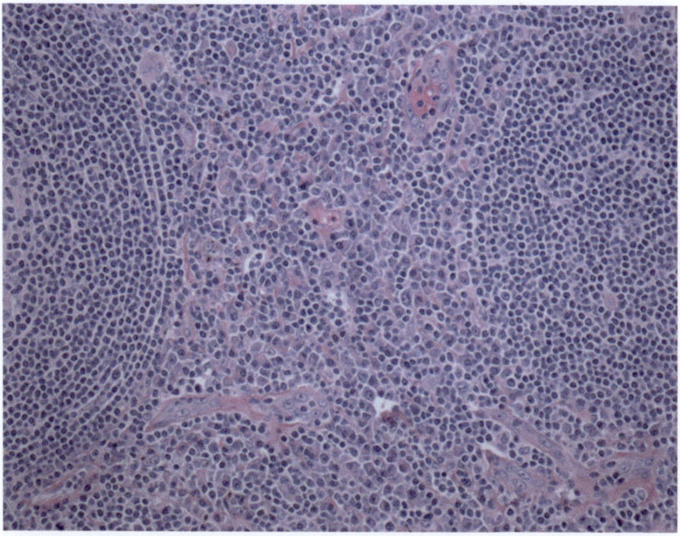

Castleman disease. Sheets of plasma cells in the interfollicular areas of the plasma cell variant

Human Immunodeficiency Virus Lymphadenitis

Snapshot

- Lymph node enlargement due to human immunodeficiency virus (HIV) infection

Clinical Features

- Lymphadenopathy can occur during the acute and/or chronic phase of HIV infection
- Associated with decreased CD4+ T-cells (AIDS when <200/mm^3)
- Often seen in conjunction with other infectious lymphadenitidies such as *Mycobacterium tuberculosis, Histoplasmosis*, etc.

Morphology

Three patterns have been described:

Pattern A—Acute phase. Enlarged lymphoid follicles, possible folliculysis, occasional interfollicular hemorrhages and clusters of monocytoid B-cells in sinuses can have multinucleated Warthin-Finkeldey cells

Pattern B—Chronic phase. Begin to have follicular effacement with fibrosis, decreased numbers of lymphocytes, vascular proliferation, increasing numbers of plasma cells

Pattern C—Atrophic phase. Follicles are atrophic and hyalinized (may have central “lollipop” arterioles; blood vessels are significantly increased; lymphocytes are further decreased

Differential Diagnosis

- *EBV lymphadenitis* (can resemble Pattern A with reactive follicular hyperplasia; serologic testing for HIV and EBV can differentiate)
- *Toxoplasma lymphadenitis* (can resemble Pattern A with clusters of monocytoid cells, but HIV should not have epithelioid histiocytes)

- *Other viral lymphadenitis* (many viral infections can have mild distortion of lymphoid architecture (similar to Pattern A) without identification of the causative virus)
- *Angioimmunoblastic T-cell lymphoma* (can resemble Patterns B and C with increased vascular proliferation; however, should have follicular effacement and often scattered large B-cells)
- *Castleman disease* (can have hyalinized follicles with "lollipop" arterioles similar to Patterns B and C but should not have lymphocyte depletion; also confirmed with HIV antibody testing)

Kaposi Lymphadenopathy

Snapshot

- Lymphadenopathy caused by an HHV-8-positive vascular neoplasm

Clinical Features

- Caused by HHV-8
- Can be found sporadically or in immunosuppressed individuals (often with AIDS)
- Kaposi sarcoma can involve lymph nodes, skin, and internal organs (most commonly the GI tract)
- Is often multifocal

Morphology

- Lymph nodes are generally enlarged and often matted
- Tumors evolve from the capsule into the lymph node parenchyma
- Neoplastic vascular proliferations are composed of bland spindle cells and have slit-like spaces containing red cells
- Red cell extravasation is also present
- The neoplastic endothelial cells often contain PAS-positive hyaline globules within the cytoplasm
- Admixed plasma cells are frequent
- CD34, CD31, and usually Factor VIII will stain the endothelial cells
- HHV-8 immunohistochemistry is positive

Differential Diagnosis

- *HIV lymphadenitis* (Pattern C can have prominent vascular proliferation but should be negative for HHV-8 staining)
- *Angioimmunoblastic T-cell lymphoma* (can exhibit increased vascular proliferation; however, should have follicular effacement and often scattered large B-cells without spindle cells)
- *Castleman disease* (can have hyalinized and vascularized follicles; however, should not have spindle cell proliferations or lack of lymphocytes)

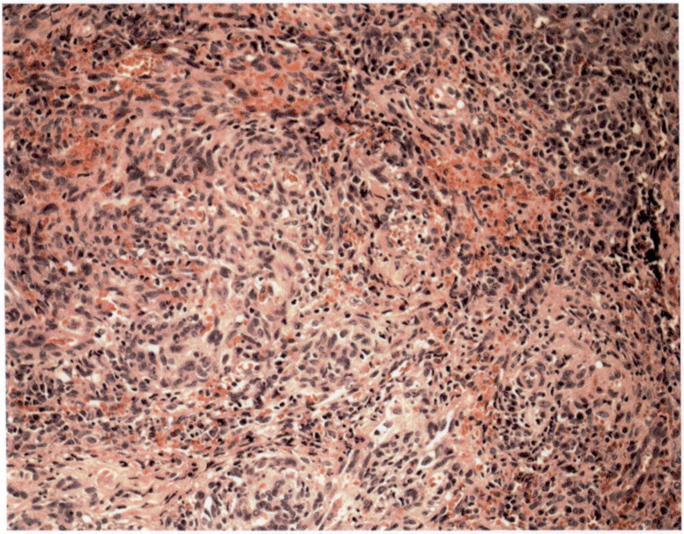

Kaposi lymphadenopathy. Lymph node showing a proliferation of spindled cells, capillary spaces, and red cell extravasation in Kaposi sarcoma

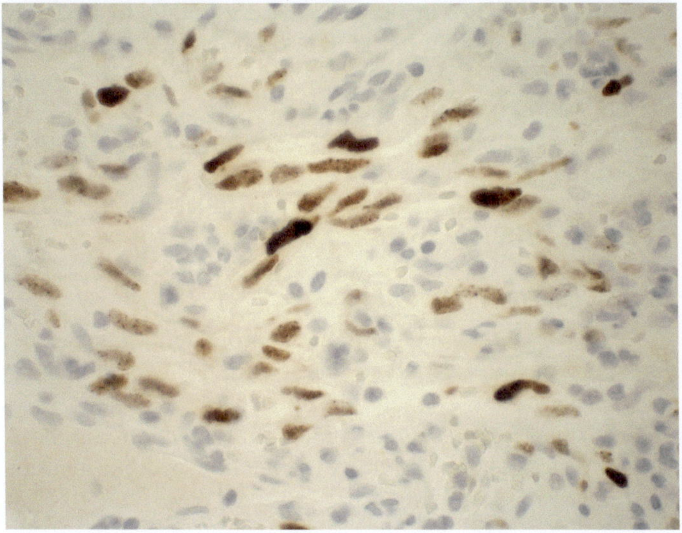

Kaposi lymphadenopathy. Positive HHV8 immunostain in Kaposi sarcoma

Epstein-Barr Virus Lymphadenitis

Snapshot

- Lymph node enlargement due to EBV infection
- Also referred to as infectious mononucleosis-associated lymphadenitis

Clinical Features

- Caused by HHV-4 (Epstein-Barr virus)
- Typically seen in younger patients
- Causes fever, lymphadenopathy, splenomegaly, pharyngitis
- May have peripheral blood leukocytosis with atypical lymphocytes

Morphology

- Mild distortion, but not total effacement, of normal lymphoid architecture
- Paracortical expansion by a heterogeneous cell population
- Immunoblasts are increased, can occasionally form sheets
- Some large immunoblasts may resemble Reed-Sternberg cells
- May exhibit focal necrosis
- EBV+ immunoblasts are CD45 and CD30-positive, CD15-negative
- EBV detected by IHC (LMP1) or in situ hybridization (EBER RNA)

Differential Diagnosis

- *Toxoplasma lymphadenitis* (less prominent paracortical expansion and a triad of monocytoid B-cells, follicular hyperplasia, and epithelioid histiocytes)
- *Other viral lymphadenitis* (many viral infections can have mild distortion of lymphoid architecture without identification of the causative virus)

- *Large cell lymphoma* (usually only large lymphocytes are present in sheets, and there are a variety of cells seen with EBV lymphadenitis)
- *Classic Hodgkin lymphoma* (true Hodgkin Reed-Sternberg cells are negative for CD45, with a cherry red nucleolus, while EBV immunoblasts have more basophilic nucleoli)

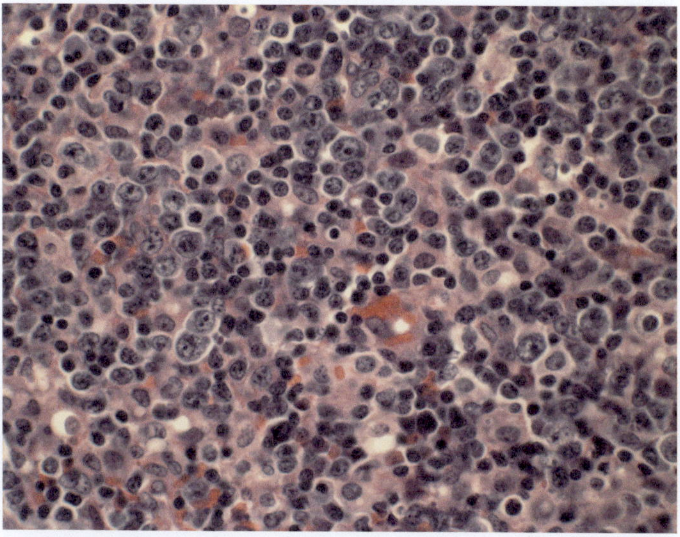

Epstein-Barr virus lymphadenitis. Lymph node containing increased large immunoblasts

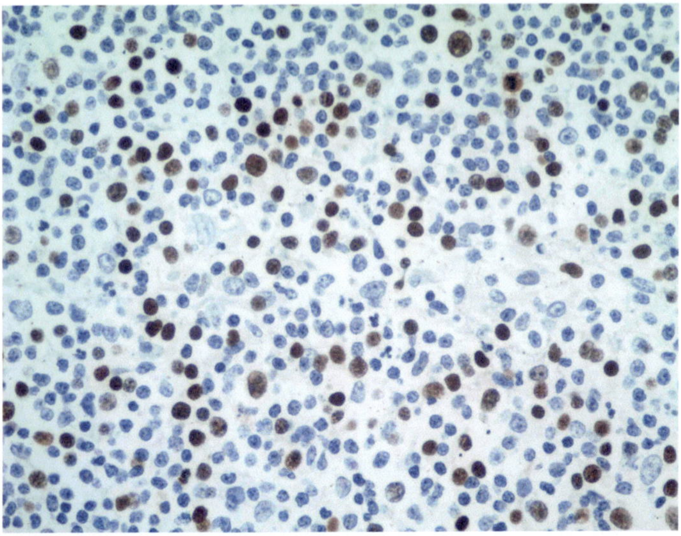

Epstein-Barr virus (EBV) lymphadenitis. EBV encoded RNA (EBER) in situ hybridization stain highlights positive cells in acute EBV infection

Cat-Scratch Lymphadenitis

Snapshot

- Granulomatous lymphadenitis due to the bacteria *Bartonella henselae*

Clinical Features

- In immune competent hosts, cat-scratch disease manifests as regional lymph node enlargement associated with fever, aches, and malaise, possibly with conjunctivitis
- In patients with immunodeficiency, cat-scratch disease may be disseminated and cause multiorgan failure

Morphology

- *B. henselae* is a Gram-negative coccobacillus (catalase and oxidase-negative)
- Nonspecific early changes including follicular hyperplasia and mild distortion of architecture
- Vascular proliferation and sinuses containing monocytoid B-cells
- In established disease, there are stellate abscesses with necrosis and neutrophils, surrounded by palisading histiocytes
- Silver stains (such as Warthin-Starry) or specific immunohistochemical stains may highlight *Bartonella* organisms

Differential Diagnosis

- *Other bacterial lymphadenitis* (can also cause suppurative disease and may be difficult to differentiate without culture of the organism)
- *Fungal lymphadenitis* (cryptococcus or histoplasma can be stained to highlight yeast forms)
- *Kikuchi-Fujimoto disease* (areas of necrosis are present; however, there is an absence of neutrophils and Warthin-Starry stain will be negative)

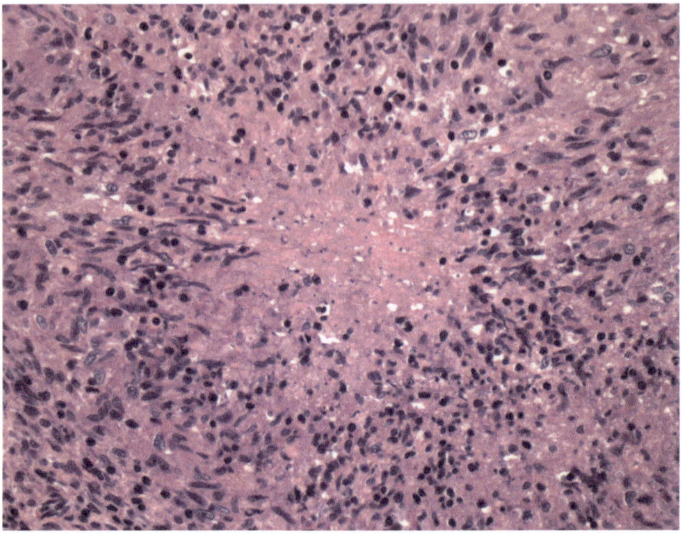

Cat-scratch lymphadenitis. Large abscess with central necrosis is present

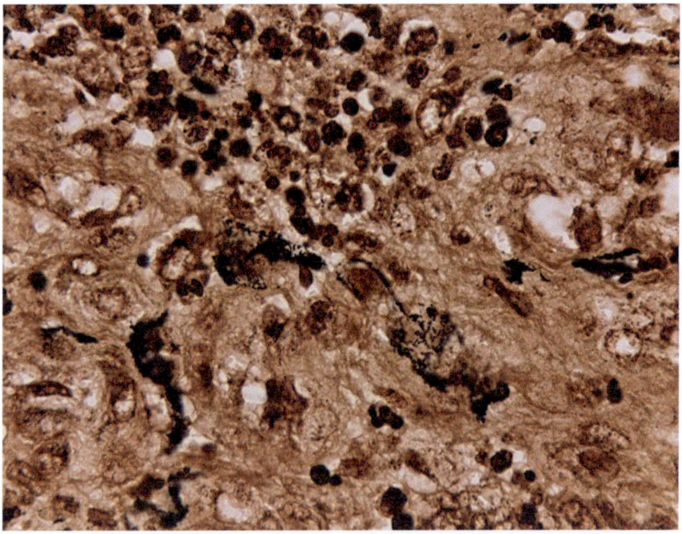

Cat-scratch lymphadenitis. Warthin-Starry stain highlights *Bartonella* organisms

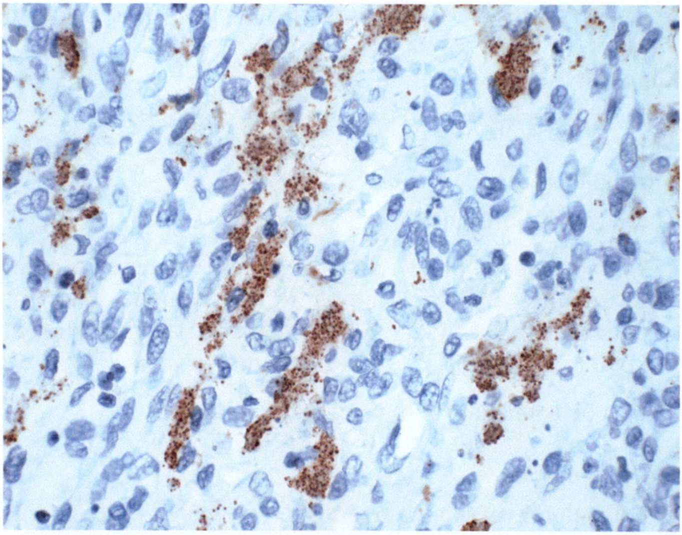

Cat-scratch lymphadenitis. *Bartonella* immunohistochemical stain may also be used to highlight the bacteria

Toxoplasma Lymphadenitis

Snapshot

- Lymphadenitis due to the parasite *Toxoplasma gondii*

Clinical Features

Three general presentations:

- *Toxoplasma* lymphadenitis in an immune competent host
- Disseminated toxoplasmosis in an immune deficient patient (e.g., secondary to bone marrow transplantation)
- Fetal toxoplasmosis from vertical transmission

Can be confirmed with serological studies

Morphology

- Follicular hyperplasia, aggregates of monocytoid B-cells are present, and scattered epithelioid histiocytes are classic morphology
- Granulomas and necrosis are not typically present
- Rarely, clusters of trophozoites within macrophages may be seen
- Organisms may be highlighted by immunohistochemical stains

Differential Diagnosis

- *EBV lymphadenitis* (can resemble with reactive follicular hyperplasia, but should not have epithelioid histiocytes; serologic testing for toxoplasmosis and EBV can differentiate)
- *Classic Hodgkin lymphoma* (true Hodgkin and Reed-Sternberg cells are negative for CD45 and generally have a cherry red nucleolus; should not have clusters of monocytoid B cells)
- *Sinus histiocytosis with massive lymphadenopathy* (will generally have histiocytes demonstrating emperipolesis)
- *Leishmaniasis* (can rarely infect lymph nodes and may have very similar histology; serologic testing can help differentiate)

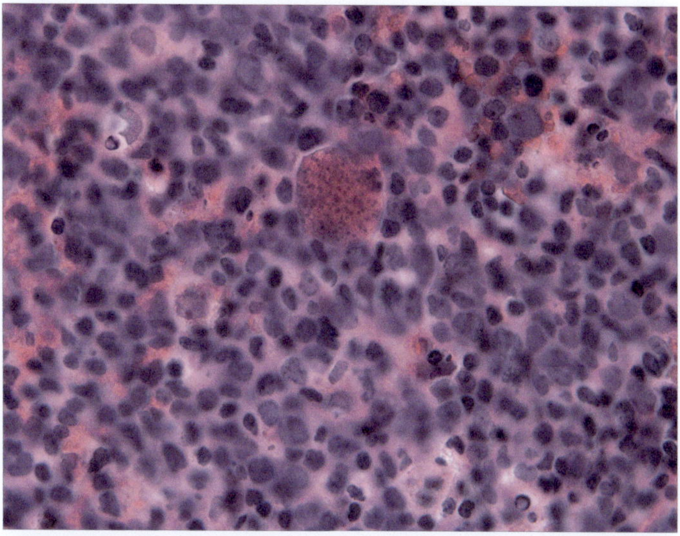

Toxoplasma lymphadenitis. Group of trophozoites is present within a macrophage

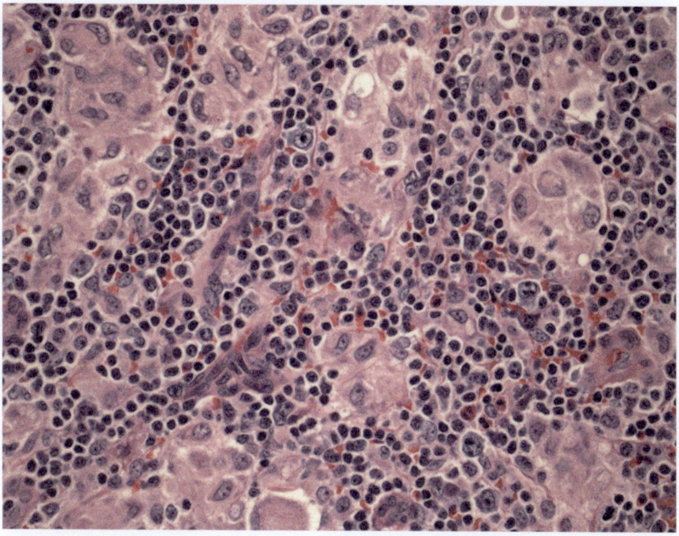

Toxoplasma lymphadenitis. Scattered epithelioid histiocytes present throughout the lymph node

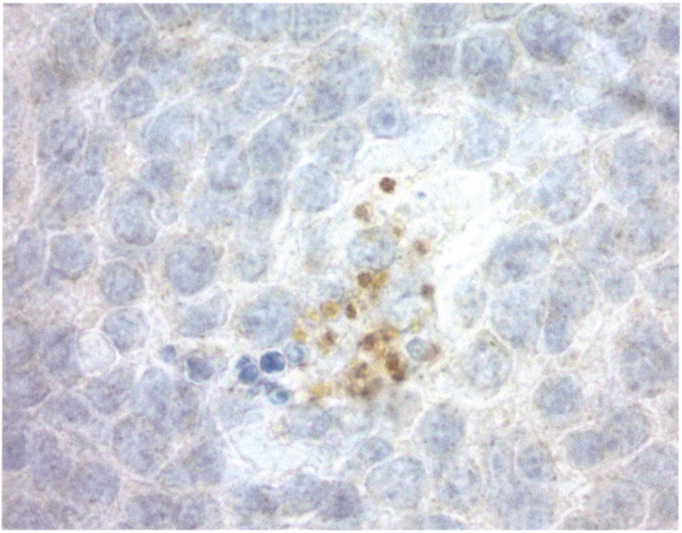

Toxoplasma lymphadenitis. Immunohistochemical stain for toxoplasma

Mycobacterial Lymphadenitis

Snapshot

- Lymphadenitis caused by *Mycobacterial spp. (M. tuberculosis, M. avium-intracellulare [MAC], M. haemophilum, M. Scrofulaceum)*

Clinical Features

- Occurs in the general population and in patients with underlying immunodeficiency, most commonly HIV-related

Morphology

- Partial to complete node effacement, often with vascular proliferation and plamacytosis
- Caseating granulomas with concentric epithelioid histiocytes, and Langhans-type giant cells (*M. tuberculosis*)
- Noncaseating granulomas more typical of *M. avium complex (MAC)*
- Beaded curved acid-fast bacteria detected with AFB stains; MAC are often more numerous and stain positive with silver stains (GMS) and PAS

Variant

- *Histiocyte-rich mycobacterial spindle cell pseudotumor*
  – Numerous intracellular acid-fast bacteria in lymph nodes (usually due to *M. avium complex (MAC)*

Differential Diagnosis

- *Sarcoidosis* (granulomas are noncaseating and acid-fast bacilli are absent)
- *Kikuchi lymphadenitis* (necrosis and histiocytes can be seen; however, no well-formed granulomas or acid-fast bacilli are present)
- *Histoplasma infection* (silver stain will generally highlight the yeast, and serum antigen testing usually positive for the causative organism)

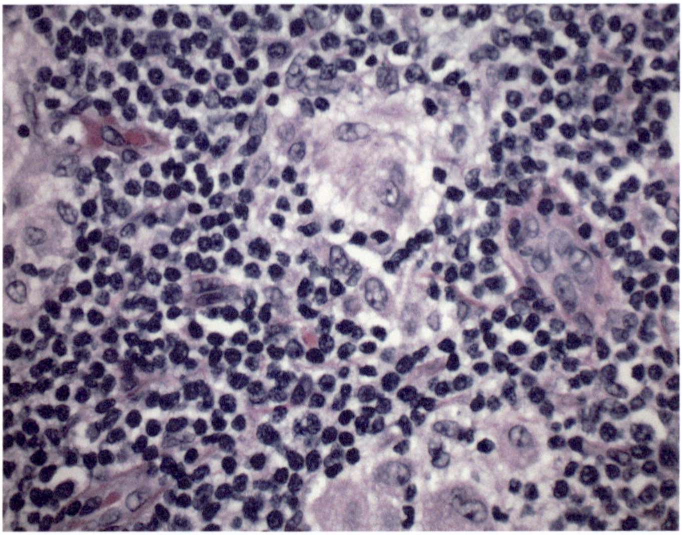

Mycobacterial lymphadenitis. Lymph node containing epithelioid histiocytes in an early mycobacterial infection

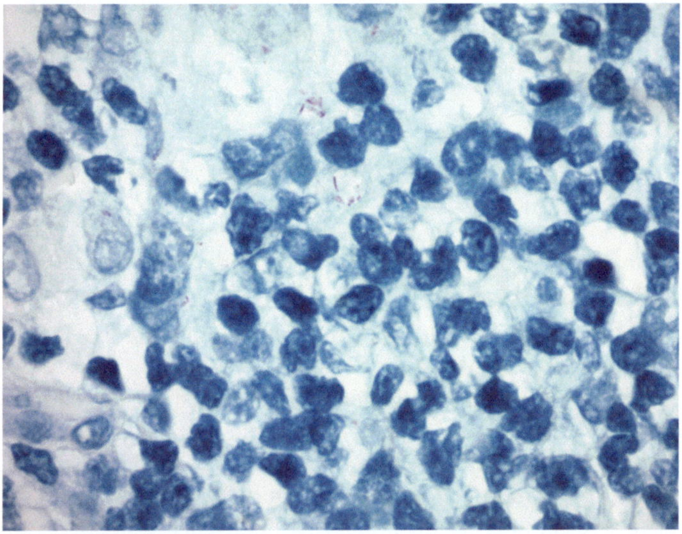

Mycobacterial lymphadenitis. Acid-fast bacillus (AFB) stain highlighting rare acid-fast bacilli

Syphilis Lymphadenitis

Snapshot

- Lymph node enlargement caused by *Treponema pallidum* infection

Clinical Features

- Caused by the spirochete *T. pallidum*
- Can be transmitted through sexual contact or vertically
- Clinical syndrome of primary (chancre), secondary (lymphadenopathy and rash), and tertiary (neuro-) syphilis

Diagnosis

- Follicular hyperplasia with numerous secondary follicles and interfollicular immunoblasts
- Thickened fibrotic lymph node capsule
- Prominent plasma cell proliferation may form sheets
- Noncaseating epithelioid granulomas or single multinucleated giant cells
- Warthin-Starry stain highlights spirochetes
- Serologic testing for *T. pallidum* for confirmation

Differential Diagnosis

- *Mycobacterium tuberculosis* (can have areas of caseating necrosis, AFB stain is positive)
- *Sarcoidosis* (granulomas predominate with no significant increase in plasma cells)
- *Follicular lymphoma* (*BCL2-positive* follicles)

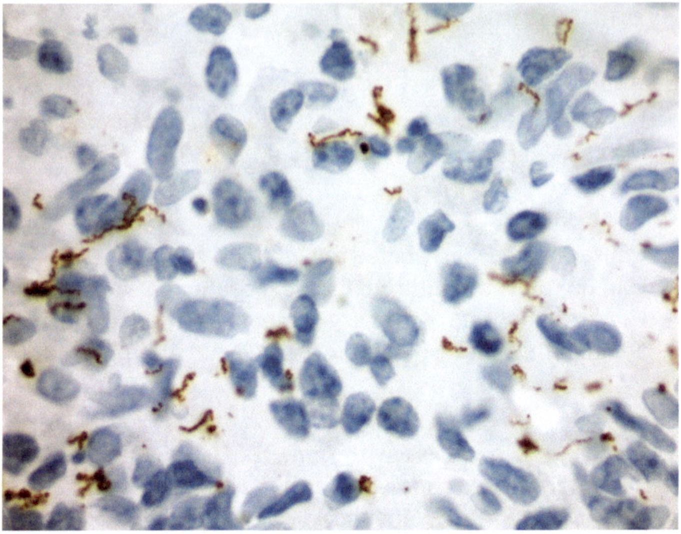

Syphilis lymphadenitis. Syphilis immunohistochemistry highlighting spirochetes in a lymph node

Lymphogranuloma Venereum Lymphadenitis

Snapshot

- Lymph node enlargement caused by Chlamydia trachomatis

Clinical Features

- *Chlamydia trachomatis* bacteria cause sexually transmitted lymphadenitis and proctitis
- Generally latent for 7–12 days followed by a painless herpetiform ulceration on the genitalia
- Lymphadenopathy occurs weeks to months later
- Can cause fever, headaches, body aches

Diagnosis

- Geographic necrosis with epithelioid histiocytes and multinucleated giant cells
- Macrophages may have vacuoles containing *Chlamydia* organisms
- Organisms are Gram-negative with Brown-Hopp and other tissue gram stains
- Also positive for Warthin-Starry stain
- *Chlamydia* can be detected with PCR or antibody testing in the clinical laboratory

Differential Diagnosis

- *Cat-scratch lymphadenitis* (can look identical; distinguished by clinical laboratory testing or identification of a primary *Chlamydia* lesion)

Herpes Simplex Virus Lymphadenitis

Snapshot

- Lymph node enlargement caused by HSV infection

Clinical Features

- Can be caused by either HSV-1 or HSV-2
- HSV-1 more common in children and adolescent populations
- Lymphadenitis is rare, but can be seen in association with hematologic malignancies

Diagnosis

- Typically causes nodular or diffuse paracortical lymph node expansion with compression of follicles
- Can have areas of necrosis with neutrophilic debris and infected multinucleated cells with groundglass chromatin
- Immunoblasts may be prominent and numerous
- Immunohistochemistry or in situ hybridization for HSV may be helpful
- Electron microscopy can identify viral particles

Differential Diagnosis

- *Mycobacterium tuberculosis* (can have areas of caseating necrosis; however, generally will also exhibit granulomas)
- *Cat-scratch lymphadenitis* (may have areas of necrosis; however, no HSV inclusions are present and Warthin-Starry may highlight bacilli)
- *Kikuchi-Fujimoto disease* (necrosis with absence of neutrophils and without viral inclusions)

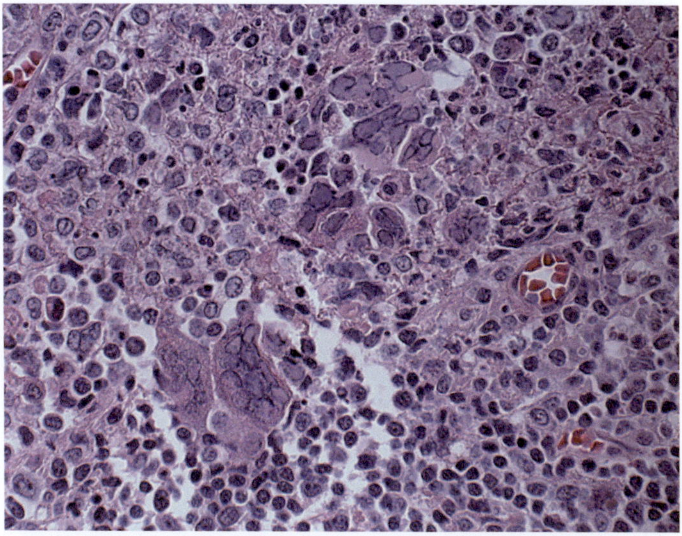

Herpes simplex virus lymphadenitis. Large multinucleated cells with glassy nuclear features of the herpes simplex virus infection

Lupus (SLE) Lymphadenopathy

Snapshot

- Lymph node enlargement associated with systemic lupus erythematosus (SLE)

Clinical Features

- Constitutional, skin, and musculoskeletal symptoms associated with SLE are frequent
- Lymphadenopathy can be localized or generalized
- Associated with more active disease and high anti-dsDNA titers

Morphology

- Follicular hyperplasia with increased vascularity and plasmacytosis
- Necrosis is often present but may not be associated with an inflammatory response
- Necrosis may be surrounded by lipid-laden macrophages
- Hematoxylin bodies present
- Granulation tissue may also be seen

Differential Diagnosis

- *Kikuchi-Fujimoto lymphadenitis* (neutrophil-poor geographic necrosis with nuclear debris, no hematoxylin bodies, numerous immunoblasts)
- *Cat-scratch lymphadenitis* (palisading granulomas with necrosis)
- *Toxoplasma lymphadenitis* (clusters of epithelioid histiocytes, often within germinal centers)

Suggested Reading

Textbooks

Foucar K, McKenna RW, Peterson LC, Kroft SH. Tumors of the bone marrow. (AFIP atlas of tumor pathology, 24/Series 4.). Silver Spring: American Registry of Pathology; 2017.

Foucar K, Chabot-Richards D, Czuchlewski DR, Hunt Karner K, Reichard KK, Vasef MA, et al. Diagnostic pathology. Blood and bone marrow. 2nd ed. Philadelphia: Elsevier; 2018.

Hsi ED. Hematopathology. 3rd ed. Philadelphia: Elsevier; 2019.

Ioachim HL, Medeiros LJ, editors. Ioachim's lymph node pathology. 4th ed. Philadelphia: Lippincott Williams & Wilkins/Wolters Kluwer; 2009.

Jaffe ES, Arber DA, Campo E, Harris NL, Quintanilla-Martinez L, editors. Hematopathology. Philadelphia: Saunders/Elsevier; 2017.

Medeiros LJ, Miranda RN. Diagnostic pathology: lymph nodes and extranodal lymphomas. 2nd ed. Philadelphia: Elsevier; 2018.

O'Malley DP, George TI, Orazi A, Abbondanzo SL. Benign and reactive conditions of lymph node and spleen. (AFIP atlas of nontumor pathology, 7/Series 1). Washington, D.C.: American Registry of Pathology; 2009.

Orazi A, Weiss LM, Foucar K, Knowles D. Knowles' neoplastic hematopathology. 3rd ed. Philadelphia: Lippincott Williams & Wilkins/Wolters Kluwer Health; 2014.

Swerdlow SH, Campo E, Harris NL, Jaffe ES, Pileri SA, Stein H, et al., editors. WHO classification of tumours of hematopoietic and lymphoid tumors. 4th ed. Lyon: International Agency for Research in Cancer; 2016.

© Springer Nature Switzerland AG 2019

S. D. Hudnall et al., *Pocket Guide to Diagnostic Hematopathology*, https://doi.org/10.1007/978-3-030-10630-0

Review Articles

Chapter 1 Chronic Myeloid Neoplasms

Chronic Myeloproliferative Neoplasms

Barbui T, Thiele J, Gisslinger H, Kvasnicka HM, Vannucchi AM, Guglielmelli P, et al. The 2016 WHO classification and diagnostic criteria for myeloproliferative neoplasms: document summary and in-depth discussion. Blood Cancer J. 2018;8(2):15.

Czader M, Orazi A. Acute myeloid leukemia and other types of disease progression in myeloproliferative neoplasms. Am J Clin Pathol. 2015;144(2):188–206.

Reiter A, Gotlib J. Myeloid neoplasms with eosinophilia. Blood. 2017a;129(6):704–14.

Myelodysplastic/Myeloproliferative Neoplasms

Calvo KR, Price S, Braylan RC, Oliveira JB, Lenardo M, Fleisher TA, Rao VK. JMML and RALD (RAS-associated autoimmune leukoproliferative disorder): common genetic etiology yet clinically distinct entities. Blood. 2015;125(18):2753–8.

Patnaik MM, Parikh SA, Hanson CA, Tefferi A. Chronic myelomonocytic leukaemia: a concise clinical and pathophysiological review. Br J Haematol. 2014;165(3):273–86.

Patnaik MM, Tefferi A. Chronic myelomonocytic leukemia: 2016 update on diagnosis, risk stratification, and management. Am J Hematol. 2016;91(6):631–42.

Zoi K, Cross NC. Molecular pathogenesis of atypical CML, CMML and MDS/MPN-unclassifiable. Int J Hematol. 2015;101(3):229–42.

Myelodysplastic Syndromes

Arber DA, Hasserjian RP. Reclassifying myelodysplastic syndromes: what's where in the new WHO and why. Hematology Am Soc Hematol Educ Program. 2015;2015:294–8.

Bejar R, Steensma DP. Recent developments in myelodysplastic syndromes. Blood. 2014;124(18):2793–803.

Bennett JM. Changes in the Updated 2016: WHO Classification of the myelodysplastic syndromes and related myeloid neoplasms. Clin Lymphoma Myeloma Leuk. 2016;16(11):607–9.

Cazzola M, Malcovati L. Prognostic classification and risk assessment in myelodysplastic syndromes. Hematol Oncol Clin North Am. 2010;24(2):459–68.

Cazzola M, Della Porta MG, Travaglino E, Malcovati L. Classification and prognostic evaluation of myelodysplastic syndromes. Semin Oncol. 2011a;38(5):627–34.

Cazzola M, Malcovati L, Invernizzi R. Myelodysplastic/myeloproliferative neoplasms. Hematology Am Soc Hematol Educ Program. 2011b;2011:264–72.

Cremers EM, Alhan C, Westers TM, Ossenkoppele GJ, van de Loosdrecht AA. Immunophenotyping for diagnosis and prognosis in MDS: ready for general application? Best Pract Res Clin Haematol. 2015a;28(1):14–21.

Czader M, Orazi A. World Health Organization classification of myelodysplastic syndromes. Curr Pharm Des. 2012;18(22):3149–62.

Glaubach T, Robinson LJ, Corey SJ. Pediatric myelodysplastic syndromes: they do exist! J Pediatr Hematol Oncol. 2014;36(1):1–7.

Glauser TA, Sagatys EM, Williamson JC, Burton BS, Berger C, Merwin P, et al. Current pathology practices in and barriers to MDS diagnosis. Leuk Res. 2013;37(12):1656–61.

Hasegawa D. The current perspective of low-grade myelodysplastic syndrome in children. Int J Hematol. 2016;103(4):360–4.

Hyjek E, Vardiman JW. Myelodysplastic/myeloproliferative neoplasms. Semin Diagn Pathol. 2011;28(4):283–97.

Komrokji RS, Zhang L, Bennett JM. Myelodysplastic syndromes classification and risk stratification. Hematol Oncol Clin North Am. 2010;24(2):443–57.

Lindsley RC, Ebert BL. Molecular pathophysiology of myelodysplastic syndromes. Annu Rev Pathol. 2013;8:21–47.

Malcovati L, Cazzola M. Recent advances in the understanding of myelodysplastic syndromes with ring sideroblasts. Br J Haematol. 2016;174(6):847–58.

Meers S. The myelodysplastic syndromes: the era of understanding. Eur J Haematol. 2015;94(5):379–90.

Mufti GJ, Bennett JM, Goasguen J, Bain BJ, Baumann I, Brunning R, et al. International Working Group on Morphology of Myelodysplastic Syndrome. Diagnosis and classification of myelodysplastic syndrome: International Working Group on Morphology of myelodysplastic syndrome (IWGM-MDS) consensus proposals for the definition and enumeration of myeloblasts and ring sideroblasts. Haematologica. 2008;93(11):1712–7.

Nguyen PL. The myelodysplastic syndromes. Hematol Oncol Clin North Am. 2009;23(4):675–91.

Patnaik MM, Tefferi A. Refractory anemia with ring sideroblasts and RARS with thrombocytosis. Am J Hematol. 2015;90(6):549–59.

Pellagatti A, Boultwood J. The molecular pathogenesis of the myelodysplastic syndromes. Eur J Haematol. 2015;95(1):3–15.

Porwit A. Is there a role for flow cytometry in the evaluation of patients with myelodysplastic syndromes? Curr Hematol Malig Rep. 2015;10(3):309–17.

Steensma DP. The changing classification of myelodysplastic syndromes: what's in a name? Hematology Am Soc Hematol Educ Program. 2009:645–55.

Stetler-Stevenson M, Yuan CM. Myelodysplastic syndromes: the role of flow cytometry in diagnosis and prognosis. Int J Lab Hematol. 2009;31(5):479–83.

Tiu RV, Sekeres MA. Making sense of the myelodysplastic/myeloproliferative neoplasms overlap syndromes. Curr Opin Hematol. 2014;21(2):131–40.

Valent P, Orazi A, Büsche G, Schmitt-Gräff A, George TI, Sotlar K, et al. Standards and impact of hematopathology in myelodysplastic syndromes (MDS). Oncotarget. 2010;1(7):483–96.

Vardiman JW. Myelodysplastic syndromes, chronic myeloproliferative diseases, and myelodysplastic/myeloproliferative diseases. Semin Diagn Pathol. 2003;20(3):154–79.

Zhou J, Orazi A, Czader MB. Myelodysplastic syndromes. Semin Diagn Pathol. 2011;28(4):258–72.

Chapter 2 Myeloid Neoplasms with Germline Predisposition

Czuchlewski DR, Peterson LC. Myeloid neoplasms with germline predisposition: a new provisional entity within the World Health Organization Classification. Surg Pathol Clin. 2016;9(1):165–76.

Chapter 3 Acute Myeloid Leukemia and Related Precursor Neoplasms

Adams J, Nassiri M. Acute promyelocytic leukemia: a review and discussion of variant translocations. Arch Pathol Lab Med. 2015;139(10):1308–13.

Arber DA. Revisiting erythroleukemia. Curr Opin Hematol. 2017;24(2):146–51.

Arber DA, Orazi A, Hasserjian R, Thiele J, Borowitz MJ, Le Beau MM, et al. The 2016 revision to the World Health Organization classification of myeloid neoplasms and acute leukemia. Blood. 2016;127(20):2391–405.

Bhatnagar N, Nizery L, Tunstall O, Vyas P, Roberts I. Transient abnormal myelopoiesis and AML in Down Syndrome: an update. Curr Hematol Malig Rep. 2016;11(5):333–41.

Bueso-Ramos CE, Kanagal-Shamanna R, Routbort MJ, Hanson CA. Therapy-related myeloid neoplasms. Am J Clin Pathol. 2015;144(2):207–18.

Charles NJ, Boyer DF. Mixed-phenotype acute leukemia: diagnostic criteria and pitfalls. Arch Pathol Lab Med. 2017a;141(11):1462–8.

Chen YC, Mapp S, Blumenthal A, Burgess ML, Mazzieri R, Mattarollo SR, et al. The duality of macrophage function in chronic lymphocytic leukaemia. Biochim Biophys Acta. 2017;1868(1):176–82.

Cremers EM, Alhan C, Westers TM, Ossenkoppele GJ, van de Loosdrecht AA. Immunophenotyping for diagnosis and prognosis in MDS: ready for general application? Best Pract Res Clin Haematol. 2015b;28(1):14–21.

Döhner H, Weisdorf DJ, Bloomfield CD. Acute myeloid leukemia. N Engl J Med. 2015;373(12):1136–52.

Foucar K, Anastasi J. Acute myeloid leukemia with recurrent cytogenetic abnormalities. Am J Clin Pathol. 2015;144(1):6–18.

Ganser A, Heuser M. Therapy-related myeloid neoplasms. Curr Opin Hematol. 2017;24(2):152–8.

Khan M, Siddiqi R, Naqvi K. An update on classification, genetics, and clinical approach to mixed phenotype acute leukemia (MPAL). Ann Hematol. 2018a;97(6):945–53.

Leonard JP, Martin P, Roboz GJ. Practical implications of the 2016 revision of the World Health Organization classification of lymphoid and myeloid neoplasms and acute leukemia. J Clin Oncol. 2017;35(23):2708–15.

McNerney ME, Godley LA, Le Beau MM. Therapy-related myeloid neoplasms: when genetics and environment collide. Nat Rev Cancer. 2017;17(9):513–27.

Shumilov E, Flach J, Kohlmann A, Banz Y, Bonadies N, Fiedler M, et al. Current status and trends in the diagnostics of AML and MDS. Blood Rev. 2018;32(6):508–19. pii: S0268-960X(18)30023-7

Wang SA, Hasserjian RP. Acute erythroleukemias, acute megakaryoblastic leukemias, and reactive mimics: a guide to a number of perplexing entities. Am J Clin Pathol. 2015;144(1):44–60.

Wang W, Wang SA, Medeiros LJ, Khoury JD. Pure erythroid leukemia. Am J Hematol. 2017;92(3):292–6.

Wilson CS, Medeiros LJ. Extramedullary manifestations of myeloid neoplasms. Am J Clin Pathol. 2015;144(2):219–39.

Wong E, Juneja S. Acute myeloid leukaemia and myelodysplastic syndromes with 50% or greater erythroblasts: a diagnostic conundrum. Pathology. 2015;47(4):289–93.

Chapter 4 Mastocytosis

Chiu A, Orazi A. Mastocytosis and related disorders. Semin Diagn Pathol. 2012;29(1):19–30.

Doyle LA, Hornick JL. Pathology of extramedullary mastocytosis. Immunol Allergy Clin N Am. 2014;34(2):323–39.

Horny HP. Mastocytosis: an unusual clonal disorder of bone marrow-derived hematopoietic progenitor cells. Am J Clin Pathol. 2009;132(3):438–47.

Metcalfe DD, Mekori YA. Pathogenesis and pathology of mastocytosis. Annu Rev Pathol. 2017;12:487–514.

Chapter 5 Blastic Plasmacytoid Dendritic Cell Neoplasm

Facchetti F, Cigognetti M, Fisogni S, Rossi G, Lonardi S, Vermi W. Neoplasms derived from plasmacytoid dendritic cells. Mod Pathol. 2016a;29(2):98–111.

Pagano L, Valentini CG, Grammatico S, Pulsoni A. Blastic plasmacytoid dendritic cell neoplasm: diagnostic criteria and therapeutical approaches. Br J Haematol. 2016;174(2):188–202.

Shi Y, Wang E. Plasmacytoid dendritic cell neoplasm: a clinicopathologic review. Arch Pathol Lab Med. 2014;138(4):564–9. Review

Chapter 6 Myeloid/Lymphoid Neoplasms with Eosinophilia and Rearrangement of *PDGFRA, PDGFRB, FGFR1*, or with *PCM1-JAK2*

Reiter A, Gotlib J. Myeloid neoplasms with eosinophilia. Blood. 2017b;129(6):704–14.

Savage N, George TI, Gotlib J. Myeloid neoplasms associated with eosinophilia and rearrangement of PDGFRA, PDGFRB, and FGFR1: a review. Int J Lab Hematol. 2013;35(5):491–500.

Vega F, Medeiros LJ, Bueso-Ramos CE, Arboleda P, Miranda RN. Hematolymphoid neoplasms associated with rearrangements of PDGFRA, PDGFRB, and FGFR1. Am J Clin Pathol. 2015;144(3):377–92.

Chapter 7 Acute Leukemias of Ambiguous Lineage

Béné MC, Porwit A. Acute leukemias of ambiguous lineage. Semin Diagn Pathol. 2012;29(1):12–8.

Charles NJ, Boyer DF. Mixed-phenotype acute leukemia: diagnostic criteria and pitfalls. Arch Pathol Lab Med. 2017b;141(11):1462–8.

Khan M, Siddiqi R, Naqvi K. An update on classification, genetics, and clinical approach to mixed phenotype acute leukemia (MPAL). Ann Hematol. 2018b;97(6):945–53.

Porwit A, Béné MC. Acute leukemias of ambiguous origin. Am J Clin Pathol. 2015;144(3):361–76.

Weinberg OK, Arber DA. Mixed-phenotype acute leukemia: historical overview and a new definition. Leukemia. 2010;24(11):1844–51.

Chapter 8 Precursor Lymphoid Neoplasms

Cortelazzo S, Ferreri A, Hoelzer D, Ponzoni M. Lymphoblastic lymphoma. Crit Rev Oncol Hematol. 2017;113:304–17.

Loghavi S, Kutok JL, Jorgensen JL. B-acute lymphoblastic leukemia/lymphoblastic lymphoma. Am J Clin Pathol. 2015;144(3):393–410.

Ohgami RS, Arber DA, Zehnder JL, Natkunam Y, Warnke RA. Indolent T-lymphoblastic proliferation (iT-LBP): a review of clinical and pathologic features and distinction from malignant T-lymphoblastic lymphoma. Adv Anat Pathol. 2013a;20(3):137–40.

Paolini S, Gazzola A, Sabattini E, Bacci F, Pileri S, Piccaluga PP. Pathobiology of acute lymphoblastic leukemia. Semin Diagn Pathol. 2011;28(2):124–34.

Paul S, Kantarjian H, Jabbour EJ. Adult acute lymphoblastic leukemia. Mayo Clin Proc. 2016;91(11):1645–66.

You MJ, Medeiros LJ, Hsi ED. T-lymphoblastic leukemia/lymphoma. Am J Clin Pathol. 2015;144(3):411–22.

Chapter 9 Mature B-Cell Neoplasms

Adam P, Bonzheim I, Fend F, Quintanilla-Martínez L. Epstein-Barr virus-positive diffuse large B-cell lymphomas of the elderly. Adv Anat Pathol. 2011;18(5):349–55.

Agbay RL, Jain N, Loghavi S, Medeiros LJ, Khoury JD. Histologic transformation of chronic lymphocytic leukemia/small lymphocytic lymphoma. Am J Hematol. 2016;91(10):1036–43.

Bogusz AM, Bagg A. Genetic aberrations in small B-cell lymphomas and leukemias: molecular pathology, clinical relevance and therapeutic targets. Leuk Lymphoma. 2016;57(9):1991–2013.

Cheng CL, O'Connor S. T cell-rich lymphoid infiltrates with large B cells: a review of key entities and diagnostic approach. J Clin Pathol. 2017a;70(3):187–201.

Galletti G, Caligaris-Cappio F, Bertilaccio MT. B cells and macrophages pursue a common path toward the development and progression of chronic lymphocytic leukemia. Leukemia. 2016;30(12):2293–301.

Harmon CM, Smith LB. B-cell non-Hodgkin lymphomas with plasmacytic differentiation. Surg Pathol Clin. 2016;9(1):11–28.

Hartmann S. From a pathologist's point of view: histiocytic cells in Hodgkin lymphoma and T cell/histiocyte rich large B cell lymphoma. Pathol Res Pract. 2015;211(12):901–4.

Hsi ED, Lorsbach RB, Fend F, Dogan A. Plasmablastic lymphoma and related disorders. Am J Clin Pathol. 2011;136(2):183–94.

Jiang M, Bennani NN, Feldman AL. Lymphoma classification update: B-cell non-Hodgkin lymphomas. Expert Rev Hematol. 2017a;10(5):405–15. Review

Li S, Young KH, Medeiros LJ. Diffuse large B-cell lymphoma. Pathology. 2018;50(1):74–87. Review

Ondrejka SL, Hsi ED. Pathology of B-cell lymphomas: diagnosis and biomarker discovery. Cancer Treat Res. 2015;165:27–50.

Patel S, Xiao P. Primary effusion lymphoma. Arch Pathol Lab Med. 2013;137(8):1152–4.

Phillips EH, Fox CP, Cwynarski K. Primary CNS lymphoma. Curr Hematol Malig Rep. 2014;9(3):243–53.

Roschewski M, Wilson WH. Lymphomatoid granulomatosis. Cancer J. 2012;18(5):469–74. Review

Said J. Diffuse aggressive B-cell lymphomas. Adv Anat Pathol. 2009;16(4):216–35. Review

Said J, Lones M, Yea S. Burkitt lymphoma and MYC: what else is new? Adv Anat Pathol. 2014;21(3):160–5.

Salaverria I, Martin-Guerrero I, Wagener R, Kreuz M, Kohler CW, Richter J, et al. A recurrent 11q aberration pattern characterizes a subset of *MYC*-negative high-grade B-cell lymphomas resembling Burkitt lymphoma. Blood. 2014;123:1187–98.

Skinnider BF. Lymphoproliferative disorders of the gastrointestinal tract. Arch Pathol Lab Med. 2018;142(1):44–52.

Steidl C, Gascoyne RD. The molecular pathogenesis of primary mediastinal large B-cell lymphoma. Blood. 2011;118(10):2659–69.

Wotherspoon A, Attygalle A, Mendes LS. Bone marrow and splenic histology in hairy cell leukaemia. Best Pract Res Clin Haematol. 2015;28(4):200–7.

Xie Y, Pittaluga S, Jaffe ES. The histological classification of diffuse large B-cell lymphomas. Semin Hematol. 2015;52(2):57–66.

Chapter 10 Immunodeficiency-Associated Lymphoproliferative Disorders

Cesarman E. Pathology of lymphoma in HIV. Curr Opin Oncol. 2013;25(5):487–94.

Chadburn A, Abdul-Nabi AM, Teruya BS, Lo AA. Lymphoid proliferations associated with human immunodeficiency virus infection. Arch Pathol Lab Med. 2013;137(3):360–70.

Chapter 11 Mature T- and NK-Cell Neoplasms

Broccoli A, Zinzani PL. Angioimmunoblastic T-cell lymphoma. Hematol Oncol Clin North Am. 2017;31(2):223–38. Review

Cheng CL, O'Connor S. T cell-rich lymphoid infiltrates with large B cells: a review of key entities and diagnostic approach. J Clin Pathol. 2017b;70(3):187–201.

Cortés JR, Palomero T. The curious origins of angioimmunoblastic T-cell lymphoma. Curr Opin Hematol. 2016;23(4):434–43.

de Wolf-Peeters C, Achten R. Gammadelta T-cell lymphomas: a homogeneousentity? Histopathology. 2000;36(4):294–305. Review

Dojcinov SD, Fend F, Quintanilla-Martinez L. EBV-positive lymphoproliferations of B- T- and NK-cell derivation in non-immunocompromised hosts. Pathogens. 2018;7(1):28. https://doi.org/10.3390/pathogens7010028

Eberle FC, Song JY, Xi L, Raffeld M, Harris NL, Wilson WH, et al. Nodal involvement by cutaneous CD30-positive T-cell lymphoma mimicking classical Hodgkin lymphoma. Am J Surg Pathol. 2012;36(5):716–25.

Ferreri AJ, Govi S, Pileri SA. Hepatosplenic gamma-delta T-cell lymphoma. Crit Rev Oncol Hematol. 2012;83(2):283–92.

Foppoli M, Ferreri AJ. Gamma-delta T-cell lymphomas. Eur J Haematol. 2015;94(3):206–18.

Foss FM, Girardi M. Mycosis fungoides and Sezary syndrome. Hematol Oncol Clin North Am. 2017;31(2):297–315. Review

García-Herrera A, Calonje E. Cutaneous Lymphomas with Cytotoxic Phenotype. Surg Pathol Clin. 2017;10(2):409–27.

Gru AA. Pathology of T-cell lymphomas: diagnosis and biomarker discovery. Cancer Treat Res. 2015;165:51–95.

Jiang M, Bennani NN, Feldman AL. Lymphoma classification update: T-cell lymphomas, Hodgkin lymphomas, and histiocytic/dendritic cell neoplasms. Expert Rev Hematol. 2017b;10(3):239–49.

Lan TT, Brown NA, Hristov AC. Controversies and considerations in the diagnosis of primary cutaneous $CD4^+$ small/medium T-cell lymphoma. Arch Pathol Lab Med. 2014;138(10):1307–18.

Lansigan F, Choi J, Foss FM. Cutaneous T-cell lymphoma. Hematol Oncol Clin North Am. 2008;22(5):979–96, x. Review

Lin WC, Moore JO, Mann KP, Traweek ST, Smith C. Post-transplant CD8+ gamma-delta T-cell lymphoma associated with human

herpes virus-6 infection. Leuk Lymphoma. 1999;33(3–4):377–84. Review
Lisby G, Konstatinov K, Vejlsgaard GL. Retroviruses and cutaneous T-cell lymphoma. Curr Probl Dermatol. 1990;19:50–68. Review
Lunning MA, Vose JM. Angioimmunoblastic T-cell lymphoma: the many-faced lymphoma. Blood. 2017;129(9):1095–102.
Ondrejka S, Jagadeesh D. Enteropathy-associated T-cell lymphoma. Curr Hematol Malig Rep. 2016;11(6):504–13.
Ondrejka SL, Hsi ED. T-cell lymphomas: updates in biology and diagnosis. Surg Pathol Clin. 2016;9(1):131–41.
Pillai V, Tallarico M, Bishop MR, Lim MS. Mature T- and NK-cell non-Hodgkin lymphoma in children and young adolescents. Br J Haematol. 2016;173(4):573–81.
Pizzi M, Margolskee E, Inghirami G. Pathogenesis of peripheral T cell lymphoma. Ann Rev Pathol. 2018;13:293–320.
Pulitzer M. Cutaneous T-cell lymphoma. Clin Lab Med. 2017;37(3):527–46.
Montes-Mojarro IA, Steinhilber J, Bonzheim I, Quintanilla-Martinez L, Fend F. The pathological spectrum of systemic anaplastic large cell lymphoma (ALCL). Cancers (Basel). 2018;10(4). pii: E107.
Sandell RF, Boddicker RL, Feldman AL. Genetic landscape and classification of peripheral T cell lymphomas. Curr Oncol Rep. 2017;19(4):28.
Shi Y, Wang E. Hepatosplenic T-cell lymphoma: a clinicopathologic review with an emphasis on diagnostic differentiation from other T-cell/natural killer-cell neoplasms. Arch Pathol Lab Med. 2015;139(9):1173–80.
Siaghani PJ, Song JY. Updates of peripheral T cell lymphomas based on the 2017 WHO Classification. Curr Hematol Malig Rep. 2018;13(1):25–36.
Termuhlen AM. Natural killer/T-cell lymphomas in pediatric and adolescent patients. Clin Adv Hematol Oncol. 2017;15(3):200–9. Review
Tse E, Kwong YL. The diagnosis and management of NK/T-cell lymphomas. J Hematol Oncol. 2017;10(1):85.
van de Water JM, Cillessen SA, Visser OJ, Verbeek WH, Meijer CJ, Mulder CJ. Enteropathy associated T-cell lymphoma and its precursor lesions. Best Pract Res Clin Gastroenterol. 2010;24(1):43–56. Review
Weaver J, Hsi ED. CD4+/CD56+ hematodermic neoplasm (blastic NK-cell lymphoma). J Cutan Pathol. 2008;35(10):975–7.

Wilcox RA. A three-signal model of T-cell lymphoma pathogenesis. Am J Hematol. 2016;91(1):113–22.

Wilcox RA. Cutaneous T-cell lymphoma: 2014 update on diagnosis, risk-stratification, and management. Am J Hematol. 2014;89(8):837–51.

Xing X, Feldman AL. Anaplastic large cell lymphomas: ALK positive, ALK negative, and primary cutaneous. Adv Anat Pathol. 2015;22(1):29–49.

Yabe M, Miranda RN, Medeiros LJ. Hepatosplenic T-cell lymphoma: a review of clinicopathologic features, pathogenesis, and prognostic factors. Hum Pathol. 2018;74:5–16.

Chapter 12 Hodgkin Lymphomas

Abdull-Gaffar B, Seliem RM. Hodgkin lymphoma with an interfollicular growth pattern: a clinicopathologic study of 8 cases. Ann Diagn Pathol. 2018;33:30–4.

Eberle FC, Mani H, Jaffe ES. Histopathology of Hodgkin's lymphoma. Cancer J. 2009;15(2):129–37.

Goel A, Fan W, Patel AA, Devabhaktuni M, Grossbard ML. Nodular lymphocyte predominant Hodgkin lymphoma: biology, diagnosis and treatment. Clin Lymphoma Myeloma Leuk. 2014;14(4):261–70.

King RL, Howard MT, Bagg A. Hodgkin lymphoma: pathology, pathogenesis, and a plethora of potential prognostic predictors. Adv Anat Pathol. 2014;21(1):12–25. Review

Mani H, Jaffe ES. Hodgkin lymphoma: an update on its biology with new insights into classification. Clin Lymphoma Myeloma. 2009;9(3):206–16. Review

Mathas S, Hartmann S, Küppers R. Hodgkin lymphoma: pathology and biology. Semin Hematol. 2016;53(3):139–47.

Savage KJ, Mottok A, Fanale M. Nodular lymphocyte-predominant Hodgkin lymphoma. Semin Hematol. 2016;53(3):190–202.

Schnitzer B. Hodgkin lymphoma. Hematol Oncol Clin North Am. 2009;23(4):747–68.

Venkataraman G, Mirza MK, Eichenauer DA, Diehl V. Current status of prognostication in classical Hodgkin lymphoma. Br J Haematol. 2014;165(3):287–99.

Chapter 13 Histiocytic and Dendritic Cell Neoplasms

Dalia S, Shao H, Sagatys E, Cualing H, Sokol L. Dendritic cell and histiocytic neoplasms: biology, diagnosis, and treatment. Cancer Control. 2014;21(4):290–300.

Emile JF, Abla O, Fraitag S, Horne A, Haroche J, Donadieu J, et al. Histiocyte Society. Revised classification of histiocytoses and neoplasms of the macrophage-dendritic cell lineages. Blood. 2016;127(22):2672–81.

Facchetti F, Cigognetti M, Fisogni S, Rossi G, Lonardi S, Vermi W. Neoplasms derived from plasmacytoid dendritic cells. Mod Pathol. 2016b;29(2):98–111.

Harmon CM, Brown N. Langerhans cell histiocytosis: a clinicopathologic review and molecular pathogenetic update. Arch Pathol Lab Med. 2015;139(10):1211–4.

Takahashi E, Nakamura S. Histiocytic sarcoma: an updated literature review based on the 2008 WHO classification. J Clin Exp Hematop. 2013;53(1):1–8.

Chapter 14 Non-neoplastic Marrow Findings

Otrock ZK, Daver N, Kantarjian HM, Eby CS. Diagnostic challenges of hemophagocytic lymphohistiocytosis. Clin Lymphoma Myeloma Leuk. 2017;17S:S105–10.

Chapter 15 Non-neoplastic Lymph Node and Spleen Lesions

Ohgami RS, Arber DA, Zehnder JL, Natkunam Y, Warnke RA. Indolent T-lymphoblastic proliferation (iT-LBP): a review of clinical and pathologic features and distinction from malignant T-lymphoblastic lymphoma. Adv Anat Pathol. 2013b;20(3):137–40.

Szalat R, Munshi NC. Diagnosis of Castleman disease. Hematol Oncol Clin North Am. 2018;32(1):53–64.

David Hudnall S, Kuppers R, editors. Precision molecular pathology of Hodgkin lymphoma: Springer; 2018.

Index

© Springer Nature Switzerland AG 2019

S. D. Hudnall et al., *Pocket Guide to Diagnostic Hematopathology*, https://doi.org/10.1007/978-3-030-10630-0

MIX
Papier aus verantwortungsvollen Quellen
Paper from responsible sources
FSC® C105338

If you have any concerns about our products,
you can contact us on
ProductSafety@springernature.com

In case Publisher is established outside the EU,
the EU authorized representative is:
Springer Nature Customer Service Center GmbH
Europaplatz 3, 69115 Heidelberg, Germany

Printed by Libri Plureos GmbH
in Hamburg, Germany